GERIATRICS FOR NURSES AND SOCIAL WORKERS

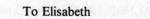

To Elisabeth

GERIATRICS FOR NURSES AND SOCIAL WORKERS

John Agate

C.B.E., M.A., M.D.(Cantab)., F.R.C.P.

*Physician, Consultant in Geriatric Medicine,
the Ipswich and Suffolk Hospitals,
and the Ipswich Health District*

Second Edition

WILLIAM HEINEMANN MEDICAL BOOKS LIMITED
LONDON

First Published 1972
Second Edition 1979

© John Agate, 1979

ISBN 0 433 00204 2

By the same Author
The Practice of Geriatrics
Second Edition 1970

Taking Care of Old
People at Home, 1979.

Text set in 11 pt Photon Times, printed and bound
in Great Britain at The Pitman Press, Bath

PREFACE
TO THE FIRST EDITION

This short book has its origins in the talks given by the author to nurses in hospitals in Ipswich and elsewhere, as well as in courses of lectures for Health Visitors and Social Workers in training at the Suffolk College at Ipswich over the years. He has often been asked for a short text to cover the same ground, and here it is. It is not intended to teach geriatric nursing care to nurses, nor yet sociology and social work methods to social workers, for these can be learned elsewhere, and best of all practically, at the bedside, the chairside, and in people's own houses. Instead the book seeks to show what it is about old people individually and collectively, what it is about their inevitable ageing and their many kinds of physical and mental illnesses, which so often brings them into the hands of social and health workers as "problems". This *is* Geriatrics, and if one understands its principles, the proper remedies are so much easier to see and to apply.

It could be argued that if one book attempts to cater for two different groups of readers, it will fail them both. The author thinks this is not necessarily so, believing that, in this field above all others, there is a vital need for nurses to understand their patients' social circumstances, and for social workers to have a firm grasp of some medical facts and parlance, to assist them in casework and decision-taking. For too long there has been a great divide between the territories of practising medical workers and social workers; perhaps this may help to bridge the gap so that our older people may be even better served by both.

* * *

The book is affectionately dedicated to my students, past, present and future, in appreciation of the stimulus provided by talking to people so clearly devoted to their job. It is a pleasure to acknowledge the help and gentle forbearance of my publishers, and in particular Mr. Owen R. Evans, the general assistance of Mrs. Rosemary Rooksby, and of Miss Susan Lee, who did the charts and drawings.

J.N.A.

Chattisham, Ipswich   January 1972

PREFACE
TO THE SECOND EDITION

It is pleasant to find a second edition of this book now called for. In the seven years since the first, geriatric medicine has made rapid strides forward and British geriatric nursing has become highly reputable and recognized as vital to the very continuance of a National Health Service, while geriatric nursing is necessary experience for all students and pupils. Not least, the social services' contribution to geriatric work has proved itself essential – as if there were any doubt of that previously – to the whole functioning of the health services. In recognition of this latter trend and in the hope of promoting still better co-operation between the two, Chapter 14 in particular, on the community care of elderly people, has been much recast and brought up to date. Since the last edition we have had major reorganizations of the Health Services, the Local Authorities and their Social Services Departments; we have adopted the metric system more widely in medicine and the S.I. units of biological measurement. I have taken this opportunity to bring the text terminologically up to date, to include some of the newer knowledge, and to correct some previous aberrations of style and phrase.

Notwithstanding a number of changes, the basic principles and philosophy of geriatric care, on which this book was first based, will be seen not to have changed one whit. I believe they will not change, whatever scientific advances we achieve, and they must be told to each new generation of those who work for the good of older people. Meanwhile, my students in the several disciplines, for whom the book was designed, continue to act as a powerful stimulus and to be, I dare say, my friends.

It is a pleasant duty to record the help and encouragement I have had from Mr. Richard Emery of William Heinemann Medical Books Ltd., and the continuing assistance of Mrs. Rosemary Rooksby with the manuscript.

J.N.A.

Chattisham, Ipswich

April 1979

vi

CONTENTS

Chapter 1

THE ELDERLY IN OUR POPULATION

Geriatrics is quite a new speciality within Medicine. No apology is needed for it, because it came into being in answer to a need, a need which had already become desperate when the National Health Service in Great Britain started in 1948. In a nutshell Geriatrics is the practical medical, nursing and general care of elderly people. It also includes the study of what old age itself means to us and them, and it is concerned too with their social circumstances: it must be, because an old person's social circumstances affect most of the decisions to be taken while he is being treated by doctors and nurses.

Gerontology is a different science – that is, it studies the processes of ageing on cells and tissues and chemical mechanisms of living things. It is more fundamentally concerned with why ageing takes place and how, perhaps, it might be prevented or slowed down.

The fact that old age is reached by a large proportion of our people is something quite new; it forces us to adopt a new outlook to much of our planning. The average age of people in Great Britain has doubled in the last 150 years, and at present about half of our men will reach the age of 70, and more than half of our women will reach 75. This is the same as saying that the "average expectation of life" of men is now 70 years, and of women over 75 years. In the middle of the last century the figure was nearer 40 years. It is probable that the average expectation in the time of Ancient Greece and Rome was not much more than 20 years, and we believe that between the coming of William the Conqueror and Queen Elizabeth I it was probably about 30 or 32 years (Fig. 1). There were, of course, old men and old women in those days, but there were far fewer of them in proportion to the whole population. The death rate amongst new born and young children and young adults was very high in those days, epidemic diseases and wars carried off large numbers, and relatively few people survived to become old. Those who did so must have been remarkably healthy and tough, or unusually lucky. Our present high average expectation of life is also found in most Western Civilization countries, but the average expectation in many other countries like India

1

and China is much lower. They do not yet have such serious problems of how to cater for a high proportion of elderly people, but these difficulties will certainly come to them before long.

The improvement in our average expectation of life came about first by improvements in water and food supplies, sanitation and public health generally, and the overcoming of the worst epidemic diseases like typhus, typhoid and plague, greatly helped as this was by the development of scientific bacteriology, which at last demonstrated the true cause of so

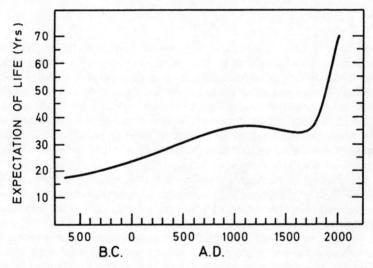

Fig. 1 The average expectation of life of newborn children at various times in history.

many diseases and made it possible to control them or to immunize people against them. Secondly, there were great improvements in maternity and child care, so that fewer mothers and babies were lost. Then there were improvements in nutrition and living and working standards, and the abolition of the worst of the occupational diseases like silicosis and industrial poisoning which killed many young men. Much later came the discovery of powerful drugs to defeat the infections which escaped control by public health methods. This is really a development of only the last 30 years. Tuberculosis is the last of the great infectious killers in this country which has almost been mastered, even though it is not properly controlled yet amongst older people (see page 99) nor is it yet in underdeveloped countries. In place of tuberculosis road traffic accidents are now the greatest killers of young people.

Our expectation of life is still going upwards and women have a clear advantage over men in living longer – on average their advantage is over 5 years. There is no sign yet of this tendency stopping. However, it is very unlikely that our expectations will continue to rise for ever, because we still have not solved the problem of increasing the total life-span of the human race, as demonstrated by its most favoured individuals. In other words it is still, as it always was, very unusual indeed for humans to live to be over 100 years old. Some very fundamental discovery in gerontology will probably be necessary before this fact of life changes. It is as if the limit of our biological age has been set and as a race we are little nearer to immortality now than ever we were.

The cause of our present problem over the number and frailty of older people is not, as we have seen, a question simply of medical treatment having become available. Some old people are living a little longer than they would have done thanks to antibiotic drugs, but the real heart of the matter is the low death rate amongst young people. So doctors who practise particularly amongst old people should not be accused of struggling to keep old people going longer and longer. This is not their object; their main wish is to help old people to be more healthy and active when they are old. Occasionally it turns out that a geriatric physician can prolong a useful, meaningful life, but that is just a bonus.

It is now possible for people who were ill or disabled early in life to live to be old: they do not so easily succumb to one of the infections which used to make them die young. Whether it is *right* to enable severely handicapped people to grow old and be a full responsibility of the health and welfare services is not a matter to be discussed in this short book. It is however exemplified by the present-day argument about whether or not infants with spina bifida should be treated surgically, as a result of which they might survive but still grow up with gross disabilities. The fact is that people can now be old and very disabled and still survive, whereas 100 years or so ago, only very healthy people normally reached a "geriatric" age. For people who have already reached retirement age the further expectation of life is scarcely any longer now than it was a century ago (Fig. 2). At this time of life the degenerative diseases become more and more important (see Chapter 4) and they have not yet been overcome. This is still the real challenge to Medicine in our time.

Though the chances of longer survival are better for the individual person, this is not necessarily an advantage to the nation, for there will be more people who are not producers (i.e. children and retired people) to be supported by the working population, either directly or through pensions and services which are paid for by rates and taxes. At this time there are about 660 "dependent" people for every 1000 people who are of an age to be working.

If "younger" old people could go on in employment longer they would be producers as well as consumers. Yet, even supposing they wished to do so, this policy would not be popular if it meant that the chances of promotion of younger people with family responsibilities was delayed. It might be possible for older people to take on relatively junior or part-time jobs again after a certain age. However, Britain is now facing a time of increased unemployment, and demands for a shorter working week and greater leisure all round. It looks as though the prospects of older people

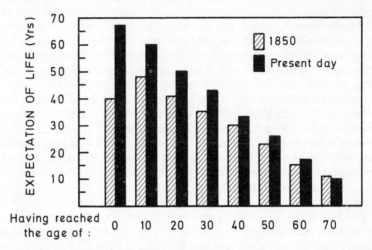

Fig. 2 The further expectation of life of people who have reached various ages: comparing the year 1850 with the present day.

finding paid work, even part-time, will diminish sharply. This again is a question too complex to deal with here.

Population figures will help to explain why the specialty of geriatrics has become necessary. In Great Britain in 1851 the number of people over 65 was one million (4.7% of the total); in 1911 it was two million one hundred thousand, in 1939 – four million two hundred thousand, and in 1947 five million (or 10.5% of the total).

By 1975 there were over seven million people aged more than 65 (about 13% of the total). The likelihood is that this number will continue to rise until at least 1991, when there may be over eight million – though it is predicted that in the last decade of the century there might be a small reduction in the total over 65. Even so, the social and medical problems are likely ultimately to increase rather than diminish because, though there will probably be a decrease in the *total* of those aged 65–75, those aged 75 and over will continue to increase, actually and also in proportion to the size of the total population. By A.D. 2001, then, there might be 40% more people over 75 than at present, and there might be 1.8 million people *over 85*. Even people over 75 have a high rate of hospital admissions, and on average they stay in hospital much longer than young people. Those aged 85 and over – the "old old" if they may be called so – are in addition likely to be quite frail as well as having a high risk of illness (see below). Although it is not universally true, those aged 85 and over are often too physically weak to care for themselves properly, even though they may not be ill. This is the outstanding problem in the Residential Homes, at the present time (see Chapter 15), and it is likely to become even more difficult. There are reasons for thinking that in thirty five years time there might be more than twice as many women over 85 as there are at present. This should make us all pause to think. As one hospital doctor has put it – "So many old ladies seem to be indestructible"!

It is necessary to consider in more detail what happens in terms of medical and nursing needs when a population grows older as ours is doing. Young adults have least disease and least need of medical atten- tion, but from later middle age onwards the proportion of people with illness and disability begins to rise sharply (Fig. 3). People aged 85 and over have a 66% chance of not being fully well, and a 10% chance of being so seriously disabled as to need a great deal of personal aid and attention from other people. Many very old persons do not have just one disease process going on, but several at once, and this just at a time when their strength is beginning to wane. The impact of this increasing frailty

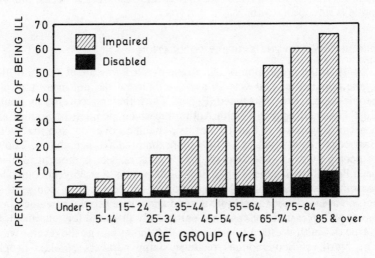

Fig. 3 The chance of being ill as the person's age increases.

and disease on the medical, nursing and social services of the country generally would not be hard to imagine if people thought more about it. It is felt by doctors in General Practice, who have many more calls on their services by elderly people than the average number of calls for other people in their practice. It is felt by Home Nurses who now spend a very large part of their time caring for the elderly. It is being felt increasingly by Health Visitors, and by hospital-based Social Workers as well as by Social Workers who are working outside the medical services. It was felt, and still is being felt acutely, by the hospital side of the National Health Service, which after the Second World War was left with a number of very old, neglected and under-staffed hospitals where the elderly were looked after, but regarded simply as the "chronic sick", for whom everyone said "nothing can be done" (see Chapter 15). There were nevertheless a few notable pioneers, and a new idea emerged – that old people could be diagnosed, treated and made active again so that they need not stay in hospital for ever. Thus a hospital geriatric specialty emerged which began to solve this problem without demanding many thousands more hospital beds – which is what everyone feared would happen. If it had not been for the coming of the National Health Service, however, this new idea could not have developed (see page 244). Before that time many elderly frail ill people were confined to the old institutions which began as the erstwhile Poor Law workhouses. The new Service made a fairer distribution of money and staff possible to all hospitals, whatever their origins. Geriatric Medicine was thus founded on the old workhouses, largely divorced from other medical activities. It has had quite a struggle to gain the recognition and resources it needs, but the battle is now being won.

GEOGRAPHY AND THE ELDERLY POPULATION

In 1970 the proportion of old people over 65 was about 12.5% of the whole population. This was an average figure: it did not mean that old people were evenly distributed (Fig. 4). Thus, the area covered by South East Thames Regional Health Authority, which includes the South East coast of England too, had 15% of its population over 65, and the South East coast resorts had up to 10% more than the average, that is, 22.5% of people over 65. The "worst" area in this respect is thought to have been Bexhill-on-Sea, which had 36% of its people over 65 years old! The reason for such an unusual distribution of old people is, of course, that certain areas, where the climate is good and where people remember they have spent pleasant holidays, are particularly favoured for retirement. It is true of South Western England also. Yet things can go the reverse way. The North of Scotland has relatively large numbers of older people because the younger people have migrated away to the South and to in-

dustrial districts with better prospects of employment. There is generally
a drift of younger people from country districts towards the towns and to
industrial districts. East Anglia has a relatively high proportion of old
people too, though we are not quite so sure why: it is perhaps because the
tempo of life is slow, the air is clean, and the population has been
toughened by a lifetime of east winds! These population differences do
mean that certain areas, certain individual towns perhaps, need a greater-
than-average expenditure on all the things which are necessary when
there are elderly people to help, i.e. Hospitals, Homes, Home Helps and

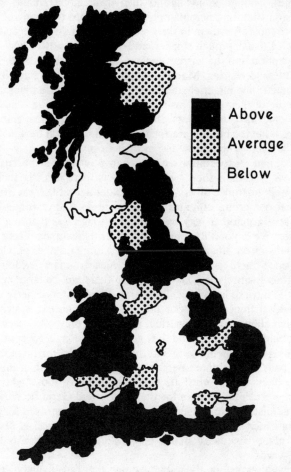

Fig. 4 Map of Great Britain showing areas where the percentage of people aged over 65 is
the average for the country as a whole, above the average, or below the average.
(After Ashley J. S. A., and Klein R. E., (1971), Modern Geriatrics, Vol. 1, p. 326.)

all Social Services. Planners often work on national or regional averages or even sometimes London averages. Here is an area of planning activity in which averages can be very misleading indeed.

RECENT POPULATION TRENDS AND THEIR EFFECTS

It will be worthwhile to examine some of the other causes and effects of the population trends just mentioned. Some of the high proportion of old people in the 1970's is explained by the high birth rate in late Victorian times. Though many infants died then, large families were very common and Victorian parents might look forward to having at least one daughter to look after them in their old age. But in the 1920's and 1930's families were usually much smaller, and so they are now. This is because of contraception and the wish of women to be released from the tyranny of constant child bearing. Many of them did and still do have jobs, want to contribute to the material standard of living of their families, and want to have a life of their own. This trend is likely to continue. Thus, today's elderly people have much less chance of offspring – now middle aged themselves – being able to care for them; and so it will be when the present middle-aged people grow old in their turn.

Since a man's expectation is less than a woman's, he survives on average less well than she does. This means there is likely to be an increasing preponderance of women of the older ages. In Great Britain now the 85-year-old group contains about twice as many women as men. Looking at it in another way we find that though less than one in ten of British men live beyond 85, one in five of British women does reach this age. It follows from this that there will be a large number of widows, especially since there is a tendency for men to marry women rather younger than themselves. Very likely then there will be large numbers of women who have to live alone. The numbers of solitary elderly women is one of saddest things about our present social scene. It is strange, too, that women should live longer than men, since they often seem to have more disabilities than men; and they go on much longer (in spite of multiple disabilities) occupying long-stay hospital wards, for instance, where they are likely to need more personal help from nurses than the men do. These are facts which must be borne in mind by those who plan the staffing of Residential Homes for the Elderly and Geriatric Hospitals. In geriatric admission wards there is a somewhat greater need for women's places than men's; in long-stay sections the proportion is about three women's places for every man's place, and nurses' work is harder in women's wards.

When widows are in their own homes they are usually very much more domestically capable than widowers are. They have had more practice and experience, and they have seldom had to make the great readjustment which retirement brings. Professional women may retire and have special problems, but housewives never retire.

HOSPITALS AND THE AGEING POPULATION

People who work in hospitals can see with their own eyes what effect our ageing population has upon their work. Except in children's wards, maternity wards and perhaps men's orthopaedic wards, old people seem to be everywhere. Statistics show that (excluding the maternity wards) people over 65 account for 22% of all admissions to general hospital beds even though they total only 14% of the total population. Many of these admissions take place into general medical and surgical wards even where active geriatric departments exist. Indeed, it has been estimated that people over 65 account for 30% of the general surgical beds, and 44% of the general medical beds occupied each day, though the proportions vary from place to place. Unless there is a change in policy, present-day trends suggest that by the turn of the century elderly men could be occupying 75% of all acute general hospital beds and elderly women 90%! Where would gravely ill younger people be treated then? This tendency is the undeniable argument for saying that all nurses should be trained in the proper care and management of elderly people and their problems. *There is no better place for this than a good geriatric ward.* One of the main functions of this book will be to show where the differences lie between the needs of the elderly and those who are younger. The same sort of admission figures apply to mental hospitals too. The elderly also tend to stay longer in hospital, so that they occupy over 40% of all the hospital beds, and 45 % of all mental hospital beds. It is well recognized that single, widowed and divorced people are heavier users of hospital beds than others, because they have less support at home in times of emergency.

There can be no doubt that large numbers of hospital beds everywhere are occupied by elderly people who do not really need to stay in hospital, but have nowhere else to go, or whose own homes are unsuitable now that they are frail or have disabilities which remain after treatment. This is a direct challenge to the Social Services. It can be fairly said that even in 1979 a good geriatric department can rehabilitate more elderly people than the social services can absorb back into the community. Patients over 65 often go back from hospital into the community needing considerable social support. One cross-section showed that on discharge of old people from all departments of a hospital 43% needed help with bathing, 29% help with dressing, and 22% help with going to the lavatory. Geriatric departments take as much care as possible not to send old people home if their needs are too great, but they are always under pressure to admit even more handicapped people who are at the start of their illnesses. This point is sometimes misunderstood by Social Services Departments. Something more must be done than at present, therefore, to meet the social needs of elderly people, and it cannot be done without sufficient money and enthusiasm.

The challenge of the slowly increasing numbers of elderly people who are ill can partly be met in two ways. The first is by the provision of fully efficient hospital geriatric departments, with good equipment, sufficient space, and staff who are well trained so that waiting lists are kept small, admissions are rapid, treatment starts at once, the patient's length of stay is made as short as possible, long-stay care is reduced, and the old person returns as soon as possible to the community. In spite of this self-evident fact, some hospital geriatric departments are short of facilities, equipment and staff.

The other method is by prevention of disease. This should start in middle life at least, and we could assist by trying to persuade people to live in such a way as to avoid diseases which could be avoided, and by detection of anything which went wrong at the first possible opportunity. At present we do not really know how to prevent much of human degenerative disease: we know it starts long before old age, and one day we may discover how, by dietary or other means, it could be got rid of. The author hopes that the chapters of this book which deal with what can go wrong with old people will help nurses and social workers to be on the watch for these things, and feel better able to deal with them supposing that they cannot be prevented.

Chapter 2

AGEING—NORMAL AND ABNORMAL

The process of growing old can be called "normal senescence". We can think of it as normal because it happens to all animals and all humans, but a frail aged person is perhaps not *as* normal as a young one. In senescent people active growth is still going on; for example, they can form new blood cells constantly and can replace some tissues if they are injured. However, generally speaking in old people (as distinct from the young), decline or "involution" is going on faster than growth. Ageing is continuous but does not go at a steady rate, nor at the same rate in all people, for this depends on many things like place and climate, and most of all perhaps on the hereditary "hand-out" we have had from generations before us. A longstanding disease like rheumatoid arthritis makes some people, but not all, age faster. So perhaps does grinding overwork and malnutrition over the years. Old age itself is *not* a disease.

In rats and some other animals it has been shown that using a diet which is otherwise well balanced but reducing the calorie intake leads to a much longer life than expected. This is interesting, but we cannot say the same is true for other species like Man. Nevertheless fat people do not generally live to be very old, for obesity causes or aggravates several diseases.

Practically speaking we recognize "young" old people, full of vigour and mental activity but also, sadly, some "old" younger people too. It is not the actual age in years which seems to matter. We should not judge people on that basis but rather how old they *look* for their years and what sort of people they *are* in their activities and behaviour.

To treat and nurse older people properly we must have summed them up, or "assessed" them, as the modern phrase is. To judge of their biological age (as opposed to their actual years of living), we must know what the process of ageing usually does to most people. Theories of *why* people age and what the chemical changes are in them which control this are interesting but they are not of day by day importance to practical people. What happens to people's various organs, to heart, lungs, kidneys, brain, eyes etc., is however very important, because it affects their performance.

11

PHYSICAL AGEING

(a) OUTWARD SIGNS

Weight and Build; Height and Posture

Any changes are difficult to judge because we still have no satisfactory physique, height and weight figures to use for averages for normal old people. Usually beyond a certain age, but not always, people grow lighter and have a smaller build. They usually lose some height: younger people normally have the same height as the distance between their fingertips when the arms are stretched out sideways (this is known as "span"). Old people's height is usually less than their span. Their posture tends to be flexed, their hips and knees rather bent, and their trunk and neck stooping. This flexed position is not really necessary unless there is disease present. Old people can usually draw themselves up when they have a mind to. Usually a faulty, stooping posture seems to be a matter of habit. Think of the uprightness of Chelsea Pensioners with their long Army training!

The Skin

The skin becomes more lax, wrinkled, inelastic, drier, and it may lack fat under the surface. It is also yellower and has brownish blemishes or even so-called "senile warts", and small purple spots – De Morgan's spots – on the trunk. Cosmetics do not make the skin younger but they do hide the blemishes. We can encourage older women to use them because it is good for morale, theirs and ours! On the backs of the hands and forearms there are frequently purple discolourations (ecchymoses) like very small bruises – which they are. They occur because of an age change in small blood vessels, and even a slight knock can bring them out. They are not evidence therefore of ill treatment, and the public should never be allowed to think so.

The Hair

An older person's hair will usually grow thinner, greyer or whiter and it may be lost altogether from the temples and the top of the head especially in men. This is largely a matter of heredity. The same "male pattern" baldness may afflict a few women. In very old people body hair is lost too. Nevertheless some old people have quite full heads of hair and a few keep their dark hair always. Some older women, because of hormonal changes, grow hair on their faces after the menopause.

Eyes and Ears

The eyes may begin to show age signs which affect their performance very early – at, say, 40 to 45 years. This change (presbyopia) means that gradually the lens cannot be brought to focus on close work. Reading glasses become necessary, and bifocal lenses are needed by many who want to be able to see close and distant things equally well without changing their glasses. Bifocals cause difficulties for some people on stairs and elsewhere, but their use can be mastered.

The so-called "arcus senilis" is a band of white material laid down at the outer edge of the iris diaphragm; it is a sign of age but has no other significance. Old eyes do not adapt so quickly for seeing in the dark, and the importance of this is obvious.

The ears lose some sensitivity for high pitched sound like bird song; this too starts quite early at, say, 40 to 45 years. Real deafness is usually due to disease but sometimes it is simply due to wax in the ears. Many old people hear very well indeed and we should neither assume they cannot hear what we say, nor should we shout unnecessarily. Good hearing depends on good mental concentration, and deaf people should watch the face of anyone speaking to them.

(b) INTERNAL SIGNS OF AGEING

The Chest, Lungs and Heart

Age changes here mean that lung function gets progressively less effective and the total space for air (which can be measured by the "vital capacity") steadily falls as the tissues become less elastic and the chest muscles less strong. Therefore breathlessness may be seen after only slight effort, but this does not necessarily mean there is any disease of lungs or heart. The heart of an old person may look just like a young person's; nevertheless it probably has less reserve of power for exertion or when the patient is ill. Still, the heart in old people can gradually enlarge to compensate for overwork, as is the case with high blood pressure.

The Brain and Nervous System

Unlike some other organs the brain can never grow in size or replace any of its cells after they have been lost for any reason. Probably vital brain cells *are* lost steadily, every day, from an early age; but as they number many many millions these losses do not necessarily have a very marked effect on the brain's performances (see below). Nevertheless, the elderly brain becomes smaller, as many organs do; and as the brain grows smaller there is more space for cerebrospinal fluid between its grooves and also more space for fluid in the ventricles within.

The rest of the nervous system itself undergoes some changes and perhaps also suffers some losses of irreplaceable cells and fibres. This may account for some of the loss of sensation, like vibration sense, and some of the changes of reflexes like ankle jerks or for the abnormal plantar responses which we find when examining older people. There is evidence too that old nerve fibres conduct impulses more slowly.

The Kidneys

The excretory power of the kidneys reduces with age. Gradually whole excretory units made up of glomeruli with their associated tubules disappear, but this produces no signs or symptoms in normal old people. Nevertheless they cannot produce urine of high specific gravity (S.G. 1020, or above) as young people can. This relative loss of kidney reserves becomes important in disease. It also suggests the necessity of supplying plenty of fluid for aged kidneys to do their job of excreting properly. Producing a lot of dilute urine is much less of a problem to kidneys than working with too little fluid. Practically speaking this means old people must drink plenty.

Other Organs

Bones change somewhat in shape and structure and become more liable to fracture. Cartilages, especially rib cartilages, may harden with calcium. Joints do not generally alter in their range of movement just because of age, and if there is restriction of movement it suggests disease is present or else that the muscles are stiff. These muscles themselves may lose power and bulk as time goes on. Rapid movements become less easy and strong movements are less able to be sustained. Some old people who always used to work hard physically and then continue to take good exercise can keep very powerful muscles; also muscles can still be built up by training, though much less so than in young adults. By contrast, putting old people to bed reduces their muscle strength very quickly indeed.

Arteries are very prone to disease, but the pure age changes in them are probably confined to growing slightly longer, so they are often found to be tortuous.

The coats of the stomach and intestines grow thinner and less active in their normal movements, but they still seem capable of full digestive function, and the liver continues to act as an efficient chemical factory or storage organ. Various endocrine glands do alter in their chemical activity but probably continue to function sufficiently to maintain an aged body even at the age of 100. Nevertheless, it is common to find changes in sugar metabolism approximating almost the state of diabetes (perhaps from lack of full pancreatic beta-cell activity), some reduction of thyroid or pituitary function and, naturally, loss of secondary sex characteristics due to steady reduction of hormone production in the testes, ovaries and other organs, as might be expected when the breeding period of life is over and sexual attractiveness is less of a driving force. Notwithstanding, it is possible for very old men to beget children, so the testes do not lose their capacity entirely. There is no real evidence that replacing the missing hormones promotes longer life or vigour, though many people have hoped that this would be so.

In an old person the blood cells are renewed regularly as always by a more restricted quantity of bone marrow, though the haemoglobin level may diminish a little and still be reckoned normal. It seems likely that the defence mechanisms of the body, in which the spleen and lymph nodes are implicated, are less efficient in old age, making older people vulnerable to infections.

Temperature Regulation

The balance of mechanisms to keep the body temperature constant may easily be upset in old age. In general, temperatures tend to fall rather than to rise, and serious illness may even lead to a fall instead of the rise one would have expected in a young person. This loss of temperature control is bound up with the most difficult problem of hypothermia which will be discussed in Chapter 5. Evidence is increasing from surveys of people at home that some old and rather inactive people often have remarkably low temperatures (as low as 35°C or 95°F) without outwardly seeming to be ill. With old patients we really need to revise our ideas about what is a "normal" temperature.

Changes in Blood Chemistry

Doctors and nurses are accustomed to think of certain basic blood levels of substances like sugar, urea, cholesterol, etc. as being "normal" values, though always there is a *range* of normality. These "normal ranges" are used in conjunction with physical examination in judging whether the patient has certain diseases. In the elderly the range of normal is often much wider than is usually understood, so that near-normal figures are misleading. For example, in old people who are apparently quite well, values of blood urea or cholesterol are obtained sometimes which would signify kidney diseases or thyroid insufficiency in a younger person. Here as well as elsewhere in geriatrics it is important to judge people's performance by the correct standards: sometimes it is not easy to be sure what standard to use. One does not base diagnosis just on laboratory or X-ray results: the clinical picture is more important than any of these.

MENTAL AND PSYCHOLOGICAL AGEING

THE NORMAL STATE

People's minds grow old just as their bodies do. In the same way as we notice that not all people of the same age are equally "old" in respect of physical attributes and performance, so we can see that some keep their mental alertness and vigour up to a great age – and some do not. Perhaps even more than physical ones, mental qualities depend on the person's capabilities in youth and middle age; people who are highly intelligent and creative probably have the best chance of fending off the ill effects of mental ageing.

Memory is one of the earliest faculties to show changes. Some degree of memory loss (amnesia) must be reckoned normal; remembering names of people and places becomes harder; there is a natural tendency to recall distant events but forget things which happened recently. Mental processes which depend on short-term memory, like adding up a column of figures, can become more difficult. Yet minor memory loss can be helped by simple devices like keeping diaries, making shopping lists or tying knots in one's handkerchief. The irritating habit of repeating a story again and again to the same hearers is just one example of a failing memory.

So much of memory depends on the grasp of the situation and the interest in the subject. The process consists of feeding in information, storing it, and being able to call it out from the store when needed. Much of the forgetfulness of older people is caused by lack of concentration or lack of interest; what is not put properly into the memory store obviously cannot be brought out of it again later.

Other mental traits which may become obvious are: (i) narrowing of interest in outside affairs and a corresponding increase of interest in oneself and one's own activities, bodily functions and shortcomings; (ii) a failure to accept new ideas – summed up by the phrase "the old ways are best" – which may not be true at all; (iii) a tendency to be pessimistic rather than optimistic, and this could be a fundamental change or it could be the result of the many disappointments of a long life; (iv) a "cooling" of the emotions, so that happy events do not seem to excite older people, and sad events are accepted with an unexpected indifference which may seem like heartlessness; (v) loss of adaptability on one hand and a tendency on the other to become a slave to routines, which have an exaggerated importance – yet which sometimes may help people to manage when their memories are becoming faulty; (vi) a tendency to become more and more like a caricature of oneself. Faults in personality may then be exaggerated; thus, a mean man becomes a veritable miser; an efficient, managing or over-possessive mother may eventually become the feared tyrant who rules the roost from her armchair. Eccentric and hysterical trends become even more obvious. It is always interesting to speculate what manner of people our patients were when they were much younger!

It is never easy to be sure how far mental changes are normal, or at what point they are evidence of disease. Too great a memory loss certainly suggests a mental disorder is developing. Yet it is vital to recognize that a sudden and unexpected mental change means, very likely, a physical disorder needing to be diagnosed and promptly treated (see Chapter 7).

Intelligence

One's basic intelligence is thought not to improve after early teenage. Measuring the intelligence of older people with the tests used for young people gives unreliable results for a number of reasons. However, it is necessary to say that there is *some* decline in intelligence in many people as the years advance. It may not be very noticeable and it may appear very late – or never. Some great thinkers have lived to be very old men and kept up their activities almost to the end. A highly intelligent old person will normally remain above normal intelligence. Naturally, the more intelligent the person the more apparent will any change for the worse be. A subnormally intelligent man may go further down the scale, but this may escape notice!

This preservation of intelligence in the majority is one of the more satisfactory truths about growing old. Besides, performance may improve in certain directions – like handling words when writing and speaking to an audience – and the range of vocabulary improves. Then, on top of basic intelligence the older person may acquire much wisdom and sagacity, and a whole life-time of experience. This is why young people so often turn to the elderly for advice, for the older person may have faced the same problems before and tell of his own responses. Besides, he will have developed useful short-cuts in doing things and in thought processes which compensate for other short-comings and slowing up.

Learning Ability

The old saying is, "you cannot teach an old dog new tricks". This is not true – not even for dogs. Certainly it is more difficult to learn later in life; it takes longer, and mistakes in learning are harder to get rid of, but learning is certainly possible. Older instructors teach older people best, and they have to go at a deliberate pace, not overtaxing their "students' " memories. Practical knowledge is easier to absorb than theoretical. If these things were not true it might be difficult to rehabilitate elderly invalids, and courses of "preparation for retirement" would be nonsensical.

General Performance

Two particular facts about senescence are worth mentioning. First, it is not possible to sustain strenuous physical effort for so long, and this is not just a matter of having weaker muscles. Therefore many men in later middle life feel obliged to look for lighter work. This is one of the serious problems ageing brings to an industrial society. It is also noticeable that older people have more difficulty in conditions of poor light.

Secondly, the body as a whole slows up in its responses. This can be seen in older games players, in old people trying to keep their balance, and especially when the elderly are in traffic. Here sensory messages about moving vehicles have to be received from the eyes, ears or nose, transmitted to the brain, and the latter's "command" has to be transmitted to the muscles for appropriate action – to move or to stand still. This two-fold transmission of nervous impulses tends to be slightly slowed in old people, but the intermediate processes of the brain, in recognizing the traffic situation and judging the correct action to take, are very much slowed up. This, no doubt, is why elderly drivers have increasing difficulty in modern road conditions and it is a very clear reason why we should all be very much more watchful for elderly pedestrians and give them plenty of time. This *slowing of sensorimotor activity* shows itself even when we are asking questions and get very slow answers from old people. It may take an old person a remarkably long time to give an answer to a question.

Special Skills

Certain special skills – those that do not require sustained or rapid, hard muscular work – remain with old people, and sometimes they are remarkably dextrous in what they do. If a skill is learned early in life and is used regularly it can survive almost indefinitely. Other faculties remain intact; for example, old professional pianists, watchmakers or needlewomen show a skill which is the envy of us all. The best "burlers and menders" (those who examine cloth for snags and put them right) in the textile trade all seem to be elderly. This, then, is another hopeful aspect of ageing which has a moral for us all: i.e. acquire a light manual skill early, use it, and it will be there to enliven one's old age.

COMPENSATIONS FOR AGEING

The inevitability of a lessening physical and mental capability may give younger people the impression that everything is in decline and that self-respect, independence and enjoyment will all vanish as people go further down the road. To some extent this may be true, but some saving graces of senescence have already been mentioned. Besides the preservation of their intelligence and personal skills, most people can look forward to gaining in wisdom, experience and even tranquillity. There is less need to rush, more time for thought, less compulsion to provide for dependants and "keep up with the Joneses", easier acceptance of one's final end. It is important for those approaching old age to have the right objectives. Continuous rest and total inactivity only suit the mentally and physically torpid. Yet, only being interested in physical activities must lead people to disillusionment – even digging or golf may be no standby in one's 80's. Things of the mind, which eventually can be followed sitting down, will last us a good deal better.

Growing old gracefully takes some thought. People should also pursue an active policy of trying to keep healthy, and start well before old age begins. Poor health in old age is an unwelcome prospect.

ABNORMAL OLD AGE

If growing old is a natural process and old age is not itself a disease – which is the only sensible way of looking at it – we can ask ourselves what sort of ageing *is* abnormal. There are very rare and tragic cases of young children looking just like old men or women. This is a disease ("Progeria") due to abnormalities of the pituitary gland. There are also the adults who are prematurely old and others who have severe mental changes making them rather like very old patients – yet they are only in their 50's or early 60's. We do not know the cause of such early mental or physical ageing, but it is abnormal without any doubt.

Otherwise, abnormal ageing, when patients are far less capable than the average for their age, is likely to be due to disease. Much of the rest of this book will be concerned with disease in old age, because this is largely what makes them need the care and help of nurses or social workers.

LOSS OF FACULTIES

Failing Vision

Changes in faculties, normally occurring or due to disease, must be understood, for they affect our method of approach to older people. Presbyopia (see page 12 above) is not failing vision; it is an alteration of vision but the eyesight remains acute. Loss of sharpness ("acuity") of vision even when wearing the correct glasses is a cause of great misery, especially as it interferes with most sedentary activities. But the first essential is to have correct glasses. Older people should have their eyes tested every two years at least; they should wear their glasses, and the lenses should be kept clean. Real loss of vision may be due to disease of the outer surfaces, e.g. conjunctivitis or keratitis, for which treatment is available, or it may be due to pressure changes within the eye (glaucoma) which can to some extent be treated; or it may be due to the lens becoming opaque (cataract) which can be treated by removing the lens and providing much thicker positive lenses in the spectacle frames. Finally, it may be due to diseases in blood vessels within the eye, or diseases of the all-important light-sensitive retina. Some of these latter changes seem to be specifically characteristics of old age. These internal eye diseases are much less easy to treat. Blindness itself in old age is a great scourge and is becoming increasingly common. It reduces some old people to deep depression and even to suicidal ideas. Few of them take real trouble to feel their way about or tap with a white stick; they seldom can learn braille or moon or any other special reading method. Blindness coming on rapidly may reduce them to sitting quite still, afraid to move anywhere. Some old people with cataracts find direct light has a hazy glare, so they take to tinted spectacles; but, otherwise, dramatic dark glasses which are worn regularly indoors rather suggest attention-seeking attitudes in their wearers!

Failing Hearing

Some high-tone hearing loss has been mentioned as one of the almost inevitable findings in old age, and certainly the chance of being slightly deaf rises with the years. Apart from the immediately curable deafness of wax in the ears, lasting deafness is due to previous diseases of the small conducting ossicles or to changes in the auditory nerve mechanism itself. By some people deafness is reckoned to be a worse disability than blindness. The deaf are seldom so serene as the blind and the sad fact is that people are always sympathetic to a blind person but much less so, generally, to a deaf one. Accordingly, deaf people feel cut off and a nuisance, and they often seem to become suspicious and even "paranoid", and it must be said that living with them and having always to raise one's voice is very trying. Very deaf people, being unable to hear their own voice production, may develop harsh "corn-crake" type of voices. Trying to talk to the deaf necessitates our speaking distinctly, with clear articulation and from right in front of them, so that they can also see lip movement. They simply will not hear chance remarks thrown at them from anywhere in the room. Yet if old people can lip read – and some can – they may unexpectedly "hear" our unguarded remarks if we speak facing them even though we are some distance away, so we must be discreet! Some partially deaf people, as most people do, hear what interests them but miss the rest. Some people seem deaf only to things they do not want to be concerned with! This we can call "selective" deafness.

Most deaf people ought to have the chance of trying a hearing aid. The very old have little prospect of learning to use an electronic aid, so deaf people must start early. Electronic aids tend to amplify all the clatter and unwanted sounds as much as the desired voices, so an ear-trumpet type of aid is often better for very old people and not nearly so unacceptable as might appear.

Loss of Sense of Smell

About one person in three over the age of 65 has difficulty in discerning rather delicate smells. Some of the quality goes out of life if one cannot smell. Besides, taste and smell are closely linked. Loss of a sense of taste may affect the appetite, and it may explain why some old people appreciate more highly spiced food than one would expect.

Other Sensations

There may be slight changes in the sense of touch, of heat or vibration, but they are not of real practical importance. The sense of pain however is difficult to judge, for some remarkable old people appear able to endure severe pain without a murmur, and others seem to react violently to quite a minor stimulus. The appreciation of pain is not something which we can measure, and whether or not it is felt excessively in the nervous system it is closely linked with complex psychological factors. The "threshold" of pain seems to be high in some patients and low in others. Putting on and inflating the cuff of a blood pressure apparatus to the usual level (say 120 mm. of mercury) is a good test, since to most people it feels an uncomfortable squeezing but nothing more painful than that. Over-reaction to this suggests a low pain threshold. Older people are much more likely to have painful "rheumatic" conditions than young people, and it is better always to give them the benefit of any doubt about the presence of pain. Some very old people in their 90's, for example, cry out as if they are being hurt whenever anyone touches them or even attempts to move or help them. It is doubtful if this really indicates pain; it is much more likely to be a general expression of resentment or a wish to be left alone.

APPROACHING ELDERLY PEOPLE

It is not easy for younger professional people who are not very used to the aged to know how they should make an approach, particularly since they may be in a position of some temporary authority, as a nurse or a social worker or a therapist is. Yet the client is perhaps several times older. This chapter, especially where it described senescence, has already pointed to some guidelines.

It is important to talk face to face and to be fairly close, so that one's voice will be well heard and the play of lip movements and expression can help in conveying the meaning (see Plate 1). It is a mistake to stand and talk downwards to older people, who, when they are sitting down, cannot look upwards easily, and may be made to feel inferior. One's speech should be distinct, fairly slow, but only loud enough to be plainly heard. Above all the patient must be given time to answer questions: with muddled or ill old people this may be a very long time indeed! Questions may have to be repeated quietly if attention is wandering. A friendly touch of the hand is usually appreciated, especially where the older person might be frightened, lonely or bewildered. Blind people need special consideration because they cannot know what is happening round them or who is approaching; one should say who one is as one passes, to keep them in the picture. This is but common humanity, and should be a rule. Talking to old people is best done as one sensible adult to another. They do not expect servility or special deference just because they are old; but on the other hand they will not appreciate liberties being taken, and they will dislike any hint of being patronized or belittled. It *cannot* be right to address and treat old people as if they were children. Treat an old person as a child ("do this, there's a good girl"!), and she may react as a child, with all that that implies. Anyway, older people react to insults or what they imagine to be insults, and yet may not speak of them openly. They are experienced and can be very wily; some of them have their own means of making their disapproval felt. Dressing old women like children with bows of ribbon in their hair surely pleases no one except nurses with too strong a maternal instinct. Normal human dignities should be preserved even at the very end of life. A patient who has a reputation for being "difficult" is often one who is being handled wrongly, and in these circumstances every person concerned should first consider whether the fault might lie with herself. The "holy terror" can become a "nice old person" when moved to a ward or a Home where the staff are more enlightened. This is just one of the many justifications for special hospital wards for elderly people.

AGEING AND "SENILITY"

Ageing we have discussed, but senility we have not. Whatever the original dictionary meaning of the word senility might have been, it has come to be used in an unpleasant sense. No one ever means anything kindly by using it, and the word would be best forgotten. Senility seems to imply all that is unsatisfactory about old age and old people; it is almost a term of abuse. A few doctors still label their patients as suffering from "senility", as if it were a true diagnosis – which it certainly is not. It is a convenient device for not looking any further for the real causes of the upset, whether they are physical or mental. The word "senile" itself is often used similarly. It has the same respectable Latin origin, but the author thinks it should only be used now as an adjective to describe some particular condition – implying something which belongs entirely to old age (e.g. senile cataracts, senile warts). It is best used, too, well out of a person's earshot as he might think of it as being used about him in its other, insulting, degrading way.

SEX IN LATER LIFE

Many people have the impression that sexual life is unimportant to old people and that it "fades out": some women believe their sex life ought to end at the menopause, and, since they believe this in advance, it may very well do so. The attitude of the young, with their idealism and their sense and possession of physical beauty, might suggest to them that sexual activity could not be satisfactory or even "decent" in older men and women. A marriage between an older man and a young woman is thought sometimes not to be quite right, even though such marriages are often highly successful. Finally, people who run Homes are apt to think that cohabitation between a man and his wife is somehow repellent "at that age": "They could hold hands," they say, "but what more do they need?" This attitude is changing, fortunately, but in the old days men and their wives in institutions were strictly separated.

Older people do not talk very freely about this subject, and older women are especially reticent – or perhaps one does not like to ask them. Yet it has been shown that 7 out of 10 healthy couples remain sexually active beyond the age of 60, and 25% are still active when the man is 75 or more. We must not of course forget that as a rule men are married to women rather younger than themselves, and many people anyway have lost their partners by bereavement. Usually it is not "failure" or even loss of interest which causes people to stop cohabiting in old age so much as the ill health of one of the partners. On the other hand, those who have always found the whole business rather embarrassing may use their age as a convenient reason for stopping.

There is nothing like anxiety for upsetting sexual activity, and some men fear that they will lose their potency: it is not in fact true, or not true till an advanced age, especially if they have always been active in that respect. If we judge potency simply by frequency, then the man does probably become slightly less potent from adolescence onwards. With women the capacity to experience orgasm does not diminish. There is usually no time of life, then, when a large group of people suddenly ceases to be sexually active, and no one ought to assume there is anything abnormal or "disgusting", or even exhausting, in the process.

We must most certainly remember that there is much more to marriage than sexual activity. It is a great stabilizing force and a source of comfort and companionship in old age; it is in fact a cause of the very survival of pairs of people who would almost certainly live less long if they were not together. Indeed, quite often it happens that a man and his wife are so much "one" that if either of them dies the other very soon follows, almost as if the will to live had left the one who survived a little. The social services and the hospitals would be very hard put to it if women did not look after their sick men, and men after their sick wives equally, very often. The decision to separate a man and his wife and send one or other into hospital as the "most sensible thing" must be thought about very carefully. It may *not* in fact be the best thing; it may imperil the lives of both. Just as mother-and-baby units are a sensible idea, it might be practical and sensible to have man-and-wife units for older people in hospital, not simply on a permanent basis, but so that a woman could look after her sick husband in a crisis when she needed more help and better equipment than she had available at home.

Above all we must rid ourselves of the idea that there is anything unseemly or abnormal about a man and wife being in the same Home together and occupying the same quarters. However, if they are not too grossly disabled, they will probably try to stay out of Residential Homes at all costs!

When the author started to bring into use "mixed" day rooms for old men and women patients in hospital (with many misgivings from the Authorities), it became immediately clear that the men and the women were behaving in a more normal and acceptable way, and taking much greater care of their appearance and their language. The experiment has been a great success, and mixed day rooms are more the rule than the exception.

Chapter 3

PATTERNS OF LIVING

Social Workers, Home Nurses and Health Visitors quickly learn from personal experience what effect poor social conditions and lack of understanding and foresight have on their work for older people. They know where the supporting services are most needed. The sad fact is that many old people have to fight an illness and bad social conditions at the same time. Good links between hospital and community were never more needed than in geriatrics.

It must be true that social factors can sometimes themselves be a cause of poor health or even serious disease: we might think at once of the so-called "diseases of deprivation" such as malnutrition. If people cannot afford food or cannot get it because they are frail and far from the shops, these are social considerations, unmistakeably. The same can be said if old people for economic reasons always buy the wrong food, grow fat, and then fall ill because of it. But not all deprivation is the fault of poverty or of selfish people not caring about their neighbours. One knows of old people who are lonely even though they have large families. There is perhaps antagonism, the children do not visit – but sometimes this was more the fault of the older generation than the younger; some of the deprivation then was of their own making. Again, some of the half-starved people are those who live like hermits and will not allow anyone to call.

Geriatric physicians are always coming across elderly people who have always lived in poor conditions yet even so have enjoyed quite healthy lives. It is when some major illness descends on them that the difficulties start and the poverty of their circumstances comes to everyone's notice. By contrast there are some well off old people too – but they also seem to fall ill with many of the same complaints.

In short, the real problem of old age so often centres round a breakdown in physical and mental health which is not really related to the way in which the old people have been living. Up to a point one can live in squalor if one prefers to without harmful effects! This may not, of course, be so true of countries where average living standards and sanitation are less good than our own. No one denies that the opposite is also

25

true—a serious illness can be managed better in a good home where help is available.

Admission to hospital often depends on such social considerations. The geriatric physician takes them very much into account when deciding if and when to arrange admission, so it always pays to let him have the true facts. A hospital team, or anyway a *geriatric* hospital team, does not resent the fact that social factors force some admissions: it is all part of the work.

Once an elderly patient has fallen ill and into the hands of the specialist team, however, it is vital that its doctors, nurses, therapists and social workers should understand clearly what the patient will face at home when she is better, even though perhaps she is still rather disabled. Geriatric departments, more perhaps than any other department except the paediatric department, must be concerned with the whole life pattern of their patients right from the time that they first meet them. Sending a patient back to an unknown home environment might mean she relapsed in a very few days. This is why most geriatric physicians consult their medical social workers personally at every stage, and why so often a reasonably fit person's discharge has to be delayed. A good modern geriatric department sets a hot pace for its local supporting services whose function is to take over on discharge.

CHANGES IN FAMILY LIFE

Large families were the accepted pattern in Victorian times. To have a large family was an insurance for one's own old age. It was usually understood that a younger daughter should stay on at home and care for her parents, and this was done, and often still is done, by devoted people at great personal sacrifice. These days there is more of a tendency to arrange for frail parents to move round various family members when all share in the care. The Victorian children are now old people. There are still many of them, and usually they themselves had smaller families. Sometimes they were used to having domestic servants; but these are no more, and even a paid companion or just "someone to come and live with us", is very hard to find. So now that they are aged there are fewer of their own people to help them. Besides, it has become quite usual for unmarried women and housewives who have brought up their families to have regular work which they do not want to give up. In many places it gets harder and harder to find anyone willing to care for elderly people at home.

As well as being smaller, today's families are more dispersed, because quick transport and expanding opportunities have made this possible. There are still families whose members mostly live in one town or one village, but the younger generation are going further afield. Thousands of young emigrants leave Britain every year. In all this movement it is usually the older generation which is left in the family house, which is probably old, inconvenient, dilapidated, and too large now for just one or two people. Even when the members of the younger generation remain in the same town they tend to migrate to the outlying districts where there are better houses – but also higher rents.

The problem of what best to do for their elderly relatives faces many families. A three-generation family, i.e. grandparents, parents and children living together, seems to be an ideal and natural arrangement – or it does so at first sight. No doubt where families are close knit and accustomed to spending their lives and even their holidays together, this idea often works. It can work too when things are deliberately planned so that an elderly parent has a room or flatlet and separate cooking arrangements for her own use, so she lives very close but partly independently. Unhappily, very few families can manage this. Suddenly deciding to form a three-generation household after the oldest member has been ill and seems too frail to go on living alone is a very different proposition, especially when it means overcrowding everybody, depriving the children of their own bedroom, or risking disagreements between in-laws. It might work, but it is often a disaster. Anyone, therefore, who advises a family to do this takes a very great deal upon herself. Even two-generation households can be full of stresses and strains. This observation does not imply that younger people should *not* give a welcome to their parents. Sometimes it works very well, but a trial period, keeping the older person's house going in case she wants to return there, is a wise first step.

The younger generation do have some moral obligations towards their parents, but they no longer have legal obligations as they used to do. Happiness seldom results for either side if the younger generation accepts greater responsibilities than it wishes to, out of a sense of guilt. We professional health and social workers should avoid implanting a sense of guilt. Unjust criticisms of Hospitals and Homes arise sometimes because a son or daughter, feeling guilty, attacks the very people who are bearing the burden of care. It is never wise within the family circle to enter into promises which may be too difficult to keep. Some old people hand over their houses and money in return for a promise of care "till they die". Some younger people say, "We promise never to let you be taken away to hospital or a Home." Who can say what circumstances might make that necessary?

Some old people's children will give up work to care for sick parents till the end of their days. Yet it would be hard to justify the only wage-earner doing this, for that would mean everyone living on State benefits. Working women often do make this sacrifice, and all honour to them: but it is reasonable to ask if the Community would not be served best if its most valuable women workers, especially its nurses, therapists, social workers and teachers went on doing their invaluable work and let the Hospitals or Homes take care of their frail or invalid parents. Blood may be thicker than water, but special skills were not meant to be wasted.

VOLUNTARY AND OFFICIAL HELP

Many people believe that there is a growing tendency for young people not to look after their elders but to say, "The Welfare State should provide" – because (they say) they are paying taxes anyway. Some do certainly take this line – perhaps more so now than in former times. Nevertheless a great many old people are kept going at home, in health and sometimes in sickness, by devoted friends or relatives. It would be a bad day for the Hospitals and Social Services Departments' Residential Homes if these supporters suddenly went on strike, for they would be overwhelmed. Members of families and other volunteers spend their own money, make journeys, cook and carry meals, and give all kinds of practical help. The country's official policy is wherever possible to try to keep old people out of hospitals and other institutions. It could not be carried out if it were not for the unofficial and unstinted voluntary help which so many people give. It is right that we should acknowledge this, and right, too, that every help and every financial assistance should be given to them in this valuable work.

At the present time about 12% of elderly people living at home receive help from either or both the Health or Social Services. Probably a great many more *should* be receiving it if everyone had his rights. There is room for both voluntary effort and official help. The most needy and most lonely or disabled should have first priority for official help, naturally; but otherwise the work of volunteers and official workers should be complementary.

THE EFFECT OF MARITAL STATUS

There is no doubt whatever that people who are alone are most vulnerable to the effects of old age and disease. It is not hard to see why. People on their own cannot see themselves through an illness which is long or serious. Statistics from many sources show that there is a greater chance of people who are unmarried, widowed, separated or divorced entering geriatric hospitals or mental hospitals, and that their chances of remaining as long-stay patients is also higher than the average. It is probable, though more difficult to prove, that people on their own are less able to withstand life's unkind buffetings. In short, whatever other advantages it has, the married state is probably best for facing old age. This is not to say that many spinsters do not keep themselves healthy and active to a very great age, for indeed they do. Bachelors are generally less viable!

It is not true that all marriages stand the test of time; sad to say, some elderly couples fall out of love and some grow very bitter indeed. Nevertheless married people do have moral and legal obligations to each other, and most of them are only too glad to give the partner all possible care and help "in sickness or in health". Discharging patients from hospital is not so often a problem when there is a wife or husband to receive the invalid back, though we must remember that both may be frail and in poor health.

A well-known situation occurs in geriatrics when one partner has to be admitted and the other must come too or be admitted to a Home temporarily. Together these two "semi-isolates", as they are called, just manage to get along; take one away and the *ménage* collapses.

THE EFFECT OF LOCALITY

Elderly town dwellers have many advantages over country people because shops, libraries, churches and clubs are nearer at hand and transport arrangements are better. The various social services which ought to be provided, especially Home Helps, are also likely to be more easily available in towns, though it is good to see Meals-on-Wheels services now developing in so many country districts.

People in the country may face very great difficulties because their cottages are old, damp, without sanitation and sometimes even without piped water supplies. Hot water systems and baths are unusual to find. People often cook on coal ranges or use oilburning stoves; their public transport is deplorable; the social services are spread thinly and even the Home Nurse may serve several parishes and have to come several miles. Country dwellers nevertheless have some advantages – clean air, peace, room to grow vegetables, more obliging neighbours perhaps, coupled with a closer knit, friendlier community. Big cities teeming with people are often lonely places for old people, for it is quite normal not even to know one's neighbours. In villages curiosity gets the better of shyness!

Isolation by distance together with bad housing very often makes admissions to hospital urgently necessary for elderly country dwellers, though the same illness might need less drastic steps in a town. For the same reason the prospects of discharge of a partly disabled old country person may be less good too. This very fact alters the pattern of geriatric hospital work in country areas, and may affect the number of beds required.

It is quite common now for elderly workers who have saved money for their own home to leave the district they have always lived in and retire to the seaside (see Chapter 1), or to some place where they usually spent their holidays. The points in favour of this are a quieter, pleasanter and perhaps less polluted environment. There are many points against it. Uprooting is more difficult in later life, and old, deep roots are most valuable to some people. By moving one might have to leave behind one's family and staunch friends; new friends would be harder to make now, and they would not feel the same sense of obligation. So this kind of retirement can turn out to be lonely, and many people come to regret their move. When they fall ill or finally are widowed their state is pathetic.

HOUSING

Since the chances of being frail and handicapped increase with the passage of time, it follows that older people need warm, comfortable, well lit, safe and trouble-free places to live. So often bad housing tips the scale the wrong way, whereas a good house makes independent living still possible. Bad housing in the country has already been described and in towns it is often little better. Seeking out an older patient on a visit the doctor looks for the house in the row which has the peeling paint, the overgrown front garden, the heavy curtains and the bell which does not work. Inside, that house is often dark, cheerless, cold, cluttered up, full of heavy furniture and loose mats, with awkward steps and primitive kitchen and sanitary arrangements. The risk of a serious accident in such a home is frightening to think about. Yet some old people do manage in spite of all the difficulties to keep their homes bright, clean and fairly safe. We do not have to search far for the reasons for not doing so: lack of funds; lack of foresight; lack of energy and finally apathy, these all play their part. Cold houses carry a risk of hypothermia (see page 59), bronchitis and pneumonia; damp seems to add to the possibilities of rheumatic symptoms; outside lavatories do not encourage continence; dark, drab rooms increase the chance of depression. People who are in lodgings or are acting as companions to other people, or who occupy rooms in private hotels are in a very vulnerable position. They are liable to get their marching orders if they fall ill or need too much personal aid.

The solution to bad housing is *rehousing*. It ought not to be necessary to think at once of a move to a Home. There are many possible alternatives before that step: a bungalow or flatlet on an estate – probably one which was built especially for older tenants; a good bedsitting room in a larger house subdivided and run by a Housing Association (of which there are many); an almshouse if it has been brought up to date; or a small house or a bungalow grouped with others in a Council or voluntarily provided "sheltered housing" development with a warden within call, heating provided effortlessly from a central boiler house – all these have their particular merits for particular people. There cannot really be much doubt that one of the surest ways of solving the mounting difficulties of old people is to provide first-class living conditions and let them be as independent as possible. This duty falls mainly on the Housing Departments of local Councils. It is probably wiser to build much more sheltered housing than to go on building one new Residential Home after another. Some old people finally do have to be taken "into care", as some deprived children do; most would prefer to run their own lives still if only it were made possible.

MONEY

Retirement almost always reduces living standards. Some people have saved carefully or invested some money; more and more are qualifying for pensions from their service or their employers, and the State contributory pensions systems are quickly being improved to make life more bearable in later life. However some people never could save, and some never had the chance. For most of them there is the Retirement Pension and the various supplements to which they may be entitled – even if in times past many of them refused to apply for supplements because they made the mistake of thinking of them as "charity". More than one-third of the elderly people in Britain depend entirely on the State for their income. Pensioners of all types are at the mercy of inflation: wages rise, prices rise, and eventually State pensions have to rise, but they always lag well behind the increases in wages of working people. There is a great deal to be said for linking them to a cost-of-living index.

Retirement pensions, then, are very small and numbers of old people are barely able to manage at all. They can, if they are very careful, pay the rent and fuel bills and have enough over for just adequate food without luxuries. This leaves hardly any margin over for clothes, entertainments or domestic replacements, and any unusual happening may strain their resources very severely. A sudden cold snap means spending more on heating and cutting down on food; or it means going cold and eating as usual. Financial arrangements as stringent as these work out only if budgeting is well done and the shopper can look around for bargains; but some old people do not spend their money wisely and some are too disabled to "shop around". Some are too proud to accept the unpopular and less expensive kinds of meat, for example, even though these are known to give good food value. It is quite possible in these circumstances to be undernourished. Not replacing old electrical apparatus leads to risks of serious accidents; economizing with fuel increases the chance of respiratory infections and other diseases. In bad times old people go to bed just to keep warm, and that in itself is undesirable (see Chapter 5). In these and other ways, apart from the misery it causes, a low income could lead to disease which might be avoided. Many people want to help themselves by taking simple part-time work, though our present official pension arrangements do not give them much encouragement; but not every old person can do this anyway. Many younger people, with one eye on inflation say, "Saving? What's the use?". But there are ways of saving which go some of the way towards off-setting inflation. For the sake of a more comfortable time later, therefore, it seems a wise thing to do. Anyway, who can doubt that old age is easier to face if one is reasonably comfortably off?

LONELINESS

A few people wish to live alone; most others who are alone have it thrust upon them by circumstances. We have already seen what effects this is likely to have when a major illness strikes them down. Isolation itself may be harmful. Eating alone is dull; cooking for one person is a trouble, and many solitary people bother less and less about getting proper meals. Anyway budgeting is easier for a group than it is for individuals.

The more isolated people are, the less they feel the need to take trouble with their housework, to keep clean and well-groomed. If no one calls, they say to themselves, "What does it matter?". Though some keep up their high personal standards, many become untidy, slovenly, even dirty, in a way which would not happen if they were in company. They may also become morose and resentful of other people. It is even possible that loneliness eventually results in mental deterioration and disease like depression or paranoia, for normally people talk and sharpen their wits on other people. It seems fair to assume that if mental capabilities are not used they will deteriorate, just as physical capabilities do. It is known that admissions to mental hospitals of lonely, deprived people are high, and that keeping up mental activity wards off mental change.

It is not easy to remedy loneliness, and some old people do not like "interference", as they might call our attempts to befriend them. Clubs, day centres and visiting by friends are a great help to people who will accept these ideas. Doctors, nurses, health visitors and everyone who could visit in any official capacity must recognize that the lonely are just the people most at risk of disease and deprivation. Visits of a semi-social type, just for a talk but keeping a professional eye open, help in the detection of these things, for the patient seldom complains directly.

* * *

From what has been said in this chapter it might appear that social circumstances are very much to blame for making older people ill. If it really were so, we might have a better chance of preventing disease. The fact remains that even if everyone lived in the lap of luxury there would still be a great deal of disease. Infection, cancers and degenerative conditions unfortunately have little to do with social conditions.

Chapter 4

PATTERNS OF DISEASE

Children and adolescents, young and old adults – they are all people; but as *groups* of people they are different, with different outlooks and different needs. Paediatrics came into existence as a specialty because illness and its problems in the very young were shown in so many ways to be different from illness later. Now, for the other end of life, Geriatrics has become a special branch of medical practice because the patterns of illness change, and the type of care provided has to be subtly different too. This is not to say that any good nurse or social worker would not be able to care for either of these different groups, for it is the basic act of caring which matters most. Nevertheless care will be most effective where the similarities and differences are properly appreciated. Some people say, "We all have elderly patients, so of course we all practise geriatrics now". This is only half the story; treating old people just as one would treat someone in middle life, without altering methods or tactics to fit the circumstances, is *not* practising geriatrics. Walking with an old dog, even driving an old car require altered tactics too.

Geriatrics can almost be said to be an attitude of mind: the attitude needed for treating old patients with their particular ills. The purpose of this chapter then is to describe how the patterns of disease change. People who imagine that a disease keeps to a standard pattern at all ages of the patient – just because it is caused by a particular kind of virus or bacterium, for example – are apt to make mistakes. They reckon without the changes which have taken place within the ageing body and its defence mechanisms. These differences often force us, whether we like it or not, to take a different line in treatment, or even to take "liberties" of which other doctors and nurses might not at first approve.

Some old people are in perfect health for their years – that is, if they were well endowed with good genes at birth, and have been lucky and sensible since. Many others arrive at old age carrying with them the scars of several battles; that is, battles against various diseases and injuries, and sometimes the aftermath of old deprivations too. At least we hope today's children will grow old without signs of physical deprivation.

Up to 30 or 40 years ago people usually died young if they were afflicted with certain crippling diseases or chronic infections. Being unfit, they were liable to catch other infections like pneumonia and could not throw them off. Now sulphonamides, antibiotics and good nursing have changed the scene, so they can survive and often do, to be quite old. A good example of such a survival was a dwarfed man in his middle 70's who had rickets as a young child and still showed very distorted bones and chest. Another example would be an old person who still carried in her X-rays signs of scarring from chronic pulmonary tuberculosis which may have been making her breathless; she finally overcame the illness, perhaps, after years of being in and out of hospitals, when the modern drugs appeared. Sometimes people's disabilities have existed so long and yet changed because of contractures, deformities, etc. that it is hard to be sure what the original diagnosis was.

MULTIPLE DISEASE

In later life it is common for patients to suffer from several diseases at once. In the young this would be unusual, and medical students are in fact encouraged to try to fit all the clinical evidence into one diagnosis. In geriatrics this just cannot be done. Multiple disease is the rule rather than the exception. An average "score" is 4 to 5 diagnoses at once. For example, the cause of heart failure could easily be coronary artery disease *plus* bronchitis, *plus* anaemia, all of which need treatment. A patient might have a slowly growing cancer of the breast (which she might have been hiding for months) and be sent to hospital with signs of a stroke. A cerebral secondary cancer? Perhaps, but it might just as easily be due to a simple stroke, because strokes are very common anyway.

The likelihood of several diseases occurring at once may seriously complicate treatment. A patient who already has one artificial leg and then develops even a mild stroke on the other side of the body will find it very hard indeed to walk again. Similarly, a man could suffer a coronary thrombosis and soon afterwards develop a cerebral thrombosis; the heart attack means he should rest, and the stroke means he requires active exercises as soon as possible. Therefore in geriatrics treatment is often a compromise and necessitates the taking of a middle course. Time-honoured rules may have to be broken. It is best in fact to avoid rigid rules. Several diseases occurring together often make a simple situation difficult, so that hospital admission may be needed. Thus, a man who lives alone and who attends to his own colostomy without help will be in terrible difficulty if he sprains his wrist and has to have it put into a sling. In some casualty departments one hears statements like, "We do not admit a patient with a dislocated shoulder once we have reduced it". When the patient is old such 'rules' may have to be swept aside. All the diseases present must be listed, and the effects of one on the others must be carefully thought out. A good geriatric department should record not only the various formal medical diagnoses, but also the everyday problems which beset the patient (and his helpers). Thus "immobility", "urinary incontinence" or "aphasia" are formidable problems, whatever the precise medical cause of them. Such a "problem orientated medical records" system can be a great help to the whole geriatric team.

CANCER

It has been hinted already that cancer is not always so disastrous in old age as it is in the not-so-old. Yet cancer is more likely as one grows older; indeed, it has been calculated that the risk of cancer is doubled for every eight years we live. However, after the age of about 70 or 75, many cancers become less common or if they appear they spread less rapidly. A few, a very few, even appear to get smaller, perhaps because their blood supply is not sufficient for growth of the tumour. At all events one does not necessarily rush immediately to treat cancer in an old person. The rest of that patient's troubles have to be assessed too, and the risk of surgery (for instance) weighed up. Perhaps the surgical risk is thought to be excessive; perhaps the elderly patient himself declines to accept drastic treatment; perhaps he might die of some other complaint anyway before the cancer could develop far. All this calls for cool judgement based on probability. With a younger cancer patient the issues are much clearer.

RECOVERY AND HEALING

It is often supposed that old tissues will not heal well, and that old people's recovery from illness must be slow. Sometimes these ideas prove correct but just as often they do not. Surgical wounds heal well in very aged people. Even open wounds and ulcers will heal extraordinarily quickly if they are kept clean and non-infected (which can be quite a problem with old people at home), and if the blood supply is good and the patient is well fed. You cannot build bricks without straw: so, you cannot heal your wounds without blood, protein and vitamins. Fractures will unite firmly and quickly too, but the problem here is often an insufficient blood supply to the bone. Even fractures through cancerous deposits, so-called "pathological" fractures, heal quite quickly.

General recovery from illness need not necessarily be very slow either. Many patients with pneumonia are up and about in a few days – to some people's astonishment. But if an old person is already at a low ebb, is fighting several acute conditions at once, has had a poor appetite, is anaemic and under-nourished, then his recovery will indeed be slow. This is why adequate convalescence is so important to old people and nutrition must be maintained. The appetite, in particular, takes a long time to return after a severe illness.

The duration of an illness (and therefore the length of time a bed is occupied in hospital) seem often to depend on incentives. Young people have every incentive to be up and away; there's money to earn, a family to look after, things to do. Older people often have no positive incentives; lying in bed means (they hope) that people will come to minister to them; being in hospital is (for some) a much nicer life than fending for themselves in their own homes. This is a sad reflection on social conditions.

Finally, we must remember that "recovery" in later life does not usually mean being made fit for active paid work. In other words, the objectives are different, but regaining independence of movement and domestic capability are still amongst them.

PSYCHOLOGICAL FACTORS

As has just been hinted, incentive, otherwise often called "motivation", is important, and it fails all too easily. Stress diseases, like gastric and duodenal ulcers are rather less common because there is less of ambition, compulsion and "drive" to bring them on, but general anxieties if anything multiply. Some old people show strong hysterical tendencies, though usually they were people who reacted like this earlier in life. Hysteria needs careful, firm handling.

Some unhappy old people are so resentful of the world and all its works – even of the things which nurses and others are trying to do to help – that they will co-operate in nothing. In its most serious form this amounts to an attitude of complete silence, a cutting off of all contact, a refusal to eat or drink, the condition of total "negativism". It is very difficult to overcome this even by showing great patience and kindness. Occasionally, a sad, embittered, nihilistic old person will die apparently wishing it to happen that way, refusing to allow any personal approach whatever. She just, as the saying is, "puts up the shutters". When this happens, the question of forced feeding or other extreme measures might be raised, because it could be argued that the patient does not realise how life-threatening her behaviour is; but perhaps she does know. In practice in geriatric departments there are few people who would think any sad, disillusioned elderly patient, intent on departing in this fashion, should be forcibly prevented from doing so.

PHYSICAL REACTIONS TO DISEASE

The special ways in which the aged body reacts to the "insults" heaped on it by disease make up one of the absorbing interests of geriatric work.

Sometimes the reaction seems very slight, and this suggests that the body's defences are not very powerful. This is a difficult point to prove scientifically. Yet even in young people failure of the body to react quickly and strongly to a bacterial invasion is a danger signal.

In older people it is unusual for the temperature to rise; if it does rise it is seldom much beyond 39°C at most. In the elderly a high, swinging fever is a most unusual reaction to infection, though when it does happen it suggests a large hidden collection of pus in a lung or round a kidney. Again, bed-shaking rigors are exceptional, the most common cause being infection of the upper renal tract. Much more commonly pneumonia occurs with only a slight temperature rise or none at all. Waiting for it to appear means unjustifiably endangering the patient's life. Alterations of pulse or respiratory rate are much more sensitive signs of something being wrong (Fig. 5). Observing promptly a change in the respiratory rate or its rhythm when the patient is at rest is of far more importance in geriatrics than careful charting of the temperature. Good nurses develop an instinct for changes in breathing, and should report anything of the kind to the doctor quickly.

By contrast, a *fall* of temperature in response to infection or disease is quite usual. Below 35°C a patient is moving towards the dangerous state of hypothermia (see Chapter 5). It happens so often that anyone working with old people should have a low reading thermometer always available, because other thermometers of the standard type give misleading figures. In a case of doubt placing a thermometer in the patient's rectum is far more valuable than using one of the conventional places. What this measures is the so-called "core" temperature of the body, which is the true temperature. In research work with normal people, who might object to having their temperature taken rectally, it was found that asking for urine to be passed into a big bottle through a funnel in which a thermometer lay, enabled the core temperature to be satisfactorily recorded.

Young bodies have fever as an early warning of danger. If older ones do not, at least they have another useful sign instead. This is mental confusion. The aged brain is very sensitive in this respect, perhaps because its blood supply at best is only just adequate, and any extra demands on the body as a whole deprive the brain. Whatever the explanation, almost any disease is apt to be accompanied by some fall-off in its performance, or by actual confusion. In young people with urgent illness we speak of their "delirium". With old people in the same circumstances we tend to say they are "confused" – or worse. *So, a sudden change in mental state ought always to be taken as a direct pointer towards a physical disease.* Confusion is in fact one of the most common of all first symptoms. It is not a good reason for taking steps towards admitting a patient straight to a mental hospital, especially if there is a geriatric admission ward available. Some older people who already have longstanding mental

deterioration may have further confusion over and above it when they
are physically ill, but that is a different question.

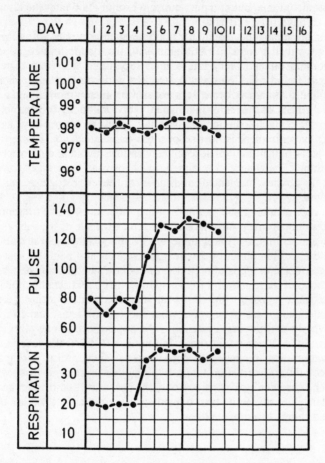

Fig. 5 A typical "T.P.R." chart of an elderly patient with pneumonia. Note: absence of
fever.

Body reactions are modified in many other ways. Sepsis should
classically be followed by local swelling, pain and heat, then perhaps
signs of lymphatic spread (lymphangiitis), and a group of enlarged,
tender glands should appear in the lymph drainage area. In older people
there is seldom a glandular reaction like this.

Many old people who are gravely ill give little outward sign of it, and
complain of nothing which is clear-cut. The risk of a mistake in diagnosis
is therefore high. People may even wander listlessly about their houses

for hours or days with "grumbling" pneumonia, obviously not well, but not very obviously ill. Listening to their chests reveals very uncertain signs of pneumonia, but at a post-mortem examination later the disease is shown to have been extensive.

Other old people develop acute abdominal emergencies without much pain and with the signs of peritonitis, say, from a perforated appendix only coming on at a very late stage. Very often a greatly distended bladder is found quite by chance, and the patient never complained of any difficulty in passing urine. It is not so very uncommon to find a fracture of the neck of the femur in a patient who took to her bed for no clear reason; she omits to mention that she had a bad fall several days ago! In younger patients there is no risk of these happenings going unreported, but an older patient may philosophically endure pain and discomfort and say nothing. The chance of a missed diagnosis is all the greater when the patient is already demented and does not even recognise her own symptoms.

One very characteristic example of age-differences in the presentation of disease is coronary thrombosis. We tend to think of it as an acutely painful and dramatic crisis with severe gripping central chest pain. Not so in old age; only about one patient in five feels any pain; the rest have fainting attacks, or signs of a stroke, or sudden mental confusion, or the appearance of gangrene of a toe, or many other unexpected happenings; yet the basic cause is the heart attack. Here, as in other geriatric situations, things are not always what they seem. Thus, diabetes often starts slowly and the first evidence is the appearance of one of its many complications. Mucous diarrhoea is found, but the real cause is gross constipation with impacted faeces. Bacterial endocarditis perhaps has no fever and no heart murmur; a hyper-active thyroid gland shows no goitre and the eyes look normal – only the heart rate and rhythm give the clue. Pale-skinned people turn out not to have anaemia. The list of unexpected things is almost endless!

SYMPTOMS

It follows from what has just been said that certain symptoms which are quite meaningful in young people are unreliable later in life. Cough is not so very common. If old people *could* cough better they might recover from chest infections more easily. Meanwhile their sputum is seldom produced for us to see. Breathlessness is an uncommon symptom of heart or lung disease, strange to relate. If old people sit still they never exert themselves enough to be breathless. On the other hand excessive fatigue is a valuable symptom of anaemia or of heart failure. Headache is a rare symptom, but when it occurs it is important – which is the opposite of headache in younger people! Palpitations are rarely complained of, though heart irregularities are exceptionally common. Constipation on the contrary is a constant worry to everyone. Sometimes it is important, and sometimes it is not. The only sure way of finding out is to do a rectal examination, which should be a routine matter anyway when a new geriatric patient arrives at a surgery, a clinic, or in a hospital ward.

In general it can be said of old people's symptoms that they are fewer than expected; therefore when they are spoken of they ought specifically to be reported to the doctor, for they may be the first and only clue that he will get. The whole of current medical practice rests on the simple idea of the *self*-reporting of symptoms. Patients normally go to doctors to relate their problems. However, it is known in geriatric work that this method often fails, and the early stages of illness are missed, as older people think their symptoms are just evidence of old age, or because they hesitate to "bother" their doctors with what might be regarded as something trivial.

GROUPS OF DISEASES

We can now list the broader classes of illnesses to be expected in later life. Diseases brought into old age and cancer have both been discussed, though they are not the most common. The largest group is made up of *degenerative diseases*, of which arterial disease and degenerative arthritis (osteoarthrosis) are commonest. Arteries supply all organs, so arterial disease can make itself felt everywhere – in the heart, the brain, the kidneys, the eyes, the legs and feet, the intestines even. Disease due to failure of endocrine glands like diabetes or hypothyroidism may be linked with degenerative changes, but this is far less certain. *Infections* are common; some are specific like Herpes zoster; some are less specific but extremely common, like bronchitis and pneumonia, cystitis and pyelonephritis. One group of diseases can be classed together as *diseases of deprivation*: these include malnutrition in all its forms, deprivation of water and sometimes of warmth, and even deprivation of affection and incentives.

There is besides an unfortunate series of disorders which result from treatment methods, because older people often react unfavourably to certain drugs or methods of therapy even though they were necessary for us to use. We should always try to see that the treatment does no harm.

Finally there is a large group of *mental disorders* which are due to age changes, degenerative disease, or so-called functional disease in old people. Therefore there is plenty of work facing geriatric hospital teams, and much research is needed on these diseases and their prevention.

DISABILITY VERSUS DISEASE

Most doctors when they were students, and most nurses too, have been taught to think of diseases as single entities, leading them to expect certain quite clear-cut, recognizable symptoms and signs. These diseases may be grouped together in our minds, like the blood diseases or heart diseases are, and this is a convenient classification for remembering facts. Yet each "disease" for most of us is one idea on to which we put a label, and then we all think we know where we stand. In fact most signs of a disease are the signs of the reaction of a body to some abnormal happening. Several similar sets of symptoms may be brought about by different abnormal happenings. A simple example is that either high blood pressure or an abnormality of the aortic valve of the heart can both start up attacks of urgent breathlessness in the middle of the night. The skill of diagnosis depends largely on being able to show the differences between rather similar happenings and so put a finger on the cause. This might be simple enough if diseases came one by one, and if by finding the cause the doctor could put the matter right once for all. With young people this is often possible, though not always. With old people, as we shall see repeatedly, there is often a mixture of many diseases all at once, and the cures may not be complete when every effort has been made. Diagnosis is therefore much more difficult.

In geriatric work therefore we need always to have in mind what the *disabilities* (handicaps) are as much as the diagnosis itself. A diagnosis is the idea on which the doctor bases his first treatment. A disability is what the whole team faces as a problem to overcome before the patient can resume his place in Society – and sometimes it remains so great that he can never do so. In a long-drawn out case the original diagnosis, though important at the time, may fade into insignificance. So the disability has become the all-important thing. This can be illustrated as follows:–

The *diagnosis* of Mrs. Evans's case may be:
   a) Old cardiac infarction.
   b) Recent right hemiplegia from cerebral thrombosis.
   c) Diabetes with cataracts.

Mrs. Evans's *disabilities* could be:
   a) She cannot exert herself in rehabilitation – which is therefore slow.
   b) She cannot use the right arm at all – with all that means.
   c) She is weak in the right leg – and walks with an aid, slowly.
   d) She cannot see out of the right half of her visual field.
   e) She cannot express herself properly in speech.
   f) She needs insulin but she cannot handle a syringe with one hand and she cannot see to measure her own dose.
   g) She tends to be incontinent at night.

Adding up the disabilities, Mrs. Evans, living alone, cannot manage, and must stay in hospital; but if Mrs. Evans lived with a kind, intelligent sister she might be managed quite well at home if a little domestic help was provided. The bare diagnosis gives not more than a hint of this, and the same bare diagnosis could involve a different set of disabilities!

It is therefore essential that all members of a geriatric team should have their eyes fixed clearly on the disabilities and the objectives in each case and just as important that the social workers involved should understand them too. It is as well to list these disabilities at intervals to judge progress, potentialities and prospects. The argument can indeed be taken one stage further. We should really be interested in *abilities* even more than *disabilities*. Disabilities are sad; abilities are reasons for rejoicing. One kind is a subtraction from the whole person, the other can be a series of additions as steady rehabilitation goes on.

There are many elderly patients who, when discussing their condition say, "Doctor, I can't do this; I can't do that; I can't do the other!". The author's reply is often simply this, "Mrs. J. I am not so interested in what you cannot do as what you *can* do!". This sounds a little brusque and heartless but it in fact summarizes the spirit of geriatric rehabilitation. Often the patient suddenly sees the difference and starts to think positively, and she may next time say with triumph, "Today, Doctor, I walked five steps alone!". To foster this aim even geriatric "disability" charts can be turned into "ability" charts for all to see. The word "can't" should be banished from geriatric wards, and nurses and social workers should quietly discover for themselves, or by referring to a senior nurse, what true disabilities remain. Old people at home, wishing to stay there, may make light of these disabilities. Old people in hospital (perhaps wishing to stay there?!) are sometimes too pessimistic about their abilities. Visiting relatives are often the most pessimistic of all. They hear what the patient says, they see her in bed (because it is evening visiting time), and they assume she is always so. The only way to convince a sceptic is to show him what an elderly patient is capable of doing, by day, dressed perhaps, and walking about in her own clothes.

Chapter 5

SPECIAL HAZARDS AND HAPPENINGS

Anyone who falls ill is to some extent in danger, but elderly people are doubly so, first because of the illness and secondly because being old, ill and inactive involves them in risks of a particular kind like contractures, bedsores and other horrors. The first part of this chapter deals with these special risks; the second with some of the other conditions, like little "attacks" and fainting fits which lead to insecurity and accidents.

It seems to be an instinct of all sick animals to lie down and rest; humans are no exception, and not so very long ago it had become almost a rule of doctors and nurses to insist on rest for most diseases. This idea no longer found so much favour when it was discovered that certain complications of surgery result from too much immobility. Geriatric physicians know that rest is harmful to elderly people even though they are not surgical patients. Now almost everywhere older people are encouraged to get up and on to their feet as quickly as possible as part of regular good geriatric policy. Some non-medical people still think this is a harsh policy, but they do not understand how serious the risks are otherwise. Minds and bodies cease to work properly if they are not kept in regular use, and the more elderly they are the greater the risks of disuse. Surely it must be pointless to insist on rest for one part of the body if that causes damage to others? Sitting in a chair during the day, provided that it is a suitable chair, is far better than lying down continuously; taking a few steps every hour or two is better than sitting down all the time. Preserving only a little mobility shortens the illness, and older people simply cannot take the risk of an unnecessarily long illness. The rule in geriatric wards should be that the patient gets up automatically, for part of the day at least, unless the doctor specifically forbids it. A geriatric patient "safely" tucked up in bed is not safe: she runs risks there – and falling out of bed is only one of them.

THROMBOSIS OF THE VEINS

Clotting of blood in the deeper veins of the legs is a well-known risk of

44

general and gynaecological surgery; it occurs almost as often in medical wards; recent research tells us that it does indeed occur so often as to be frightening, and anything we can do to prevent it is worthwhile. Thrombosis is caused by stasis, from lack of the pumping action of the leg muscle movements which normally send the venous blood back to the heart. This tendency is aggravated by infection, injury and cancer. Since old people suffer from varieties of paralysis, or lie quite still for hours on end, and since they often have reduced circulation of blood because of heart failure, the stage is all set for venous thrombosis. Following on the thrombosis the clot may become detached, so it passes to the heart, and is driven thence immediately into the lungs causing a sudden urgent attack of breathlessness, cyanosis and perhaps chest pain. The attack is often fatal. This sequence is known as thrombo-embolism. It is one of the most common causes of sudden death in old age. Warning signs are swelling of one leg (or more swelling in one than the other), blue discolouration and coldness, oedema of the leg, and pain in the calf and along the inner side of the thigh. Sometimes a leg threatened with thrombosis is warmer than expected. These are signs which ought to be repeatedly looked for in old people who are confined to bed. Unfortunately quite a large number of cases of thrombosis occur without any outward signs appearing whatever, and the cause of the sudden death is only shown at a post-mortem examination. There are now methods of detecting a thrombosis in a vein at an early stage before the limb begins to swell. One method depends on the Doppler principle, and one on the detection of fibrinogen, a blood protein, "labelled" with a radioactive isotope. If such methods could be widely used in older people's wards they might save many lives. Pulmonary embolism, the final dangerous stage of this process, will be dealt with elsewhere (Chapter 8); it may be repeated if the first attack is not fatal, and lead to a long, dangerous illness.

This sinister condition, thrombo-embolism, really must be prevented; the more active the patient, the better the chance of prevention. Leg and foot movements must be practised frequently in bed, and leg-swinging take place over the edge. A bed cradle helps, because the legs are then not restricted; pillows should not be put under the knees or thighs, though a pillow or "wedge" under the calf or heels for preventing pressure sores (see page 207) is much less of a risk. Breathing exercises and plenty of fluids reduce the likelihood too, but neither of these are popular with elderly patients.

The treatment of thrombo-embolism is to start a course of anticoagulant drugs like Heparin or Warfarin, with most careful laboratory control of the coagulation process. This is simple in hospital but so much more difficult outside hospital that all patients having such drugs should probably be admitted as inpatients first, to be stabilized. Treatment may have to continue for weeks afterwards as an outpatient if pulmonary embolism has occurred, to reduce the risk of recurrences. Prevention or prompt detection of venous thrombosis saves many lives.

Thrombophlebitis is a different condition. It is an inflammation of the superficial veins, showing as discolouration, swelling, tenderness and warmth. It needs treatment with antibiotics rather than anticoagulants, and soothing local applications. It does not carry the risk of embolism and for this reason is much less serious.

PNEUMONIA

Everyone knows that old people lying down are prone to get pneumonia from a combination of infection and poor aeration of the lungs. This used to be called "hypostatic" pneumonia; now it is usually called bronchopneumonia. It can occur also after inhaling food or drink. Pneumonia is only mentioned here in order to list it amongst the hazards of lying in bed. (See also page 256.) It seems clear that pneumonia can go round a ward full of frail old people like an infectious disease, especially in the winter. It is a telling reason for trying to keep people out of hospitals and at home.

CONTRACTURES

Joints which do not move may get stuck fast; this can happen with astonishing speed. Sometimes contractures are due to arthritis, the joint being held flexed too long because that is the least painful position. Sometimes a stroke or other paralysis so weakens the muscles that they cannot straighten the joint. Then the corresponding flexor muscle shortens, and the joint capsule and ligaments thicken and fibrose. Some very old people have permanent flexion contractures of the hips and knees because they insist on sitting during the day and lying during the night with their knees always up, never straightening their legs. In cases like this there is no other bone, joint or muscle disease to blame, and one can only think that it is the faulty position which these very aged people adopt all day and all night; there seems no other explanation for it. Such catastrophes can be prevented if one takes a firm enough line, and makes people straighten their limbs often.

A disabling contracture of the shoulder joint is called a "frozen shoulder", and immobilizing that joint with a sling is always risky. The most distressing of contractures is the common fixed "drop foot" caused by pressure of bed clothes tightly tucked in for long periods. A bed cradle really is essential for nearly every geriatric patient.

Contractures can be prevented by movement; where active spontaneous movement is impossible, then everyone concerned must be ready to move the patient's limbs regularly (i.e. passive movements). Doctors and nurses should do this as well as therapists, and members of the family can be shown how to do it at home (see page 133). Suitable splinting may be needed to stop flexion deformities, but if it is not removed at intervals it may even be a cause of contractures forming. If a contracture seems unavoidable – as sometimes seems to happen in acute rheumatoid arthritis – then the joint must be put into the most useful position. Generally speaking this means straight for legs and partially bent for an arm. The correction of contractures is difficult, lengthy, painful and not without risk – so prevention is all the more important. It is done with a series of applications of plaster of Paris cylinders, cut behind the bent joint every week or so, the gap opened a little, and plaster reapplied. Sometimes one has to resort to surgical operations like tenotomies and then plaster cylinders, and success is by no means certain.

PRESSURE SORES

Pressure sores (bed sores: decubitus ulcers) are a source of danger and distress to patients and a great worry to conscientious nurses. A nurse may be severely criticized because of bed sores appearing, and, since these sores are almost all preventable – given enough effort and care (and enough staff available) – there is a certain rough justice in this. Besides, treatment of an established sore is long, hard, and costly in nursing time; so prevention is essential.

A clear understanding of the causes will help to dispel the anxiety about pressure sores which exists everywhere in nursing circles – and sores are so serious a matter that anyone who is indifferent to their having made an appearance cannot be considered a good nurse. A very, very few patients are so frail and ill and near death that they are disintegrating, and even the weight of the bedclothes breaks their skin. Such sores are almost unavoidable. For the rest, the "patient's poor general condition" is really not a sufficient explanation.

The appearance of a succession of pressure sores in a ward suggests either a deficiency of technique and understanding or a lack of good team work. General medical and surgical wards, busy as they are with emergencies and refined techniques, are not always blameless in the matter of pressure sore prevention, which is a question of basic nursing care. If nurses in geriatric wards allow pressure sores to develop less often (though their work load is certainly no lighter!), it is because they are so highly aware of the risks and the need for prevention.

A few so-called pressure sores are caused by repeated friction of a constantly moving limb across the sheets. They are in fact friction sores or minor dry burns. Apart from these, it is possible to say that other pressure sores are due to one thing only – unrelieved pressure (or body weight). Pressure sores occur most often in places where weight is transmitted through a bony prominence close under the skin with very little cushion of muscle or fat available between the bone and the skin, i.e. at the sacrum, the outer side of the hips, the heels, or dorsal spine and scapular areas; but other places are not always exempt.

Certain parts of the body like the soles of the feet are specially designed to take pressure. Normally, relief of pressure takes place automatically, even in sleep, by the patient's spontaneous movements. We all shift about in bed for this very reason. The movements take place reflexly in answer to the stimulus of discomfort. But if pain cannot be felt because the patient is in coma, or sensation is cut off because of paraplegia, then the risk of sores is very much greater. Many elderly patients are paralysed or cannot shift because of pain, so they cannot do anything to relieve their own pressure discomforts. Those who are stuporose or heavily drugged, or very demented, do not heed the warnings their own skin sends to them.

Important work by Professor Exton-Smith and others showed experimentally that the number of movements made by a patient at night is closely related to the number of pressure sores. In other words the more frequent the movements, the fewer the sores. In short, it is possible to predict which patients, because they move so little, are the vulnerable ones. These need much more attention than other patients. A practical scoring system which helps in this respect is given in Appendix 3 (page 275). The risks are greatest during the hours of night time, unfortunately, when there are fewer pairs of hands to give the necessary help. If regular attention is required at certain intervals it is wrong not to give it because the patient is sleeping. A good motto is: "Better broken sleep than a broken back".

Naturally there are other factors which increase the likelihood of pressure sores; of these, crumbs in the bed and wrinkles in the sheet are probably the least important. The vital factors can be listed as follows; malnutrition (especially deficiency in protein and vitamin C); anaemia (itself a cause of tissue malnutrition); fall of blood pressure; venous thrombosis; insufficient arterial circulation in a limb; severe tissue wasting (from carcinoma, etc.); obesity (because more weight goes through the pressure point); devitalization of tissues by intramuscular injection; heavy sedation; abrasion of skin by dragging rather than lifting the patient; maceration of skin by urinary incontinence and soiling. Yet none of these reasons approaches anywhere near the importance of unrelieved pressure.

A combination of unrelieved pressure and a thrombus in the inferior vena cava can result in the appalling disaster of a black necrotic pressure sore the size of a plate appearing in one night.

Immobilization after amputation of one leg in an old person for gangrene involves a serious risk of a pressure sore on the opposite heel; anyone who lets this happen would have a great deal to answer for, because it might result in a bilateral amputation, which is a great disaster.

Pressure sores involving superficial skin loss only are painful to the patient but relatively not dangerous; they should heal quickly and will not cause scarring. Much more serious are deep pressure sores. They usually appear with little warning. The pressure causes clotting in the small blood vessels and death of the underlying muscle and fat, this making a deep, sterile abscess which eventually bursts through the skin and leaves a deep cavernous ulcer with a slough and undermined edges. It is seldom painful because the whole skin thickness and much more besides are lost and these deeper tissues have no pain nerve endings. Deep ulcers may go right down to the bone. They are easily infected, slow to heal, cause scarring, and are themselves a direct threat to the patient's life, regardless of what else is wrong with him.

Elderly hospital patients who are discharged quickly or who die quickly probably have little time to develop pressure sores; even so, one-third of pressure sores develop in the first week, and two-thirds within two weeks of the admission. This, then, is particularly the time to be watching and working to prevent them.

The problems of preventing and treating these pernicious effects of pressure are discussed in more detail in Chapter 13. It is still fair to say that mechanical devices, though very helpful, are no substitute for the vigilance and careful routines which come from sound training and an acknowledgement that a pressure sore might be taken as a reflection upon the capability of nurses. The nurses for their part should always be able to feel that they have the active support and interest of the doctor in the case, who should understand the causes as well as they do, and help in prevention by allowing the patient to be as active as possible and by avoiding unnecessary sedation.

We have lately discovered that restriction of a patient's intake of protein, commonly done when there is kidney failure with an increase in circulating waste products like urea, is an unwise policy for it greatly increases the risk of developing huge pressure sores.

DEHYDRATION

This is one of the diseases of deprivation (see Chapter 4). It is also one of the hazards of being ill. We have seen already (page 14) that elderly kidneys with small reserves need ample water to do their work. Many older people, especially women, have a habit of drinking very little. This is often for "domestic" reasons. Imagine the problem of an outside lavatory or garden privy in bad weather. Some old people with a tendency to incontinence imagine they will lessen the chance by drinking less; in fact they will increase it if their bladder becomes infected as a result, which is all too likely.

When old people go to bed for illness they may be too feeble to get up to make themselves drinks. If they have diarrhoea or are vomiting, dehydration will come on all the quicker, and a very serious deficiency of water and of salt will quickly occur.

Very often those who care for elderly invalids do not understand the vital need for fluids. Their own instincts and fears of incontinence may suggest cutting down the intake. It has even happened that old people have been allowed to become dehydrated in hospital wards; unthinking, busy staff put a jug on the locker of an apathetic, listless patient instead of filling a glass and putting it to her lips, while cups of tea stand cold on the bed table. Making sure that patients drink enough is a constant battle, but it has to be won and the time is well spent.

Simple Lack of Water

Lack of water happens as above, or perhaps when a great deal of fluid is lost in diabetes or nephritis with frequency and polyuria. The patient is thirsty, dry tongued, has little but concentrated urine and inelastic skin; but his blood chemistry results are normal and he can take ordinary drinks safely.

Lack of Water Combined with Lack of Salt

This is much more serious. It could be caused by diarrhoea, vomiting, burns, diabetic ketosis or too much treatment with diuretics. The patient might look like the patient above but be listless, have a low blood pressure, disturbed blood chemistry, and even lapse into coma. He may not be able to take fluid through his stomach and intestines, and giving fluid alone without any salt would make matters worse. The distinction is really a biochemical one, and needs laboratory tests, but there is a good rule: if a dehydrated patient has thirst, then it is safe to give water alone. Many dehydrated patients cannot be saved except by using a nasogastric tube, and some have to have intravenous fluids; many cases need urgent hospital admission – not so much for the illness which led to the dehydration as for the dehydration itself. It is a common cause of geriatric hospital admissions.

Loss of Potassium

Loss of potassium is a special case, though caused in much the same ways, especially by prolonged use of diuretics. A patient in this state is usually listless, very weak and collapsed, seems almost paralysed, and is in danger of cardiac complications. Yet if he is given back his lost potassium he will recover dramatically. This condition needs urgent treatment and laboratory control is important.

INCONTINENCE

Higher animals, and certainly humans, have a desire to be continent and a basic dislike of excretions. The higher centres of the brain exhibit control (i.e. inhibition) over the basic mechanisms of excretion, which are themselves controlled by spinal reflexes. Thus micturition and defaecation normally take place by release of the higher control. If the higher control is taken away, then the reflexes may act on their own. Higher control could be lacking because of coma, or physical cerebral damage, or simple "senile" dementia. Control could be cut off because of damage to the spinal cord pathways, as in paraplegia; then the bladder or bowel would empty automatically as soon as it was full. Thus we see several reasons for incontinence which have no direct cause in the bladder or in the rectum.

Incontinence of Urine

Apart from the above there are a great many local causes of incontinence, including infection, bladder stones or cancer, disease of the prostate gland in men, and many others. There is also *stress incontinence*, mainly in women, caused by local muscle weaknesses combined with raising of the abdominal pressure by effort or coughing. This is sometimes a late result of the damage caused by childbirth.

Impaction of constipated faeces in the rectum is another common "local" cause of urinary incontinence. It can fill the lower pelvis, and prevent the bladder from filling normally. The link between incontinence and infection of the urine is not so exact as one might think. Infection does not help anyone with a tendency towards incontinence (or "bladder weakness" as some patients say) to be continent, because it causes frequency and urgency. Infection, especially in women, may be the *result* of continual incontinence rather than its cause. This sounds a contradiction, but it is true. The female urethra is short, and bacteria harboured or growing in the wet skin areas ascend to and infect the bladder.

Defining incontinence is not easy. We might say it was passing urine at unsuitable times or in unsuitable places; we have most of us known patients who used a hat or a flower pot! But is a person continent who is "dry" only because a nurse reminds him of his duty every two hours – a technique which is part of "habit" training for continence? The author has coined a phrase for the condition in which a patient only remains continent as long as nurses attend to his wants at intervals, or remind him to take himself to the lavatory. The phrase is "nurse controlled continence". It is scarcely true continence, but it is a good deal better than uncontrolled incontinence, and is therefore a state worth striving for.

In practical terms women are much more often incontinent than men, and incontinence at night is more frequent than daytime incontinence.

There is more incontinence in a geriatric hospital ward than at home, for the incontinence may be the "last straw" which led to the patient's admission, so incontinent patients tend to accumulate in the wards.

A great number of cases of incontinence in old age are due to cerebral damage from strokes or to dementia. Both these latter types could justifiably be called "cerebral incontinence" because the higher control is now lacking. Cases of incontinence due to stroke often improve as the stroke improves, but incontinence in established dementia very seldom gets any better except sometimes with habit training. If sedatives are prescribed for night use there is a greatly increased chance of bed-wetting.

A few geriatric patients are incontinent for psychological reasons, like fear or anxiety or even apathy. Some seem to give up control of their bladders just as they surrender themselves, body and soul, to be "looked after"! Some react to feelings of being unwanted by being incontinent – their thought being that any attention perhaps, even exasperation, from a relative is better than being ignored. Just a few patients, fortunately a very few, are purposely incontinent to "get their own back" on a relative or on a nurse. Perhaps they feel they cannot retaliate in any other way.

Except for the few patients mentioned last, the rest are incontinent without really being able to help it; there are sufficient physical or psychological reasons. Those who are aware of their mishaps are distressed and feel guilty; those who are not aware or try to deny that they have been incontinent are very likely to have cerebral damage. Knowledge of this must surely prevent us being angry with old people who wet themselves. Nor can we expect normal behaviour if we do not answer their calls for help promptly, or if we put an ambulant patient with urgency into a bed furthest away from the lavatory.

Incontinent people need our encouragement and skill; we must be cheerful, encouraging when they manage better, and above all we must be patient. Another point is of great importance; certain old people tend to regress psychologically – that is, they become more child-like and dependent, even to the point of becoming incontinent like infants. If we encourage this regression by talking to them like children, scolding and "punishing", they will be worse. Yet, put a fairly sensible old person into her own clothes, sitting up in a comfortable day room and treat her as a responsible adult, and there is a good prospect of her becoming continent again. The nursing management of incontinence is discussed fully in Chapter 13 (page 209).

Faecal Incontinence

The various kinds of causes already outlined apply to faecal incontinence too. Practically speaking again, the commonest causes apart from diarrhoea and the use of purgatives are, first, gross constipation, impaction and "overflow" of faeces; secondly, "cerebral" causes due to brain damage or dementia. This may respond to habit-training, or even careful use of constipating drugs like codeine and regular enemas.

CONSTIPATION

One might truly say that constipation is a gastro-intestinal disorder, or else a dietary one. It is a great source of anxiety to countless old people and a direct cause of physical problems too. Keeping elderly patients inactive so much aggravates constipation that it must be called one of the hazards of the bedfast state.

Many old people have a "complex" about their bowels. This neurosis was probably implanted in their childhood, and they have been made miserable by it ever since, even though they have lived long and have come to no harm. They are constantly fretting and are begging for medicine, or dosing themselves, and sometimes refusing to believe they have had a motion that very day.

In spite of this, constipation is very much a problem to many, and it must not be glossed over as unimportant. Rectal examinations are the only deciding factor in a doubtful case. The cause is often a faulty diet with too little fluid and roughage (see page 66); sometimes it is a symptom of a lower bowel cancer, or there are other local causes; sometimes the patient, if very old, is so frail that she has not the muscular strength to defaecate, and soft, almost fluid faeces may be slowly ejected from an accumulated mass.

The results of constipation are not usually what the patients think they will be, but several of them are important. First, there is the risk of faecal impaction and then a slimy mucous diarrhoea (called "spurious diarrhoea") appears as the hard mass sets up irritation; next, restlessness and even mental confusion, which can be relieved by clearing the bowel; thirdly, retention of urine because the pelvis is full and the bladder distorted; fourthly, the risk of intestinal obstruction which may have to be dealt with surgically.

To treat constipation the first steps are reassurance, activity and a proper diet, which could have bulk-producing aperients like Agarol or Celevac added to it. There is a great variety of other aperients, from stool-wetting substances like Dioctyl Medo or Normax, which are Dioctyl sodium sulphosuccinate, or lower bowel stimulants like Dorbanex or Dulcolax, given as tablets or suppositories. One of the best and safest is the old standby, senna, given as the purified tablet or granules of Senokot.

It is dangerous to purge old people severely. In the end enemas are often needed, and severe constipation may require daily treatment like this even for two or three weeks. Digital removal is the last resort and sometimes this requires an anaesthetic. Further consideration of treating constipation will be found in Chapter 13.

OVER-DEPENDENCE AND LOSS OF MORALE

Illness makes most of us dependent upon someone, but long illness in old people can destroy their will to be independent or to leave hospital, or even in extreme cases to leave their beds. However ill or pathetic a patient seems at first, we ought to have one eye to the future, encouraging her to do whatever she can to help herself, and optimistically helping her to look ahead to a time of not being ill. Over-protection breeds dependence in the patient's mind. She may *say* she is looking forward to getting up, or leaving hospital, for example, but if we do not seize the right moment it will be lost. In the end she may try excuses or even develop new symptoms. A truly "institutionalized" patient is a sad sight to see.

UNEXPECTED HAPPENINGS

Older people are very liable to have "attacks", faints, unexpected falls and a variety of other happenings, which are as hard for them to explain as they are hard for us to analyse. All of these "attacks" make the patient feel insecure and make her friends anxious. Some are dangerous in themselves or could cause an accident. We must therefore be aware of these events and their significance. The doctor will be looking out for clues; so anyone who sees an old person in an attack will be of great help if she is able to describe exactly what was observed. The important things to notice are the patient's colour, movements, breathing, the rate of the pulse or any irregularity; if it is possible to take the blood pressure then and there, so much the better. His immediate safety comes first, but the next priority should be careful observation of the kind of attack.

EPILEPTIC ATTACKS

It is quite possible for a person who has had epileptic fits all through life to have them still in old age. However, fits coming on for the first time could be evidence of some serious disease within the skull, so investigations are needed. Most commonly it turns out that these fits are a sign of cerebral arteriosclerosis, but other things must be ruled out. Fits in later life are rather like fits in young children: they are a pointer to some serious happening. For example, a fit is one of the ways in which a stroke or a heart attack first appears.

Major epilepsy ("grand mal") usually starts with sudden unconsciousness with rigid muscles, breath-holding and a blue colour, followed by jerking movements which gradually subside, and the patient recovers sooner or later. Sometimes the jerking can be seen to start in one hand or a corner of the mouth, and this can be a vital observation. The essential thing in fits is to keep the airway clear.

Minor epilepsy ("petit mal") is momentary, where the patient stops what she is doing, looks vacant, and then carries on. This does not seem very common in old age, but when it does appear the "attacks" can last much longer than in younger people.

HYSTERICAL FITS

Hysterical fits are quite different, and they are not uncommon. Sometimes they are the hysterically-inclined old patient's way of registering a protest against something which displeases her. Yet this is not "put on"; for a hysteric does not consciously understand the reasons behind the attack. Such a fit is never true to the pattern of epilepsy – so it is likely to be noisy, dramatic, with strange movements, or writhing on the floor, but the patient does not hurt herself. Dramatic "turns" like this – if one is certain what they are – are treated by giving a sudden shock or, best of all in old age, by turning and walking away – then the patient usually stops at once and gets up! In each individual case medical advice on how to react to the situation is needed. Hysterical shaking attacks can be seen in some institutionalized patients; the deep-seated, unconscious reason is a wish to seem an important and "serious case", needing indefinite care.

SIMPLE FAINTING

Fainting (syncope) happens commonly, as a result of pain, oppressive heat or psychological stress, or sometimes as a symptom of severe anaemia or unexpected internal bleeding. Apart from in these latter cases recovery is quick, but often not so quick as in young people. Fainting should not be dismissed lightly in later life, because it usually has a specific reason, and treatment may be needed.

POSTURAL HYPOTENSION

Very close to simple fainting is so-called postural hypotension. There are many reasons why the blood pressure falls in old people. When it does so the patient often feels giddy or actually "faints" when he or she stands up. Sometimes it happens even when the patient sits up, though when she is lying down all is well. This condition makes people feel ill and most insecure, and in the attacks they may fall and break bones. The diagnosis depends on someone having blood-pressure-taking apparatus handy at the time of the attack, or comparing the blood pressure taken lying and standing, and that usually means someone else must hold them upright. Some cases are caused by too energetic use of drugs against high blood pressure. Some such attacks can be put down to a failure of the normal pressure-maintaining reflexes, perhaps because of cerebral artery disease. Sometimes these patients are found to have too little salt circulating in the blood, and the adding of extra salt to their diet or drinks helps to put matters right. Apart from the cases with special causes like cardiac infarction, persistent hypotension can be treated, but it is a lengthy and elaborate matter of drugs, gradual "tipping", abdominal binders and elastic stockings. People who have this disability *must* get out of bed by stages, and spend time with their legs dangling over the side of the bed, holding on to something before they stand up.

"LITTLE STROKES"

Patients with cerebral artery disease are liable sometimes to have attacks when they lose their speech, or have a weakness of a limb or loss of vision, perhaps with giddiness or a faint, but the attack passes very quickly. These are more properly known as transient ischaemic attacks (or "T.I.As."). They are of course alarming to everyone; sometimes they are an early first sign of a more serious and lasting stroke.

HYPOGLYCAEMIC ATTACKS

Attacks such as these, with coldness, sweating and rapid unconsciousness, occur in diabetic patients who are being given too much insulin or not eating the full diet prescribed for them. Attacks can also occur with the various tablets used for treating diabetes by mouth. The special importance of these attacks later in life is the fact that often heart attacks and strokes come on at the very same moment, with serious consequences. Hypoglycaemia therefore must be particularly avoided, and it is best for most older diabetics to "show" just a little sugar in their urine when it is tested to stay on the safe side.

CARDIAC ATTACKS

There are a number of dramatic events which make good observers think of heart disease. The most dramatic of all are Stokes-Adams attacks in which the patient goes unconscious for a few seconds during which no pulse at all can be felt. This usually happens in people with a heart conduction defect, and most of them have had a persistently slow pulse of, say, 35–45 (complete heart block). When the heart starts again the patient flushes, wakes up and carries on as before. Sometimes the heart does not start again. Because of this and because of the risk of falls and broken bones, these attacks are potentially dangerous and make patients very anxious, but they can be treated by drugs or cardiac pace-makers. Indeed, pace-makers have often been used with great success in people of a great age and have helped them to lead useful lives free of symptoms and discomfort.

Cardiac infarction and pulmonary embolism themselves cause various attacks, faintings, falls of blood pressure and even epileptic fits. Sudden changes of cardiac rhythm also produce alarming sensations with a suddenly rapid or irregular pulse. The importance of feeling the pulse in any unusual attack cannot be stressed too much.

GIDDINESS

Attacks of giddiness (vertigo) are one of the most common of all old people's symptoms. They find these feelings very difficult to describe. The older the patient, the greater the chance of vertigo; women are more affected than men. There are a great many possible causes, and often we never get to the root of the matter. Wax in the ears, ear disease, high blood pressure, low blood pressure, certain drugs like quinidine and aspirin and sedatives, all these are amongst the causes – it is impracticable to list them all.

There are links between vertigo and deafness, and one particular type is Ménières Disease. It is an acute and violent type of giddiness found in deaf people, in which the patient feels she is spinning, she vomits and every movement seems a nightmare. It is due to disease of the inner ear, but it may be treatable with certain new drugs. Other lesser forms of vertigo are most difficult to deal with; they are important both because they distress people and because they make them frightened of falling and un-willing to move about.

DROP ATTACKS

Sometimes after experiencing some falls patients say they were stand-ing up and suddenly their legs "simply gave way". They find themselves on the floor without having lost consciousness, but they cannot rise without help. Sometimes (they say), they struggle until there is something against which to put their feet, and then they can get up and continue as if nothing had happened. These quite common attacks have never been properly explained, but are known simply as "drop attacks". They give no warning; they are very disconcerting, and very difficult to treat.

FALLS AND ACCIDENTS

Falls

Old people have been shown to sway much more than young adults. It is as if they gradually lose the fine control of posture they taught themselves as young children when learning to walk. Their sense of balance becomes uncertain and their posture-holding reflexes are slow. This was described as follows by one patient: "Once you're going, you've got to go!" Besides having their natural handicaps they are liable to any of the various sudden attacks which have just been described in these last few paragraphs. It is not surprising that falls among old people are exceedingly common. People who are eighty have eight times the chance of dying from an accidental fall as people who are sixty.

One has only to watch older people getting out of chairs or walking cautiously about to see how afraid of a fall they are. Their fear keeps some of them rooted to their chairs when we want them to walk. Fear on their behalf is felt by nurses in hospital, where falls are a worrying problem. A deliberate fall in a relaxed position is usually harmless, but old people are the reverse of relaxed in these circumstances! Injuries are common, and their results are serious, even fatal sometimes in the long run. If falls are less common at home it may be because there is furniture close by to hold on to, and every nook and cranny is well remembered. Yet, on the other hand, old people's dwellings are usually full of hazards – loose mats, trailing flexes, odd steps, poorly lit stairs and passages, and a great clutter of belongings everywhere. A large proportion of accidental falls takes place on staircases.

It would be fair to say that the environment is to blame for many old people's falls. Nevertheless with some attention to detail these risks could be lessened, and Local Authorities have powers to adapt houses to make things easier and safer for handicapped people. If we want old people to be active and yet avoid falls, we should be reminding them among other things to wear their glasses, get good shoes, clear out the clutter, avoid loose mats, turn round slowly, take care with stooping, use walking sticks, hold on to solid objects if they need to, and use many other little tricks. Frailer people can mostly dress sitting on the edges of their beds, and go downstairs slowly backwards, or even forwards, sitting, sliding on their buttocks – which may be a little undignified, but is safe!

Other Accidents to Old People

Our older people are involved in accidents, whether falls or for other reasons, much more often than they should be. They figure very frequently in road accidents as pedestrians. One in every twenty of their deaths can be attributed to an accident of some kind. Domestic accidents are even more common: three-quarters of all fatal home accidents involve people over 65. Apart from falls, there are burning and scalding accidents. Naturally people who live alone are especially vulnerable. Accidents, even when not fatal, are a great source of anxiety and loss of confidence. They are also the cause of large numbers of hospital beds being occupied, at great expense and labour. Accidents to old people should be thought of as caused by three factors – (a) senescence and loss of faculties; (b) disease; (c) faults in the environment. The first two may respond to doctors' efforts; the last affords a splendid chance for Home Nurses, Health Visitors, Social Workers, and people's friends to act together in the practice of a little simple but rewarding Preventive Medicine. Every visit to an older person at home should be done with an eye open for domestic hazards.

HYPOTHERMIA

This is a somewhat mysterious condition in which the body loses heat, being unable to maintain the strict temperature it requires for normal working. It has been known for many years that even young men exposed to intense cold for long periods have a severe fall of temperature. Yet only in the last 15 years or so has it become clear how widespread this condition is among the elderly (and young infants). Research in old people's own homes showed that it is quite common to detect body temperatures round the 35–36°C mark instead of the usual 37°C. At that lower temperature these people may not even seem ill and are not complaining much of the cold. Hypothermia as a medical abnormality means, then, a temperature below 35°C, though a figure even as low as that should make us watchful. Temperatures have been recorded as low as 21°C and there have been many cases in the range 24–32°C. It was calculated a few years ago that in one three-month winter period 9,000 people might have arrived at the hospitals of Great Britain with temperatures below 35°C, though in most cases this was not suspected and some other illness was the cause of their arrival.

It used to be thought that all these cases were the result of falling and lying in the cold – hence the former name "accidental hypothermia". True cases of this kind do occur, if old people fall and break a leg on an icy path and then lie there because they cannot move. The same thing can happen even after falling at night in a cold bedroom if the victim has not the wit to pull her bedclothes down on top of her. Cold British bedrooms have rightly been blamed for other misfortunes too (see page 95)

However there are other circumstances in which hypothermia appears. First, there may be a serious illness, which, instead of raising the temperature, lowers it – as in sudden and dangerous pneumonia. This usually means the outlook is very grave. It can also happen in heart attacks, after using certain drugs (e.g. chlorpromazine), and during strokes. The author had an elderly man sitting dressed by a roaring fire in a ward, when he was seen to be unwell, was put to bed, and there it was found that he had early signs of a stroke and a temperature of 33°C. Other cases happen for no clear reason. A very old person, sitting quite still in a chair for hours is sometimes found to have severe hypothermia. It is as if in some cases the heat regulating mechanisms are suddenly thrown out of action and with no warning whatever.

Hypothermia causes many deaths and is dangerous in proportion to the fall of the temperature. It is therefore imperative that anyone who deals with old people should know of it and be wary in suspicious circumstances. It is vital that wardens of Homes and people's good neighbours and relatives should also be told what to watch for. Usually in a cold room, and being very inactive also, an old person becomes slow and slurred in speech, with a slow pulse, seems a little confused, does *not* shiver, is perhaps drowsy but does *not look cold*. The face and hands often look warm and red or purple-red, which throws everyone off the scent. The extremities feel cold, but so do the hands of many people in cold weather. A crucial point is that the places which are normally always warm, like the abdominal wall or the inside the thighs, are cold – cold as marble. Yet by this stage matters are already serious. A clinical thermometer of the normal kind reads, say, 35°C – its lowest mark – but it will go no lower even though the body temperature is less. This gives an entirely false impression of there being no urgency. If in these circumstances a low-reading thermometer – covering the range of say 24–40°C – is used a much lower true figure will be shown. Any low reading must be checked by placing the low-reading thermometer in the patient's rectum for five minutes. Home Nurses, Health Visitors, Doctors, Geriatric Hospitals and Homes will all find that to use a low-reading thermometer in old people's cases, especially in winter, is an insurance against a missed diagnosis which could be fatal. Some very old people even have recurrent hypothermia and can be at great risk whenever it is cold.

Emergency treatment for hypothermia is still very unsatisfactory. Young people can be quickly warmed and come to no harm, but at present we believe that rapid warming is very dangerous for old people in this state; sudden death often takes place. Warming should be carefully controlled at about 1°F rise in an hour (Fig. 6), by putting a few blankets on the patient, keeping the room quite warm (say 27–29°C) but *not* applying any heat to the patient direct. Intravenous fluids and hydrocortisone are used, with other drugs, but there are still many deaths just at the stage when one hopes the worst is over.

The practical answer to hypothermia is two-fold: first, we must do all we can to help old people to keep warm by good housing (see Chapter

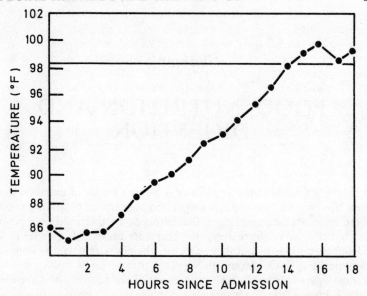

Fig. 6 A typical temperature graph of a patient with hypothermia being allowed to warm up slowly.

14) and good clothes, enough money to buy fuel, plenty of hot food, etc. and above all by encouraging them, even bullying them, to move about and generate some of their own internal heat. Secondly, by always being on the alert for this condition, which comes on slowly to take us unawares, and which is so very dangerous. Then we might catch it before it reaches a low level. With care, in the temperature range 32–35°C it may be possible to warm the patient up at home; at any lower temperature the full emergency resources of a hospital with a laboratory are needed, but sadly it may in the end be the cold, long ambulance journey which helps to seal the patient's fate.

HYPERTHERMIA

Heat stroke ought perhaps to occur in old people whose temperature regulation is not all it should be. In fact it is not a significant geriatric disorder here, but in the United States of America many cases have been reported.

Chapter 6

FOOD, NUTRITION AND DIGESTION

In theory we could judge a man's or a woman's state of nutrition if we knew the "normal" or average weight and appearance of healthy people of the same sex, age and height. But in this as in other things old people vary greatly, as we have seen, and there are no reliable standards for judging their state of nutrition. Doctors' height/weight tables were not constructed to take account of very old people. Later in life, too, the average figures obviously take no account of the people who have died, and it is known from life insurance records that one's chances of survival are better if one is not overweight. Generally speaking in old age there is more fatty tissue and less of the lean "active" tissue. It can be argued that if the active tissues are less but the fat increases, then people are eating more than is strictly necessary. There is no doubt that this happens quite often in retirement, when less work is being done, yet people are keeping to their old eating habits.

It is never easy to say at what point obesity begins. Nor is it even easy to be sure whether or not a thin person is truly undernourished. There are some great advantages in being thin and wiry!

The real essential in a healthy diet is that it should be well balanced as between the necessary groups of foodstuffs.

CALORIE REQUIREMENTS

For the average man in retirement 2,300 Calories a day should be sufficient if he walks about and keeps up his gentle activities; the equivalent figure for women is a little less than 2,000 Calories a day. For people who spend most of their time sitting down the figures are 2,000 for men and 1,750 for women, and the "basal" levels for people who are quite inactive are 1,500 and 1,250 Calories a day respectively. Probably very old people in their eighties and nineties need less than the "younger old". Nevertheless it is interesting that old bodies *can* use up large numbers of Calories per day if working very hard, as happens for example with old women working in the fields on alpine mountain sides. Nevertheless, Calories are only part of the nutritional story.

PROTEIN, FAT AND CARBOHYDRATE

The total bulk of protein in old people's bodies, which is mainly in their muscles, usually diminishes, but what remains still needs steady replacement – as parts of all muscles and all other cells do. Therefore 1 gramme per kilogramme of their own body weight of good protein, principally in the form of meat, fish and eggs, is still needed every day. When old people are ill, or feverish, or anaemic, or have healing wounds or pressure sores, the need is a good deal more. There is no evidence at all that normal old people cannot digest and use up large quantities of protein, and this is a most attractive and palatable, if expensive, kind of food.

Estimating the body's need of fats raises certain difficulties; certainly some fat is regularly needed but there is a good deal of controversy about the part which fats might play in causing arterial disease – and this is one of the scourges of old age, as we shall see. The fat in animal (dairy) produce are so-called "saturated" fats, while those in some vegetable oils are largely "unsaturated". One school of thought believes that saturated fats are most likely to lead to artery disease. If it were true the moral would be obvious – take care with animal fats and use vegetable oils when possible. Not everybody believes this, for the evidence is conflicting. Indeed, another school of thought blames refined sugar for the high prevalence of artery disease in civilized countries.

Carbohydrates are what provide the main source of energy for work and movement. In short they are required, not for bodybuilding or replacement as fat and protein are, but are needed to make up the calories. They are also the cheapest kinds of food available and often the easiest to manage because they keep well and often need least elaborate preparation. They are *not* however an adequate substitute for fat and protein, even though when taken excessively they are converted into extra body fat.

MINERALS

The human body needs a supply of certain mineral salts which are got from food. One of them (common salt) is added in cooking for flavour anyway, but there is usually no shortage of it in the diet. Two minerals, calcium and iron, are particularly necessary, but are often found to be in short supply. Calcium is needed among other things to maintain the health and strength of bone, and there is some evidence that a deficiency here leads to "senile osteoporosis", the cause of many painful bent backs and a special liability to fractures in old age. (There are other possible causes too!) Probably one gramme a day of calcium is needed, this coming mostly from milk, cheese and bread.

Iron is often lacking in old people's diets, or is lost by minor bleeding from the intestinal tract going unnoticed. The body can only absorb small quantities of iron at any one time; so if a deficiency has developed it is not easy to make it good even with iron tablets. Iron comes from meat and green vegetables, and some old people have no liking for these things or for some long-forgotten reason were warned earlier in life not to eat them – so they never did. It is small wonder that many of them develop anaemia. It is always difficult to provide enough iron in hospital diets especially if some patients have food fads. The daily need of iron is about 10 to 12 mg.

Other minerals are needed too in minute quantities but this does not seem to cause difficulty. There is some evidence that giving zinc salts in small doses by mouth helps wounds and "chronic" ulcers to heal, but we have little evidence so far of any true deficiency of zinc.

VITAMINS

For years there has been much talk of possible vitamin deficiencies; some of it tends perhaps to be exaggerated. Besides the well-recognized true deficiencies, we may hear mention of "sub-clinical" deficiencies, which means there are no very definite signs of disease but there is a general hint of the patient just being "not up to the mark". Normal younger adults on well balanced diets in Great Britain should not be deficient of any vitamins. If certain deficiencies are a reality, they might be expected to occur in old people with too little money or mobility, whose diets are restricted, and in those with very strong likes and dislikes or strange behaviour or mental abnormality. We really do need more accurate scientific evidence. It is all too easy to blame the vitamin deficiencies for the happenings of normal senescence like lassitude, weakness, poor appetite, faulty memory, or even bleeding under the skin of the hands (see page 12). But these symptoms affect so many old people. It would be comforting to think that we could all be made healthier by being given general vitamin supplements, but this seems to be a vain hope. If so, then it is doubtful if vitamin pills should be handed out except to people we might suspect of being on inadequate diets. In talking of "deficiency" states we would perhaps be wisest to include only those signs which we can all see and agree about. As to the "sub-clinical" states – we can keep an open mind.

Nevertheless certain clear-cut vitamin deficiencies have been shown even in Great Britain. Vitamin A deficiency is not seen for practical purposes, but there is perhaps a link here with poor night vision. With Vitamin A are grouped vitamins D, E and K because they are all found in fats. Of these only lack of Vitamin D is established as one of the recognizable deficiencies of old age. Rickets only occurs in children, but evidence is building up that osteomalacia due to dietary lack of vitamin D, causing abnormalities of bone, is occurring in Great Britain just as it certainly does occur in India and elsewhere. Other examples arise in people who have difficulty in digesting fats (the "malabsorption syndrome") (see page 73). Sunlight causes Vitamin D to be made in the skin from natural sources, and as old people keep themselves so well covered and out of the sun, they are doubly at a disadvantage. Vitamin D comes naturally from eggs and fish and has been added to margarine – yet in spite of its cheapness and high food value many old people will not eat margarine, not taking to its taste or, unhappily, because of food snobbery.

Vitamins of the "B" series, and Vitamin C, are water soluble. Vitamin B1 (thiamine) deficiency is clear-cut in the disease called beriberi, but this is very rare in Britain. It is possible that in old people lack of this vitamin contributes to mental confusion; large doses are given sometimes in treatment – but with very limited success. The daily need is about 1 mg a day. Riboflavine deficiency is sometimes the cause of sore tongue and sores at the corners of the mouth, and eye changes. The daily need is about 1.5 mg. Deficiency of this kind might be a pointer to other Vitamin B deficiencies.

Lack of Vitamin B12 is basically a cause of Pernicious Anaemia, but the vitamin in the diet has to be combined with a substance (intrinsic factor) which comes from the normal stomach lining, and it is this factor which is absent in many older people who develop pernicious anaemia. Vitamin B12 levels in the blood are often low in old people as judged by normals in young people – but is this the correct standard to use? The daily requirement is only one millionth of a gramme. Several research workers found a link between a low blood level of Vitamin B12 and "senile" dementia, but others denied this. It is an open question still. The same can be said of folic acid deficiency and dementia. Folic acid is also needed in the proper production of red blood cells. There are some areas in Britain where folic acid deficiency has been reported.

Vitamin C (ascorbic acid) deficiency (or scurvy) does occur, particularly towards the end of the winter in people on strange diets lacking in fruit, potatoes and other vegetables. Particularly vulnerable people are those undernourished, undomesticated bachelors and widowers, and this form of scurvy has actually been named after them ("Widowers' scurvy")! They are found to have swollen gums, skin signs, large areas of bleeding under the skin, and sometimes bleeding into joints. Vitamin C is also needed for normal healing, and indeed some old people's wounds or ulcers do heal slowly. The daily need is 25 to 50 mg. Slow cooking of vegetables and potatoes destroys the Vitamin C, and a long wait in a heated trolley will do the same. It is for these reasons that a proper Vitamin C level in the diet in Hospitals and Homes is hard to maintain, especially if they are using processed foods. Old people could get their Vitamin C from oranges and lemons, but they seldom eat them unless someone will help them. If would be possible and not very costly to provide all patients and residents with daily ascorbic acid tablets "just in case": a nicer way would be to offer them all fresh or canned orange juice.

ROUGHAGE

Roughage, mainly cellulose from fruit and vegetables, is an essential part of a balanced diet. It is needed for normal intestinal movement and bowel action. Sadly, many old people refuse to eat these essential foods. Sometimes it is because they no longer have teeth, nor have had for many years. Even if they will not eat vegetables, wholemeal bread would help to put matters right, and bran can be added to cakes or taken as a cereal.

* * *

From what has been said so far, some points of special importance emerge for nurses and all people who look after the elderly, even though there are still uncertainties about some of these dietary matters. Older people may know very little about food values and vitamins, and their shopping and cooking habits may have become very limited and stereotyped. Here is a good opportunity for unobtrusive health education by Health Visitors and Home Nurses. Older people must be persuaded to "balance" their diets, and especially to be careful how much carbohydrate they eat. They need advice about the cheaper forms of good protein, and special protective (vitamin-containing) foods like fruit, fruit juices, margarine and brown bread. From the practical nursing standpoint it is important that their food should be served appetisingly, in fairly small-sized portions, cut up if necessary (but not always minced or puréed), hot, and with as little delay as possible. More will be said about this in Chapter 13.

In catering for old people it is not the quantity so much as the quality which tells. Giving them what they really need is therefore not cheap. Hospitals and Homes which budget at a much lower figure for the elderly than for others are not doing the senior people justice. Those who think that older people eat very little and point out the waste on their plates, should perhaps ask themselves whether the food has been wasted because it was not of a kind which they could eat.

MALNUTRITION

UNDERNUTRITION

We should be on our guard against assuming that many old people are undernourished because they have low incomes and look rather thin. Some are very sensible and eat well in spite of a low income, and some people with a spare kind of build are extremely healthy. Malnutrition does occur in certain individuals, and the gaunt, haggard look of the extreme case leaves us in no doubt; but there are several kinds of debilitating diseases in old age where the victims' diet has nothing to do with their appearance. The truth is that we have no good yardstick to use. Anaemia goes hand in hand with general malnutrition, but not all anaemic patients, of course, are malnourished.

Amongst the causes of undernutrition mental illness ranks high, for badly muddled old people do not look after themselves. Loneliness is important too (see page 32). Lonely people quickly become bored, depressed and apathetic and this leads to self-neglect; but things can happen the reverse way round, namely, that malnutrition *leads* to apathy and depression. Malnutrition is hardly ever reported by the patient herself. It is something which has to be sought for in people's own homes, and the worst examples occur in just the sort of individuals who do not encourage visitors. Here is a challenge to the tact and persistence of a good Health Visitor, working from within a doctor's practice perhaps, and forewarned of possibly finding malnutrition by the patient's circumstances – age, loneliness and the remarks of neighbours who have been told to keep their distance.

The appearance of a seriously undernourished patient is one of listlessness, with a pale wrinkled skin, sunken eyes, prominent cheek-bones and temples, and usually a low blood pressure. Some have swollen legs – the so-called "starvation oedema". Certain people have a relative protein deficiency because they eat nothing but carbohydrates; they may not *look* thin, because their tissues are filled up by fluid and fat.

Treating severe undernutrition is difficult because the victim cannot tolerate a full diet, and a lethal diarrhoea may result. Some of the victims are brought so low that they will not co-operate. It is difficult to decide how far they should be driven to eat. Hospital care is needed to bring such people through. Like every other malady, malnutrition would be best prevented, not treated after it had happened. This is one of the challenges in social and preventive medicine.

OVERNUTRITION

There cannot be much doubt that in this country the state of being overweight causes more early deaths and disease than undernutrition does. It leads to or aggravates many degenerative disorders, for example heart disease, high blood pressure and artery disease, diabetes, degenerative breakdown (osteoarthrosis) of weight-bearing joints, especially the hips and knees. It is even responsible for such nuisances as unnecessary breathlessness, an added risk of falling and suffering an injury, and weeping skin (intertrigo) beneath the heavy folds of fat. Generally speaking obesity causes a great many hospital beds to be occupied and a great deal of disability to be endured at home. Many devoted daughters, husbands and wives, not to mention nurses, have reason to regret their patient's large size. Obesity is more common in women than in men. Deciding where obesity starts is difficult. It is said that obesity not only exists but needs treatment if fat causes a person to be 10% over the usual weight for his or her height and age.

The causes of obesity are many, but no one can avoid the conclusion that it results from the habit of eating more than one's body needs. Many fat people of all ages claim they eat "next to nothing"; but every ounce of body weight came past the lips, and it does no harm to point out this fact to stout people who make such claims! There are some people who do not seem to put on weight however much they eat, and there are others who have to be watchful of their weight always. No one can explain this completely. Special cases apart, there is no doubt that most obesity is the result of a lifelong habit of over-eating. Fat babies and fat children will probably be fat old people – if they last that long. The members of some families are all obese, but this may be because of the whole family's habits. The way to avoid the perils of obesity is to learn moderation in eating from the cradle onwards. Some people are "compulsive" eaters, and some eat when they are bored or unhappy. Older people who are fat are at a serious disadvantage if they need rehabilitation from a stroke or a fracture; so, it must be said, are the nurses and therapists who have to look after them!

This is not the place for a detailed account of the theory and methods of weight reduction. Basically it is a question of insisting on a diet very low in Calories, yet balanced, and with all the nutrients present. Because old people are generally inactive, losing weight is a very slow process indeed. A diet of 1,000 Calories may not be effective, and 800 Calories may have to be prescribed, which is very little indeed. Such a diet should consist of about 80 gms of carbohydrate, 50 gms of protein and 30 gms of fat. Calcium can be got from skimmed milk, while iron and vitamins must be added. This is really a matter for a dietitian to supervise. Restriction of salt and water cannot be recommended for older people, because it is too dangerous, even though it produces some apparent "results" in the early days. The forbidden foods, mainly carbohydrates, and alcohol too, are well enough known not to need listing here.

Patients' visitors are great offenders when it comes to maintaining a restricted diet. They are difficult to convince about the need; they usually think, on the contrary, that old people in hospital need "feeding up", and that food is their main source of pleasure; this could be true, but such kindness is badly misplaced, for overweight people have great difficulty in resisting dietary temptations, particularly sweets, biscuits and orange-coloured drinks full of bubbles and fattening glucose! What is more, they no longer have the main incentive which younger people have – to improve their appearance and attractiveness. They say that it is too late to start (and often they are right). They seldom have a chance to weigh themselves, and they are woefully ignorant about Calorie values and the constitution of many fattening foods and sweetened drinks. Yet if they do succeed in losing weight, they will be delighted at the greater activity and feeling of wellbeing which they will enjoy. Unless an older person is convinced of the need to slim and is fully prepared to co-operate, failure is certain. The time for prevention of obesity is very much earlier in life.

DIGESTION

APPETITE

Good digestion starts with a good appetite and efficient means of masticating food. A few old people have good appetites and their pastime is eating. We can watch them, sometimes, queuing up for meals in Homes when nobody need be in a rush! A poor appetite is the commoner thing, especially in invalids. They have lost some of the pleasure of taste and they are inactive. A small eater soon acquires a small appetite by habit, and then it is impossible for him to face normal-sized meals. Apart from acute illness, the cause of a minute appetite may be depression or negativism. Sudden loss of appetite in an otherwise well and cheerful old person might suggest carcinoma, especially carcinoma of the stomach. Otherwise it could mean heart failure, kidney or liver disease. Coaxing a reluctant old person to eat is of course a great anxiety to nurses and to everybody else. It also takes a great deal of precious time, but it is time well spent.

THE TEETH : SALIVA : DIGESTIVE JUICES

Really efficient mastication depends on having teeth. Many old people have lost their teeth years ago, or those they have left are just septic stumps. In the National Health Service good dentures are available at a small cost, but this benefit is ignored by many old people, who find they cannot get their teeth to stay in place because the bony support of their gums has receded, or because they have not one single natural anchoring tooth left. Some "do not want to be bothered" with dentures, and some even use them for cosmetic reasons only and remove them to eat – preferring to chew with their gums alone. This, unlikely as it may seem, is a practical possibility. There is no doubt that people without any teeth look older and less attractive, they talk indistinctly, and their chewing is much less efficient. We should use our powers of persuasion, before doing without their teeth becomes an unbreakable habit.

The only one of the digestive juices which significantly changes is gastric juice, and that not always. The others are produced sufficiently and are effective enough for digestion till the end of life. Lack of saliva in old age is sometimes talked about, but this is an uncommon abnormality. Most old peoples' dry mouths are a result of their mouth-open breathing habits. Nevertheless inflammation of the salivary glands with lack of saliva is common enough in illness in old age. Good mouth hygiene is vital for preventing this. Some old people seem to produce excessive saliva (ptyalism), especially if they suffer from Parkinsonism or certain kinds of strokes. Very, very old and frail people dribble constantly from open lips and jaws; they seem too feeble to prevent it.

In the stomach the juice frequently contains less acid or no acid at all. This may be a reason for difficulty in absorbing calcium, iron and Vitamin B, but it does not seem significantly to affect the ability to digest food. Since the diagnosis of pernicious anaemia and cancer of the stomach depends partly on discovering an absence of gastric juice (achlorhydria), it is important to know that it often is lacking in healthy old people too.

DISORDERS OF DIGESTION, AND THE GASTRO-INTESTINAL ORGANS

It will not be necessary here or elsewhere in this book to give an account of all the diseases, even the commoner ones, which afflict old people. For those who need them descriptions of these can be found in general textbooks. Nurses and Social Workers who work with such patients must naturally be interested in the points at which older people tend to differ from young people. If one hears old people speak of their symptoms and gets knowledge of their health problems like this, it will perhaps make it possible to tell a doctor so that something can be done more quickly. Many helpful clues to illness, passed as chance remarks, are lost sight of because their significance is not realized.

Difficulty in Swallowing

This difficulty (dysphagia) is very common and it must never be ignored. Foreign bodies sometimes get stuck, and treatment is urgently needed. Cancer of the oesophagus is an ever-present possibility. Other things are more common still. There are often pouches, twists and muscular spasms in old people's gullets which cause discomfort or pain, and the pain sometimes resembles the pain of angina very closely, so that mistakes are made. Other swallowing difficulties and discomforts are caused by the frequent appearance of a distorted portion of the stomach within the chest, this having been drawn up through a rupture in the diaphragm. This, called a hiatus hernia, is especially common in obese elderly women; it is hard to treat, yet it leads to complications as well as discomfort. Particularly, inflammation of the lower end of the oeso-phagus from the stomach acid leads to slow bleeding and the develop-ment of anaemia. Sitting up, and sleeping propped up, are ways of minimizing this risk. Cancer of the oesophagus is slow in onset, but it produces persistent and increasing difficulty with swallowing, so that in the end the patient may not even be able to swallow drinks. She can often say very precisely where the hold-up seems to be. There are surgical ways of trying to relieve this symptom, but a complete cure is very un-likely. However, the passing of a tube into the gullet to make swallowing more comfortable is not difficult, and it is hard to see why such patients should not have the relief for a few weeks or months even if they are like-ly to die of the cancer in the end.

Clearly, all forms of dysphagia need investigation. A "barium swallow" X-ray is simple and not upsetting, and because hiatus hernia is so common, all barium meals in old people are best done in conjunction with a barium swallow so that this kind of hernia shall not be missed.

One other swallowing difficulty concerns the nervous system more than the gullet. The act of swallowing is the result of reflexes controlled by centres in the lower part of the brain stem. If these centres are damaged, as they can be by neurological diseases or some kinds of strokes, the patient is in real danger of death by choking, or of taking food and drink down into his lungs. Worse still, he is acutely aware of this and will be greatly agitated. For this reason alone it is necessary and completely justified to pass a naso-gastric tube and feed the patient in safety that way for as long as is necessary. There are now on the market special tinned homogenised foodstuffs containing all the basic food requirements in liquid form, and these will pass down a very small nasogastric tube, making prolonged tube feeding much more acceptable to patients. The very narrow bore tube has to be passed in the usual way but with a stiff wire to prevent it coiling up on the way down, and the wire is removed when the tube is safely in place. The ethics of the use of tube feeding for elderly patients is discussed again in Chapter 16.

Stomach and Duodenal Ulcers

In younger people duodenal ulcer is common, and men are seven or eight times more likely to be affected than women, perhaps because of the kind of lives they lead. At later ages this wide sex difference is no longer found, whereas the chance of a woman developing a gastric ulcer is greater when she is older. So the pattern and frequency of the disease in men and women grows more similar. Ulcers are very commonly found at post-mortem examinations when there was no obvious symptom during life. Yet the surgical complications of ulcers (haemorrhage and perforation) are common enough, and it is by no means correct to assume that when either of these things happens cancer is sure to be behind it all. Non-cancerous ulcers at the pylorus can easily lead to pyloric obstruction, and this can be readily and easily treated by surgery even in quite old people.

Some extremely large benign gastric ulcers are found, especially in elderly women. In younger people, a huge ulcer in itself would often suggest a cancer, but later in life it is not necessarily the case, and the ulcer often heals remarkably quickly with modern drugs like carbenoxolone, given as tablets. An even newer drug, Cimetidine, has lately been produced for treating gastric and duodenal ulcers. Given in tablets or syrup it proves to be effective for old people, but it is still expensive. When considering the cost of drugs one must consider whether they are likely to reduce the time the patient is ill or occupying a hospital bed. By such criteria the expensive drug may prove the most economical in the long run.

Diagnosing stomach disorders accurately is important in old age because if surgical complications or repeated bleeding (haematemesis or melaena) occur, the doctor needs a clear policy – to operate or not, to go on indefinitely with transfusion or not – depending on whether a benign ulcer or cancer is known to be there. Barium meal examinations and gastric juice analysis (fractional test meal or tubeless test meal) are justifiable in quite old people but are seldom done now. These could help to decide the diagnosis.

Gall Bladder Disease

There is no real difference between gall bladder disease in younger or older people, but gall stones are very common indeed in the elderly. One person in every three over 70 years old has them, but most produce no symptoms. The problem facing old people is often whether to submit to an operation for removal of the gall bladder for recurrent inflammation or stones, or to risk second, third or fourth attacks which can be so painful. Once the pain has gone again, naturally, there is less inclination to accept a "cold" operation, for hopeful patients believe they may have been cured anyway.

Jaundice is common in geriatric patients and so are liver diseases. They do not have special characteristics which set them apart, but it is a mistake to think that jaundice always means cancer. Many cases are due to viruses (infective or serum hepatitis), and many are due to the side effects of drugs like chlorpromazine (Largactil), or chlorpropamide (Diabinese) which are so often necessary for use in geriatric patients.

Intestinal Obstruction

The special "geriatric" causes of this dangerous state are cancer, diverticulitis and hernias; occasionally severe constipation and faecal impaction are to be blamed. In any patient with abdominal pain, constipation and vomiting, obstruction has to be thought about. It is easy to come to a wrong conclusion too, because the abdominal wall of small old people is often so thin that normal intestinal movements can be clearly seen, and this in a healthy young adult would be taken as the strongest evidence of an obstruction.

Malabsorption

The conditions of excessive fat in the stools (steatorrhoea) and malabsorption are important because they are common and a frequent cause of weakness, weight loss and anaemia, so that either malnutrition for social causes or cancer could be suspected. If thin patients eat well with good appetites and yet cannot gain weight, malabsorption is very likely. Not all these cases have bulky, fatty motions. There are various complications, not least of which are anaemias and decalcification of the bones. There are many possible but complex causes; one of these is adult coeliac disease caused by the gluten in ordinary flour (to which some people are sensitive); another is a previous partial gastrectomy operation. Some people with life-long malabsorption have already adopted a gluten-free diet, because it helps them so much. However it would be a major undertaking for anyone to start such a diet late in life, because of its complications with everything having to be made with special flour.

Diarrhoea

Acute diarrhoea can be caused by eating too much fruit, or by food poisoning, dysentery or staphylococcal enteritis after using anitbiotics for an infection, or most commonly of all because of the over-use of purgatives by people who have an unreasonable worry about constipation. Diarrhoea often leads to incontinence, but it is almost too much to expect frail, ill old people with acute diarrhoea to be continent. Besides, they often become severely ill very quickly, and suffer from dehydration (see page 49).

Dysentery is endemic in some districts, and an outbreak of dysentery in an old persons' ward can be a most serious matter; it can cause deaths. Therefore all cases of sudden diarrhoea, especially if there are several cases together, must be dealt with as infectious until they are proved not to be so, and stools should be sent for bacterial culture in the laboratory as a routine matter.

Chronic diarrhoea is a symptom of a great many general diseases like diabetes and thyrotoxicosis, but also of bowel disorders, including cancer of the rectum and colon, diverticulitis, ulcerative colitis, proctitis and "spurious" mucous diarrhoea arising from chronic constipation with impaction of faeces. The "diarrhoea" of which people complain when they have a rectal cancer is often really a discharge of blood and mucus. Blood appearing at the anus is always a matter to take seriously. It is not enough just to reassure old people that it is caused by haemorrhoids without investigating any further, even though this often turns out to be the final explanation.

Chronic diarrhoea is an important matter because so many of its causes can be treated, yet are so serious if not treated. Rectal examination is a vital necessity, and it may have to be followed by sigmoidoscopy – an unpleasant but necessary item of investigation.

Chronic diarrhoea means even more misery and insecurity for old people than it would do for younger, more agile people; the problems it causes for nurses whether in hospital or the community do not need to be enlarged upon.

Prolapse of the Rectum

A not uncommon problem for very old people, especially women over 85, is to have the rectal mucosa prolapsing through the lax anal sphincter, and appearing as a soft red object which bleeds and constantly releases mucus, often faecal-stained. It is not of itself hazardous, but it is a distressing and disabling condition. Protective pads may help, but some old people feel obliged to stay in bed indefinitely because the prolapse is always "down" when they are up. It is a condition which usually responds well to a minor surgical operation for inserting a silver wire to narrow the orifice and hold the prolapse back.

Chapter 7

RHEUMATISM AND ARTHRITIS

A special chapter dealing with joint disease and the difficulties which older people attribute to their "rheumatism" would not be necessary if these were not so widespread and such a cause of pain, limited movement and general misery. We can have a daily reminder of what rheumatism and arthritis involve if we watch older people walking slowly about, bent, stiff and leaning on their sticks. They keep going with great courage, and many of them philosophically regard the pain as natural. "I must expect it, dear, at my time of life", is the sort of expression one hears. Whatever they may say, pain is not natural to ageing, and we must do what we can to cure or relieve it.

"RHEUMATISM"

Doctors and nurses employ the term "acute rheumatism" usually to mean a special and easily recognized disease, rheumatic fever, of which the worst effect is damage to heart muscle and valves (rheumatic carditis). This is not what older people mean by rheumatism, nor is rheumatic fever normally seen amongst them. They do however sometimes suffer from the later cardiac effects of childhood attacks of that disease (see page 86). "Rheumatism" to the public means painful disorders of muscles, joints and the surrounding parts of joints. It also encompasses a variety of separate conditions for which doctors have particular names, including diseases of the joints themselves, i.e. arthritis. Thus, a patient with clear-cut arthritis of the hands may tell of her "rheumatism". There is no need to correct this common and unimportant mistake. "Rheumatism" is a gentler, more acceptable notion to many people than "arthritis". It suggests a complaint which fluctuates day by day and might get better; whereas "arthritis" seems to many to indicate a most painful, crippling and even dangerous disease. We should be cautious of using the word arthritis without being sure it does not frighten our older patients; explanations are possible but the euphemism "rheumatism" does just as well.

It has to be admitted anyway that we do not yet know either the basic cause of rheumatoid arthritis, or of several of the other so-called "rheumatic" states which will be described below. When we have tried to classify all these and given them particular names, there are still a number of aches and pains in people's backs and limbs for which we have no real explanation whatever. They are more common in older people than young, and they happen more often in cold, damp conditions of living than warm, dry ones. These can be called for the moment "non-articular rheumatism" (i.e. they are nothing to do with joints themselves). This implies that X-rays have shown nothing very significantly wrong; certainly in cases of doubt X-rays of the joints are needed.

Non-articular Rheumatism

Non-articular rheumatism includes such conditions as fibrositis (myofibrositis) and muscular rheumatism, "strains" and "lumbago", torticollis or "wryneck". Feeling the painful muscles leads one to discover tender places or even "nodules" under the skin. These may not be real physical nodules but could be local areas of muscle spasm, the muscle fibres having gone into spasm perhaps to protect underlying structures. It is quite clear that these painful nodules often appear when there is spinal disease or deformity or bad alignment of joints from injury or degenerative disease; this means that fibrositis is hardly a sufficient explanation by itself for pain, especially if the pain keeps recurring. Those people who have suffered from these nodules know how acutely tender they can be, and how well they respond to physiotherapy, heat or injections. This kind of rheumatism, as well as rheumatic tenderness in capsules and ligaments of joints – especially the shoulder – are a cause of much misery, whilst a severe attack of backache may make it impossible for an old person to sit up or to get out of bed. Naturally, a medico-social crisis soon occurs in those circumstances. Pain of such a kind may be most acute when the patient tries to move, but underneath it there is a persistent severe muscular ache, which is crippling until it is relieved. It is small wonder that people who are not very active anyway cease to move about at all when their rheumatism strikes.

It is often said that old people's bodies behave like barometers; their rheumatism gets more painful when cold damp weather is on the way; this is true and it is no joke to the sufferer. It is possible that a habitual faulty position or posture makes old people more liable to these aches and pains. They are straining ligaments and muscles by making them do the weight bearing which the bony skeleton would do if only they would stand upright.

All rheumatism of these kinds are helped by heat applied to the sore region. This can be given by cautiously applying hot water bottles, electric pads, or a radiant heat lamp. Gentle rubbing with a liniment is a great comfort. Aspirin is the simplest, cheapest and one of the most effective drugs for rheumatism, but care is needed not to give it on an empty stomach, not to people who have had dyspepsia like peptic ulcers, nor to anyone who is known to be hypersensitive to this drug. There are now various new preparations which release aspirin-like drugs (salicylates) lower down the intestinal tract, by-passing the stomach, which is safer.

DEGENERATIVE ARTHRITIS

The older term used for this disease is osteoarthritis, but now there is a better word, osteoarthrosis. By tradition a word ending in "itis" is usually applied to something inflammatory. Osteoarthrosis is not caused by infection or any of the usual causes of inflammation: it seems to be a reaction to wear and tear, though this may not be the whole story. Some people consider it to be an exaggeration of the processes of ageing. If joints are out of alignment or otherwise damaged by injury, if they are wrongly or excessively used, and, most important of all, if they have had to bear too much weight because of obesity, then osteoarthrosis may follow later. This is the reason why it attacks the knees and hips in particular, as they are the large weight-bearing joints. No one has yet satisfactorily explained why the ankles usually escape, but this might be because they are highly efficient and simple hinge joints. The joints between the lower jaw and the skull (the temporo-mandibular joints) are sometimes affected, and people wonder if this could be the result of too much talking!

There is no avoiding the impression that if weight control were to be practised carefully by people all their lives, the whole pattern of geriatric medicine would be changed. As things are, many overweight people are house-bound, unable to walk far, unable to climb stairs, and in pain just because of degenerative arthritis; and thousands of geriatric and orthopaedic beds and treatment couches in physiotherapy departments are occupied by people having treatment for osteoarthrosis. Even worse, a large number of people have to give up living independently and enter Hospitals or Homes because of this joint disorder. Here then is a challenge to Health Educationalists, Social Workers and Health Visitors. By the time the first signs of the disease have appeared, the opportunity for preventing it has long passed.

Degenerative arthritis usually affects one or two joints at a time, but not a whole variety in one patient. Nor is this condition inclined to be symmetrical, as it often is in rheumatoid arthritis.

First the smooth glossy cartilage breaks up and the end of the bone is exposed and starts to wear; it creaks and is very painful. An excess of bone (osteophytes) is laid down at the edge of the joint and this interferes mechanically, so much so that all movement will be lost, the joint disintegrating, and the limb becoming shorter. A few old patients have permanently crossed legs with a "scissors gait" because of neglected osteoarthrosis of the hips. Many others, though not cross-legged, can only take steps of a few inches with great pain and tribulation. Sometimes the knee ligaments are stretched and the patient hobbles along with a gross knock-knee deformity (genu valgum). The symptoms of pain and laxity of the joints come on slowly. Pain may be felt in an unexpected area; thus, osteoarthrosis of the hip may be felt as pain in the knee. Joints begin to creak as they are moved (crepitus) and become swollen, deformed and sometimes full of fluid.

It seems very probable that people who take no regular walking exercise, or who stand in one position for long periods, start off the process of osteoarthrosis in one region of the joint, and it develops from this. It might seem to be a contradiction that exercise should be good for a wear-and-tear kind of joint disorder; yet there is good evidence that a full range of joint movement, regularly practised, without too much weight being carried, does improve the state of such a joint. Nevertheless osteoarthrosis patients are often obese, and obese patients are notoriously slow moving and not much addicted to exercise. Convincing them that treatment should consist of graded exercise rather than sitting perpetually under lamps or being treated (by massage or whatever) is difficult. Otherwise treatment consists of relieving pain by drugs, physiotherapy including short wave diathermy, and exercises. As a last resort surgery may be considered, either to free the joint, to fix it so that it shall not be painful, or to replace it with an artificial joint. Hip joints are frequently replaced these days, and replacement of diseased knees is now passing out of the experimental stage. Surgery of this kind, whether conservative or reconstructive, is expensive and it involves the patient in pain and a long struggle to win through, while the treatment departments become involved in a great deal of heavy work. The decision of whether or not to embark on a such a drastic line of treatment is difficult, for it depends so much on the patient's will to improve, her good sense, and the absence of complications like heart disease. This is characteristic of the complex decisions which have so often to be taken in geriatric work. It goes without saying that the results are best when the patient has previously co-operated in weight reduction. For those who are not so lucky as to have surgical treatment, various special walking aids may be needed. Of these the Zimmer lightweight ("pulpit") aid is one of the most significant steps forward in helping old people crippled with osteoarthrosis to become active again. It provides stability, four extra feet, and the chance to redistribute some body-weight on to the arms. Using a pair of elbow crutches is better for some. Indeed any walking aid helps to redistribute the weight differently. Most people with osteoarthrosis of the leg joints have normal, strong arms, so sticks and aids are particularly helpful to them, whereas in typical stroke patients the paralysis of the arm on the same side makes the use of walking aids much more difficult. For the same kinds of reason osteoarthritic patients get great benefit from walking practice in parallel bars, even of the portable type which can be put on any ward floor or set up in the patient's own home. The general principles of rehabilitation and the problems it particularly raises in older people will be discussed in more detail in Chapter 9.

Osteoarthrosis of the spine exists, but in a great many cases it is painless and the patient is unaware of it altogether. The osteophytes are plainly visible in X-rays, but little evidence comes from a doctor's clinical examination. In fact men who do hard manual work may have obvious X-ray signs of osteoarthrosis in their spines without having lost a day's pay. It is wisest *not* to hint to patients that they have arthritis of the spine. Any talk of trouble with the spine has a nasty ring to it, and patients become over-anxious and may develop pain and all kinds of symptoms and apparent disabilities in consequence. It is possible, after all, to lead quite an active existence with an almost rigid spine. This is not to suggest that painful backs are not disabling: they are. Nevertheless most cases of painful back are not due to osteoarthrosis of the spine.

People with any kind of chronic arthritis, not least osteoarthrosis, must try to keep their joints mobile to some extent. Otherwise they may become "set fast", and in the wrong position too. In other words, the joints have developed contractures (see page 46). It means particularly that geriatric patients with osteoarthrosis of the leg joints must not be confined to bed unless there is some dire necessity. Even a few days in bed may mean the patient never walks again. This often calls for a compromise between the rest which is needed for the other illness and the activity needed for the osteoarthrosis – but difficult decisions of this kind are part of the special fascination of geriatric medicine. Fixity (ankylosis) of the hip joint, most commonly arising from osteoarthrosis, raises certain difficulties. If the hip is bent and fixed, sitting is easy, but walking is very difficult and has to be attempted in the bent-forward position; if the hip is straight and fixed, it is virtually impossible to sit in ordinary chairs or to get out of them. Specially adapted furniture and raised lavatory seats then become a necessity, and what is provided, say, in hospital *must* be made available at home before the patient returns there. Everyone should be thinking of what aids or domestic alterations could make life easier for sufferers from osteoarthrosis.

RHEUMATOID ARTHRITIS

It used to be thought that rheumatoid arthritis was mostly a disease of younger women. Any study of geriatric patients shows that this is not true, for rheumatoid arthritis is found in men as well, and it is not in the least unusual for it to appear for the first time in women when they are quite old. In them it often seems to come on undramatically in the wrists and hands. Nevertheless most of the examples of rheumatoid arthritis seen in geriatric work arose earlier in the patients' lives and came with them into their old age, causing them to have had long-standing disabilities. There are very many thousands of rheumatoid arthritis sufferers in Great Britain, and if they live to grow old, as they very likely will under present circumstances of medical care, a large proportion will eventually find themselves, because of being so disabled, in geriatric wards. The cause of rheumatoid arthritis is not fully understood but it is essentially a whole-body disease or a reaction to some as yet obscure stimulus. Though it looks in some ways like an infection and the word arth*ritis* is used, we have no clear clues that any bacterial or virus infections may ever be to blame. There is a good deal of evidence that it is in some way a disorder of the body's defence mechanisms like the so-called "collagen diseases"; also, people with certain types of personality are more prone than others to be affected. Rheumatoid arthritis sufferers are often inwardly-turned people who always found it hard to cope with life's difficulties, but perhaps this is more true of the younger sufferers than those who develop the disease late in life. Sometimes the start of it links up with some severe psychological stress.

In the first stages there may be fever, blood changes, and glandular enlargement, and the patient is generally ill as well as having acutely inflamed joints, which are warm, swollen and tender to touch. In the "subacute" and the later "chronic" stages, where workers in geriatrics are more likely to see these patients, all the structures of a joint are affected, the capsule as well as the surfaces, and it will have become disorganized, with thickening and tightening up (fibrosis) of the capsular outer parts, destruction of the bearing surfaces, with final destruction of the whole joint, which may be bridged across by tissue and finally becomes immovable. Before this stage pain may be continuous and exceedingly exhausting, the muscles which would have worked the normal joint become wasted, whereas the joints themselves are prominent with swelling; thus they have a typical "spindle" shape. There is usually a severe anaemia present as well. Terrible deformities may result from the fibrosis, especially if the joints have been allowed to remain any length of time in unsatisfactory positions – which they often take up because this is the least painful. Deformities mean disabilities, and some rheumatoid arthritis patients are totally crippled, requiring immense time and devoted nursing care to be spent upon them.

The morale of rheumatoid arthritis patients is often low and their self confidence small. Their lives are restricted; treatment so often fails to show results; pain is ever present, and their pain is none the easier to bear because it is familiar – rather the reverse. So if these unfortunate people are sometimes bad tempered and seem to react even before they are touched, we must sympathize and remember they have so often been hurt before that they are literally afraid of what we might do.

Not all rheumatoid arthritis is incurable, but we fail to cure many cases, try as we may. Knowing this, those who in the early days of the illness allow patients' limbs to get into impracticable and distorted positions will have a great deal to answer for later. It is possible by good treatment in the early stages to relieve pain and splint the limbs, so that if the worst happens they are in the best position for use even though the joints are not freely movable. Even so, the wrists are fixed completely (and they should be in the half-way position) and the fingers are so stiff, bent and distorted that fine work is not possible. Yet the lives of severely crippled elderly rheumatoid arthritis patients are often triumphs of courage and perseverance against adversity, and they often manage to do fine needlework and feed themselves. The best position for fixing of the elbow is half flexed.

In the legs rheumatoid arthritis often affects the knees, less often the ankles, and least often the hips. The bigger muscle groups are often incredibly wasted, and it is remarkable how such patients have the strength to stand and walk at all. Indeed, walking is impossible if the knees have been allowed to become fixed in a bent position by neglect of first principles. A straight fixed knee does allow walking, providing a little "lift" is possible at the ankle joints so that the feet can pass each other. Stiff, straight knees mean that high chair seats and lavatories are needed, and chairs may have to be of special design. Some geriatric departments make a feature of mechanically straightening knees which have been contracted at an angle (even at 90°, sometimes), so that patients can walk again; but it is a slow, painful process, and not without risks in some cases. It ought not to be necessary anyway. Legs which have been artificially straightened usually have to be kept straight by light cylindrical plastic splints, which can be buckled on and taken off as need be; otherwise the limb would flex and become fixed again.

In the later stages of rheumatoid arthritis the disease process dies away and pain is slight, but the severe disability remains because fibrosis cannot be reversed. This is sometimes called "burnt out" rheumatoid arthritis, the fire of the disease having at last died down. It has been estimated that one-quarter of all rheumatoid arthritis patients who enter hospital end up severely handicapped, and that more than one in ten is entirely dependent on other people. This gives us a measure of the seriousness of this widespread disease, and the load which social and geriatric services will be required to bear.

Treatment for rheumatoid arthritis is a complex matter and tactics often have to be altered as the disease changes in severity. The number of different drugs in use suggests that they are not as efficient as we should like. Since we have no out-and-out cure available, much of the effort has to be centred on giving relief from pain, and pain which goes on for weeks and months is never easy to treat. Unfortunately, too, most of the drugs used in treating rheumatoid arthritis like corticosteroids, phenylbutazone (Butazolidin) or gold salts – even that great standby, aspirin – have unpleasant or potentially dangerous side effects. For persistent joint pain it is sometimes possible to inject the joints with certain substances, notably hydrocortisone, and get them moving again. Carefully graded physiotherapy, especially walking practice, and perhaps hydrotherapy with exercises in a pool, are most valuable to maintain mobility. Blood transfusions are sometimes the only solution to persistent anaemia in rheumatoid arthritis.

When, therapeutically speaking, we have shot our bolts, there is still a great opportunity, by using all the adaptations and gadgets invented in sections dealing with Aids to Daily Living, to make disabled rheumatoid arthritis patients more self-reliant and even largely independent once again. Some patients are too handicapped to leave hospital, but they need, and must be given within their restricted capabilities, occupational therapy of a kind to keep their interest alive and uphold their morale, which has taken so many knocks in the long, painful illness. In rheumatoid arthritis it is never allowable to say, "Sorry, nothing more can be done now". Anyway it would not be true, for there is *always* something fresh to be tried. A long medical and social plan of campaign extending forward is needed; the patient has to believe that people are deeply concerned with her illness and chances, indefinitely. In this, geriatric departments are likely to have a large part to play.

GOUT

Gout, or gouty arthritis, is far less common than the two principal joint diseases just discussed. In middle life it is a disease of men only, but later – that is, after the menopause – it can affect women also. It is a disorder often running in families, where the partial breakdown (before excretion) of certain materials in dead tissue cells, that is, nucleic acid, is abnormal. This means that an accumulation of uric acid builds up in the blood and tissues; there is too much to remain dissolved, so crystals of various uric acid salts (urates) appear under the skin, forming yellow-white nodules (as in the ears, tips of the elbows or fingers) and also in the joints, setting up an acute inflammation. Usually the first attack is very sudden, painful, and in one joint; in later attacks more joints may be involved, and some of them eventually become disorganized. Many things like cold, minor injuries or operations, a drinking bout, or the use of diuretics and other drugs seems to trigger off attacks of gout in someone who is susceptible.

The treatment of gout is first to relieve pain by the use of specific drugs like colchicine or phenylbutazone, but in the long run the plan is to reduce gradually the high level of uric acid in the body and cause the kidneys to excrete more than usual. It is a difficult task, carried out by using drugs like probenecid (Benemid). It takes many months or years to complete. The newest form of treatment tries to reduce the quantity of uric acid formed at the start, using the drug allopurinol. Strict control of the diet used to be ordered, cutting down on liver, kidney, sweetbreads and wine, but this is not now taken so seriously as in former times.

MIXED ARTHRITIS

Younger people as a rule only suffer one kind of joint disease at a time, but the older the patient is, the greater the chance of two occurring at once. Having examined some old joints and looked at their X-rays, one is convinced that two abnormalities are present side by side, like osteoarthrosis and rheumatoid arthritis in one and the same knee joint. This may complicate the treatment, but there is one golden rule to observe; arthritis (or arthrosis) always leads to disability of some degree, and a disability is itself a challenge to the geriatric team to help the patient overcome it. Many old age joint diseases are not directly curable, and patients understand this. We are not expected to give the patient back full natural function like a young athlete, but we do aim to make a life of partial independence possible for him.

OTHER JOINT CONDITIONS

There remain a variety of rarer conditions of bone, joint, muscle and ligaments which are painful and disabling. Some of them, like polymyalgia rheumatica, which affects the shoulder girdle muscles painfully, are seldom seen in young people. Many other "general" diseases also involve people's joints, making them hot, swollen and painful – in fact, arthritic. There is a host of possibilities – too varied to list here. Just one more condition needs special mention because it is common and might be prevented. Is it the condition of "frozen shoulder". This might occur when there is any painful condition round the shoulder joint, or any paralysis or any injury which causes the joint to be kept immobile or the arm put in a sling. A frozen shoulder in practical terms is one which is stuck fast, and any attempt to manipulate the limb is most painful and resented by the patient. Whenever anything untoward happens to involve the shoulder, then we must try to keep it free, by moving it, inducing the patient herself to make active movements, or at least to support the elbow away from the side. A frozen shoulder limits the usefulness of the arm and makes dressing very difficult. It can nearly always be prevented provided everyone is watchful.

Chapter 8

THE HEART, LUNGS AND BLOOD VESSELS

Diseases of the heart and blood vessels are the greatest single cause of illness in old age. Statisticians have calculated that if these could all be abolished by some miracle, people would all live, on average, an extra 8 or 10 years. Lung disease is common too, though much of it responds to treatment and disappears. In the end it is most likely to be pneumonia following on upon other medical problems which causes an older person's death. Over one-third of all men and women over 65 in England and Wales are officially certified as having died of some form of heart disease; looking at it from the geriatric standpoint, half the deaths from heart disease occur over the age of seventy; again, one out of every six older people living outside hospital is limited to some extent by symptoms of heart disease. This chapter therefore deals with a most important part of geriatric medicine, so that a broad understanding of the problems will be valuable to all who work to sustain elderly patients. In spite of the gloomy statistics mentioned above, a great many people with heart disease manage to keep going with proper treatment.

When the heart contracts it produces electrical currents which can be recorded on an electrocardiogram. Even very old hearts can behave electrically just like young ones, and they usually look just the same, young or old. In performance however, an old heart has smaller reserves, so when it is affected by disease it more quickly shows signs of stress, and may go into a state of heart "failure", though this is often a temporary state if treatment is given promptly.

CAUSES AND SYMPTOMS OF HEART DISEASE

The causes of heart disease are well known: they include congenital abnormalities, valvular disease, disease resulting from over-activity (or sometimes under-activity) of the thyroid gland, lung disease indirectly putting strain upon the heart, high blood pressure, and coronary artery disease. This latter is one of the most important ways in which artery disease makes itself felt. Anaemia, common as it is, also aggravates heart

85

disease. All of these causes can be found in old people; occasionally even congenital heart disease which has been present, undetected, throughout life, is first diagnosed in a seventy-year-old. It is very common indeed for several causes of heart disease to be present at once, making the patient's plight all the more serious. This would not be usual in a young patient. In geriatric work a patient with reduced thyroid activity (hypothyroidism: myxoedema) is sometimes found to be in heart failure, and only treatment of the thyroid deficiency will allow the heart failure to be overcome. With an over-active thyroid (hyperthyroidism) all the commoner signs of that disease may be absent, yet the heart, with rapid and irregular action, gives the clue which leads to proper treatment for the thyroid – and so the heart recovers also.

Valve disease occurs in younger people because of rheumatic fever, but it can be carried on into old age or acquired from other causes later. Of the lung diseases which embarrass the heart, chronic bronchitis and emphysema are the great culprits, and they are particularly common in industrial areas. Things have been rather better in this respect since the coming of the Clean Air Act. The combination of a major heart disorder with lung disease is often called by the Latin equivalent, "cor pulmonale".

The greatest single problem is coronary artery disease, which leads on to what is also called "ischaemic heart disease", or, more simply, a lack of sufficient blood supply, the heart being a powerful muscle needing a great deal of blood itself. High blood pressure earlier in life may have helped to bring on coronary artery disease (see page 92), but high blood pressure by itself is not so often the main cause of heart failure at 70 or 80 as it is, say, between 55 and 65.

It used to be fashionable amongst doctors of the older school to talk of "fatty heart", "senile heart" or even "tired heart". There is no real evidence that any of these things exist as such, though it may be justifiable to talk to a patient in these terms rather than go into accurate but alarming technical detail. If there is one thing which all patients know, it is that the heart is vital and irreplaceable; so even "heart trouble" is a phrase which strikes chill. We can in fact reassure many old people that in spite of this diagnosis good treatment is available and with care a very reasonable prospect of survival still remains.

In making a diagnosis of heart disease, doctors watch for certain symptoms – particularly pain, breathlessness and palpitations. Pain will be discussed below. Breathlessness in bed or in a chair is unmistakable and must be taken seriously; but the earliest symptom of trouble is most often breathlessness on making an effort. As so many older people exert themselves very little anyway, they often deny they are breathless, though some of them admit that they have to sleep propped up in bed, as breathless patients normally do. Again, palpitation as a symptom of heart disease is remarkably uncommon in old age, in spite of an irregular pulse being found so often. We might think that an irregular pulse ought to produce palpitations, but this is often not the case. So the usual symptoms often fail us in the early detection of a heart disorder. However, helpful warning symptoms are "fatigue", "weakness" or "exhaustion", and also sudden mental confusion. Where there is no other explanation, one at once suspects the heart.

CHANGES IN HEART RHYTHM

Irregularities of the pulse are very common in old people and they may come and go. These can have different explanations; they require a careful medical diagnosis backed up by an electrocardiograph. These days most effective treatment is available for nearly all of them. Therefore it is important that abnormalities of the pulse should be detected as quickly as may be. A nurse or anyone else who finds the pulse very slow or very fast, or irregular, and reports it, will be doing the patient and the doctors a great service; even if the doctor finds the pulse normal again when he comes, he will be grateful to know what it was like.

Recent research, using portable small E.C.G. recorders which go on for hours at a stretch while the patient is free to carry on normal activities, has shown how often old people's hearts change their rhythm and later return to normal without anyone really being aware of what has been happening. These rhythm changes could explain the many little mental aberrations or the unexplained falls or "attacks" which geriatric patients so often experience.

Sometimes the pulse is mainly regular but shows occasional "dropped beats" (extrasystoles); many normal people experience these, and the elderly do too; they are not as a rule of much significance, and if the diagnosis is certain the patient can safely be reassured.

Atrial Fibrillation

Amongst the many varieties of more serious rhythm changes, atrial (auricular) fibrillation is much the most common. The beat is irregular both in rate and in rhythm, and the pulse at the wrist usually has a lower rate than that felt or heard over the heart itself; not all the beats are strong enough to get through. This so-called "pulse deficit" at the wrist is used as an indicator of how well the pulse is being controlled by treatment. If the atrial fibrillation cannot be restored to normal rhythm, the next best thing is for the rate to be brought down to say 65 to 75 a minute, when the pulse rate at the wrist would probably be the same as at the apex (i.e. there would be no deficit). It is important to record, and preferably chart, both pulses. (See Fig. 7).

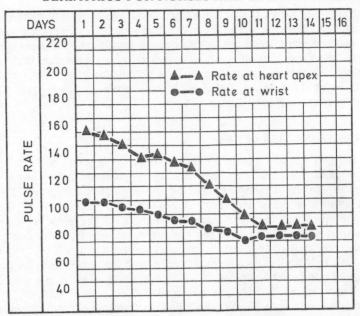

Fig. 7 Record of a patient's pulse (as recorded at wrist and cardiac apex) while atrial fibrillation is being controlled by Digoxin. Note: wrist pulse alone would have been misleading.

Some old people have a form of atrial fibrillation which is always slow, quite well controlled, and not itself serious; it is sometimes known as "senile" atrial fibrillation. Disease of the heart valves, ischaemic heart disease or hyperthyroidism are the three conditions in which atrial fibrillation is most likely to appear. When the irregularity occurs for the first time it usually marks a turning point in the illness, and from then on the patient will be more frail than before; controlling the rate and rhythm is then vital, and it needs very regular checking.

The time-honoured treatment is digitalis (usually given now as Digoxin or Lanoxin). It is important to know that many elderly people are sensitive to digitalis-type drugs and need only small doses – so the chance of toxic side effects is quite high. Amongst these are a bad appetite, nausea and vomiting, and too slow a pulse (e.g. 50 to 60). Other side effects are possible too, so if an elderly patient on this kind of drug seems to be less well, the chance of over-dosage (or occasionally perhaps too small a dosage) always has to be considered. Other newer drugs like propanolol (Inderal) and many other so-called beta-blockers are also coming into use, but they are not likely to take the place of digitalis entirely. These new drugs have helped doctors to control various disturbances of heart rhythm much better than they could in former times. Dramatic methods like electrical 'cardioversion" are seldom used for patients over the age of 65.

Heart Block

"Block" means a fault in the electrical conductivity of the heart so that it is now less efficient. The majority of cases are due to ischaemic heart disease. Though there are several so-called "degrees" of block, the only one which is immediately obvious is *complete* heart block, when the ventricles of the heart go on at their own steady rate of 35 to 45 beats a minute, regardless of what the auricles are doing, or of what demand the patient is making on her heart. Obviously this must lead to restriction of activity, for normal speeding up the heart to cope with physical effort is now impossible. As slow a pulse as this is unmistakable. Often the patient is not aware of anything wrong – and need not necessarily be told. However she may have short attacks of loss of consciousness when the heart stops beating a few seconds; it then starts up again – at which point the patient "wakes up" at once. Attacks of such a kind (called "Stokes-Adams attacks") are serious and need treatment, either with drugs like ephedrine or isoprenaline (Saventrine) or by an electrical pacemaker in the chest wall, which artificially stimulates the heart at a steady, prearranged speed by a battery working through electrodes. This is a complicated and expensive thing to do, but it may be the difference between life and death to the patient, or between mobility and inactivity. Pacemakers have been prescribed now for a number of old people; they work well, though they need regular attention and new batteries at intervals. One might think such an abnormality as complete heart block must always be serious and threaten the patient's life, yet some old people survive a surprising length of time. One patient of the author's was discovered to have complete heart block at the age of 90; he was next seen in a clinic when he was aged 95, and still had the complete heart block!

VALVULAR HEART DISEASE

Disease of the valves is much the same at all ages, except that aortic valve disease gets progressively more common with increasing age, mainly when calcium is deposited in the valves, which are roughened and fail to open and close fully. This causes easily heard cardiac murmurs. Some abnormal heart valves do not close properly, so the stream of blood flows backwards. Others are too tight and narrow, and do not allow enough blood to get through at each heart beat. Patients may go into a state of heart failure because of any valvular disease.

BACTERIAL ENDOCARDITIS

Abnormal heart valves are just the places where infection can take place by bacteria which have appeared in the blood stream – as can happen while pulling out septic teeth, passing catheters, etc. Elderly heart valves are often distorted or diseased for one reason or another even if they do not always reveal the typical signs of abnormality by the doctor's stethoscope. The circulating bacteria lodge in the valves, grow, and cause "vegetations" of clot which can break off and be passed down the arteries to various parts of the body as small emboli. The illness which results is serious and will be fatal if it is not treated with antibiotics over a long period. Therefore it is important that the diagnosis should be made in good time. In old people this is often difficult because the "normal" pattern of the disease has changed greatly, and many of the usual signs like fever, purpuric spots on the skin or "splinter" haemorrhages under the nails do not appear. Cases are quite often missed, and this is unfortunate. If everyone is thinking of bacterial endocarditis in an unusual case, when the patient perhaps has anaemia and a high pulse rate and seems unexpectedly ill, the necessary blood cultures will be done before antibiotics are used and the diagnosis will then be made. It is necessary also to take special precautions against it by giving penicillin while extracting septic old tooth stumps at any age, and not least with older patients.

HEART FAILURE

The phrase "heart failure" means something very clear to doctors and nurses, but to non-medical people "failure" might sound a hopeless situation. Yet hearts can "fail" and then be brought out of failure again. Modern diuretics and other drugs have quite altered the outlook for these patients, and it is important to be optimistic in front of the elderly sufferer. This is not to make light of heart failure, which is serious enough. Once an elderly patient has been in heart failure, he or she will probably relapse sooner or later. It is necessary to keep such a patient under regular review, for changes of treatment will be necessary from time to time. It is in this kind of case that regular "watchful" visits by Home Nurses or Health Visitors can be so helpful.

Acute infections, especially pneumonia, are very likely to throw people whose cardiac reserves are small into heart failure; the same must be said of anaemia, and of anything which artificially overloads the cardiovascular system like a blood transfusion or an intravenous infusion. These must always be given with the greatest care.

This is not the place for a detailed discussion of the diagnosis of heart failure, but certain points need to be made. Left heart (i.e. left ventricular) failure is usually caused by high blood pressure or disease of the aortic valve or ischaemic heart disease. The usual symptom is a series of sudden attacks of urgent breathlessness, especially when the patient is lying down at night and too flat. This symptom is otherwise called "cardiac asthma". Right heart (i.e. right ventricular) failure is much the more common, though in fact heart failure is often a mixture of the two states.

In right heart failure the symptoms come from back pressure of blood which the heart has failed to pump forward to the lungs; so there are various well-known signs like purplish cyanosis, the liver is distended and tender, and the legs are swollen with fluid. Most people have heard that oedema of the legs ("dropsy" to the non-medical world) is a symptom of heart disease. However, there are many other causes of leg oedema in old age. A combination of obesity and the habit of sitting all day in a chair will produce leg oedema anyway, especially in hot weather. Since this is not well understood, many elderly people are diagnosed as having heart failure – and treated energetically with powerful drugs – when they are *not* in failure. Most patients with true heart failure also have a pad of oedema over the sacrum, their hearts are large and rather rapid, and most are seen to be breathless even if they do not admit it. This diagnosis is not at all easy to make at the earliest and the most important stage, when treatment would be most effective.

The treatment itself consists of digoxin or other specific cardiac drugs, and diuretics to remove the excess fluid. What is all too often forgotten is that the patient should have a restricted salt intake, now and afterwards. This means no salt on the plate, as little as possible in the cooking, not much bread (which usually contains salt) and *no* salty foods like Marmite, Oxo, Bovril, etc. which are so often given for their "nourishing" properties for frail old people and invalids. As long as salt is restricted one need not really restrict the quantity of fluid the patient drinks; it is always risky to restrict fluids in old people. Potassium is needed as a supplement (e.g. as "Slow K") because most powerful modern diuretics cause it to be lost too fast. Lack of potassium (hypokalaemia) is a serious state for anyone to be in, not least an old person, and it also has the effect of increasing the sensitivity of the patient to digitalis. It makes people weak, listless and unresponsive. Removal of excess fluid from the peritoneal cavity (paracentesis abdominis) may be helpful. A cardiac bed is an advantage because it lets the patient rest properly almost in a sitting position. Charting of the fluid intake and output gives a good guide to progress, but watching the loss of fluid by regular weighing twice a week is less troublesome for overworked staff. Besides, a gain in weight may mean that fluid is accumulating again in the tissues some time before oedema can actually be seen. Older men can develop retention of urine if they have a rapid diuresis. Heavy old women, needing rest but disturbed by too many bed pans, may have to be catheterized, and this makes the nursing much easier too. In such a case the advantages of a catheter have to be weighed against the risks.

It is an unhappy fact that the complications of heart failure cause more deaths than heart failure itself, for some complications ought perhaps to be preventable. The worst two of these killers are bronchopneumonia and thrombo-embolism (see below and in Chapter 5), neither being easy to prevent. Antibiotics are needed at the very first hint of pneumonia, but it is not a practical possibility nor is it safe to put all patients at risk of a thrombosis in leg veins routinely on anticoagulant drugs. If geriatric patients are active and out of bed these thrombo-embolic tragedies would be less likely to happen; but heart failure patients do need their rest. As always in geriatrics, then, a compromise is necessary. In spite of everything, even patients over the age of 90 in heart failure often recover – provided they have good medical treatment and skilful nursing.

PULMONARY EMBOLISM

This urgent and dangerous condition is the outcome of venous thrombosis; there may suddenly be movement of the clot from the leg veins through the heart and out into the pulmonary artery, throwing great stress on the right side of the heart. It is a cause of many cases of sudden death or of great distress and dangerous illness in patients who have lately had operations, and in geriatric patients who have had to be kept immobile in bed, many of them being in heart failure. In severe attacks the patient is suddenly struck by urgent breathlessness and cyanosis and may go unconscious, being suddenly brought close to death's door. Lesser attacks show themselves with the pain of pleurisy and blood in the sputum, or in other ways. Doctors in fact find it difficult to distinguish between these various types of attack from coronary thrombosis and from sudden lung infections. It is vitally important in reducing the chance of pulmonary embolism to know when a deep vein thrombosis is developing so that treatment can be started. There are now ingenious new methods being developed for early diagnosis. Even more important – if the patient cannot be up – we should see that she does leg and foot exercises in bed, or if she cannot do exercises, that she has passive leg movements done by physiotherapists. However, there never seem to be enough therapists to go round, so anyone in the geriatric team with a moment to spare should try to help with patients' leg movements.

ISCHAEMIC HEART DISEASE

This means disease of the coronary arteries. In older patients the dire effects of this disease are reduced a little by the fact that the principle coronary arteries acquire channels between themselves and are able to some extent to take over each others' territory in the event of a blockage. If it were not for this we suspect the death rate from coronary thrombosis (cardiac infarction) would be much higher than it is – and it is high enough even so. Some of these deaths are instantaneous; when old people are found dead on the floor or have "died in their sleep", coronary thrombosis is a more likely cause than most others. The heart has sometimes been scarred previously from the same cause, and the scar simply tears, death following that very instant.

Cardiac infarction is so well known a condition that it might not be necessary to describe it here, were it not for the fact that the ways in which it appears in later life are very different from the usual. Less than one in five geriatric coronary thrombosis sufferers experiences the typical heart pain in the front of the chest which is the usual way for coronary thrombosis to start in middle-aged people. Sometimes there is a painless "collapse"; sometimes a stroke, or giddiness, or repeated vomiting, or sudden breathlessness, or heart failure, or even gangrene appearing unexpectedly in the toes of both feet because of a drastic fall of output of the heart. In fact there are twenty or thirty different ways in which cardiac infarction might make its presence known, and an electrocardiograph has to be routinely done, or cases will go undiagnosed.

Angina Pectoris

Angina, or cramp-like or constrictive pain in the front of the chest after effort, perhaps running up to the neck or down the arm to the hands, is experienced by older people, but not nearly so often as one would expect, considering the state of the coronary arteries of so many of them. Some people who had angina gradually get less of it, perhaps because normal senescence made them less active people. There are also other conditions causing chest pain which mimic angina (see page 71). The diagnosis is difficult to make; as a rule it is not reasonable to exercise older people hard enough to bring on an attack and then check the ECG, as is often done in younger patients to make sure of the diagnosis.

We should remember that many of our seniors know what "angina" implies and are frightened by the very word. Usually it is best not to use it in a patient's hearing. Many people have been turned into invalids unnecessarily because someone told them that they are suffering from angina or that their heart is "weak". They give up everything and live in fear of death. Surprisingly some of them survive twenty, or more years after that, so in the end the diagnosis is proved to have been wrong. It is doubtful if elderly patients should have stern warnings issued to them about "taking care" because of their heart. A genuinely abnormal heart at that age will soon tell its owner he is demanding too much of it, by developing pain or breathlessness or fatigue. He can learn to keep within the bounds which the symptoms set.

Treatment for ischaemic heart disease is not very satisfactory. The plan is to try to get the coronary arteries to dilate. Trinitrin is able to do this for a few minutes, and it is still excellent treatment though the beta-blocker drugs are proving useful too. The treatment of an attack of cardiac infarction is similar to what is used for younger patients. There is no reason why a cardiac monitor should not be used to keep watch on what is happening, but seldom do geriatric patients get admitted to intensive coronary care units. There is a limit, perhaps, to what should be provided for the aged (see Chapter 16), when expensive equipment is in such demand for younger breadwinners. It is not usual to use heroic methods of resuscitation for cardiac arrest in a known case of coronary artery disease when the patient is old, but there should not be hard and fast rules about this. It is not usual, either, to have to use morphine for heart attacks in old age, fortunately, as morphia always increases the risk of pneumonia. One coronary thrombosis may lead on to another, and it is essential for every survivor of a heart attack who is overweight to reduce his weight as soon as possible to help avoid recurrences. This advice should apply to all types of heart case, because people who are obese cause their hearts to work harder just moving their heavy bodies around.

In spite of all that has been said, it is quite usual for evidence of a cardiac infarction to be found on an ECG or at a post-mortem examination, yet there was never any suggestion of a heart attack at any time in that patient's medical history. So, old hearts often seem to endure these insults remarkably well.

The shape of old people's chests varies greatly; so does the efficiency of their chests as breathing apparatus. Some are wide and some are narrow; some are large and thick walled, some very lightly built with thin coverings. Quite commonly elderly chests are distorted in shape by former disease and by curvatures or twisting of the spine (scoliosis) or a very stooping back (kyphosis); then the whole capacity of the chest for breathing is reduced. Many older people breath poorly, using only a small part of the expansion they possess, so it is difficult to hear what is going on with the stethoscope. This is one of the reasons why X-ray facilities are so essential when chest disease is even suspected. There is no reason whatever not to X-ray the chest just because its owner is old. In a patient who turns out to have pulmonary tuberculosis (see below) this act in itself might safeguard the lives of others, especially young children.

One of the most vital skills which anyone who cares for old people can learn is how to recognize a lung infection from first signs. This is because lung infection (especially bronchitis or pneumonia) is so very common, so serious when it happens, and yet so treatable – provided treatment is started at once. The patient may look "just a little off colour" and refuse her food; she may have a slight change of colour and then begin to breathe a little more quickly, say at 24 or 26 a minute instead of 18 to 20. With this rise in breathing rate there will probably be a slight rise in the pulse rate, but (as likely as not) no change in temperature – or the temperature might fall. Good and experienced nurses develop an almost uncanny skill in detecting these small but crucial signs as soon as they occur. Generally speaking the charting of temperatures, with some exceptions, is not very helpful in geriatric wards, but recording pulse rates and respiratory rates (and these must be counted accurately) is of the greatest value.

ACUTE BRONCHITIS

This common complaint comes on rapidly, with wheezing and a high rate of breathing, and with a dry cough, some distress, but seldom any fever. The patient does not become so ill, perhaps, as the first signs would suggest, but in many cases there is a period of minor but temporary mental confusion due entirely to the infection. Always the difficulty in older patients is to decide when the trouble is simple bronchitis or when it is bronchopneumonia (see below); the first sometimes leads to the second, and the outlook is then much worse. Only in acute bronchitis with a distressing dry cough is it perhaps allowable to use sedative cough linctuses. For other chest infections the suppression of cough artificially is a risky business, for old people always have difficulty in clearing their lungs of the unwanted accumulations of phlegm, which can in the worst cases literally drown them if suction is not available. In a cold bedroom, acute bronchitis may linger on for weeks. One of the best cures is to have the bed downstairs near the sitting room fire, let the patient sit up by it most of the day and keep the fire going at night.

PNEUMONIA

In old age pneumonia is seldom confined to one or two lobes of the lung but there are times when it is a sudden illness with chest pain (pleurisy) and signs which show the doctor what the trouble is (i.e. in lobar pneumonia). It should respond to antibiotic drugs given promptly.

Much more commonly the pneumonia is *broncho-pneumonia*, which is not confined to definite areas of lung tissue. It is scattered in small patches in various parts of the lungs. Bronchopneumonia often follows on after acute bronchitis – which may merge into it imperceptibly – or after anaesthetics, or after the patient has inhaled food or vomit, and it occurs also as a complication of other severe illnesses like cardiac infarction, strokes and major fractures. Being the commonest ending to most illnesses in old age it has naturally come to be called "terminal" bronchopneumonia, the patient being unconscious at the end with a very rapid bubbling breathing. This is the "death rattle" which is so distressing to the relatives and the patient's nurses, but of which the patient herself is usually not aware. Bronchopneumonia very often affects the bases of the two lungs where fluid has accumulated, so it used to be known as "hypostatic" pneumonia. Anything which restricts movement of the chest, even simple strapping for a fractured rib, is a direct invitation to bronchopneumonia to develop.

One other form is the low-grade or "grumbling" pneumonia, in which an elderly and lonely patient, a little breathless, is found dragging herself about a cold house struggling to keep going or having a series of inexplicable falls; she is in reality ill and in immediate need of hospital care.

Bronchopneumonia is not reckoned to be an infectious illness in the usual sense, but it sometimes seems to go round an old persons' ward like wildfire. This is especially so when the patients are frail, were living protected sorts of lives at home, and then after admission became exposed to new varieties of respiratory tract bacteria against which no natural immunity was built up, as it would have been for active, busy people getting out and about. Bronchopneumonia is the main reason for a high mortality in geriatric departments between January and April every year; it also necessitates a number of urgent admissions of patients from poor home conditions at this season.

The usual mode of onset of the disease has already been described (page 38); it may be accompanied by mental confusion, equivalent to delirium. The fully developed disease is of course dramatic, with laboured, bubbling rapid respiration at a rate of 40 to 60 per minute, and deep cyanosis with the patient virtually unconscious.

Treatment is a matter of antibiotics, oxygen and support for the heart, but above all skilled nursing with the closest attention to detail, for the patient is inert and ill and liable to so many complications. The disease is perhaps the supreme test of a nurse's bedside skill.

The ethical question often arises whether or not it is reasonable to use powerful drugs in the special circumstances of the case. This will be discussed again in Chapter 16. If treatment is to be given there is no time to lose; half an hour could make the difference between life and death, for this illness can develop with astonishing speed. It is the author's policy in the "pneumonia season" to ask experienced senior nurses, when they sense bronchopneumonia to be starting, to give a preliminary dose of an antibiotic which has already been prescribed for use as necessary ("P.R.N."), before even summoning the doctor, in case he should be delayed in coming.

CHRONIC BRONCHITIS

This from the practical standpoint is a disease with cough which produces sputum, and some breathlessness when the patient tries to be active. It is in just such a case, though, that an X-ray of the chest is essential, for there are other possibilities like tuberculosis and cancer to be ruled out. Chronic bronchitis has been called the "English Disease" because we in Great Britain have the highest incidence of any country in the world, and thirty thousand deaths a year are the result. Climatic conditions are one factor, for bronchitis is triggered off by cold and damp; pollution of the atmosphere in industrial cities is another, and the fog and "smog" which results from this is highly dangerous to people with bronchitic tendencies. The death rate from this disease in South East Lancashire lately was four times higher than in Southern England, and one hundred times higher than in Scandinavia, where the air is clean and dry. The recent coming of clean air and smokeless zones in cities is helping dramatically to save lives, and prevent illness and wastage of our scarce medical and nursing resources. A man's work in dust or fumes may make him more susceptible to bronchitis. Old men who are bronchitic may have retired long since, but they still could be suffering from the consequences of the working life they had to lead. If they are smokers, so much the worse for them. There is a direct link between smoking and bronchitis, but it is sad to find how few people will give the habit up in the hope of getting relief. Cold houses and particularly cold bedrooms are bad for bronchitic patients, and the supposedly healthy British habit of sleeping in an unheated bedroom in winter with the windows wide open is a piece of dangerous nonsense! Infections of the nose and sinuses very often go down to the chest and set up bronchitis. At this stage the patient may have attacks of "acute-on-chronic" bronchitis, each being accompanied perhaps by a period of mental confusion. After each he may be left just a little worse off all round. This means there is every reason for older people to avoid colds and to take them seriously when they occur, staying strictly indoors in a warm atmosphere.

Repeated attacks of bronchitis are very likely to lead to the condition of emphysema. *Emphysema* is a state in which the lungs are over-distended, partly destroyed, and inefficient gas exchangers. People with fully developed emphysema are perpetually short of breath and wheezing, restricted in what they can do, and at the mercy of any fresh attacks of colds or bronchitis. Their chests are barrel-shaped and move very little as they strive to breath. The end result is strain thrown on the right side of the heart, and heart failure finally develops from these long-lasting pulmonary causes (see page 86); this is a form of heart failure which is very difficult to treat.

In cases where repeated attacks of bronchitis were taking place during the patient's middle life, causing absence from work, there is little chance he will grow to be an old man; further attacks of acute bronchitis or pneumonia or pulmonary heart disease will ensure that he does not. On the other hand not all unfortunate "respiratory cripples" with emphysema have a long history of repeated attacks of bronchitis when they were younger.

In the treatment of chronic bronchitis, antibiotics are used, not as a rule continuously, but at times when the sputum is greenish or yellow and seems to contain pus, to stop further lung damage from taking place. Some patients are advised to take a small preventative dose of antibiotics like tetracycline or a sulphonamide all the winter. Others are given a supply and told to dose themselves at the very first sign of a cold or an acute attack of bronchitis. When there is much wheezing an antispasmodic like ephedrine, choledyl, isoprenaline or salbutamol can help, and so can suppositories of aminophylline, but few of the older generation ever take to using the small inhalers for self-medication with antispasmodic or bronchodilator drugs which are so popular with younger sufferers and asthmatic subjects. If older people with bronchitis could only cough up their sputum they would be much better. Postural drainage should be helpful, with the help of a physiotherapist, but they cannot tolerate it for more than a few minutes, or even a few seconds sometimes. It can be seen that bronchitis is a serious problem as a potential killer, for which treatment is difficult. If we could only prevent it, by cleaner air, good housing, and an effective anti-smoking campaign, incalculable benefit would result to the community and to potential sufferers.

BRONCHIAL ASTHMA

Bronchial asthma is a condition in which the bronchioles are constricted because of an allergy plus other complex factors, and the patient seems to be fighting to breathe. This is not quite the same as "cardiac" asthma, which is a sign of left heart failure in which breathlessness is also severe. Some patients have had bronchial asthma most of their lives, and still have it when they are old. They possess a particular in-turned, anxious, nervous, self-centred temperament, and inevitably create around themselves a tense, dramatic atmosphere. No one should under-estimate the difficulties of a true asthmatic, but experience suggests that the breathlessness of many elderly so-called asthmatics has a strong psychological background, and their breathing is usually much worse when doctors and nurses are present in the room. The truth may be that real life-long asthmatics seldom survive to be old people, and that most of the elderly who are breathless in a dramatic way are suffering from bronchitis and emphysema – or else heart failure. Some true asthmatics become very addicted to their complex treatment – particularly to cortico-steroid drugs, which in the long run are likely to produce serious side-effects.

PULMONARY TUBERCULOSIS

Pulmonary tuberculosis is declining in importance. Generally speaking yearly notification has been steadily falling for twenty years, but for women aged over sixty-five the annual figure has remained the same, and for men over sixty-five it has risen. Deaths for old men from pulmonary tuberculosis are four times as frequent as for old women. This is looked on as a matter for great concern by all health authorities, because till the infection which is present in the older generation is got rid of, there will be no chance finally to get this infection rooted out of this country.

There seems every likelihood that tuberculosis exists in hostels run by the Salvation Army and others, where old men congregate at close quarters. Many of them have coughs which they call bronchitis or "smokers' coughs", and they may in reality be spreading the bacillus of tuberculosis about to all and sundry. They are not usually willing to attend the chest clinics to be kept under observation; they *might* agree to have X-rays at a Mobile X-ray Unit if it came to the hostel, and this is one good reason for keeping some of these Units in use. Older women are not always blameless; Granny's bronchitis might be undetected pulmonary tuberculosis. There have been cases where Granny's good-night kiss has meant a young child died later of tuberculous meningitis. To avoid such tragedies it is everyone's duty to persuade old people with coughs to go to have an X-ray and sputum tests if need be, until the possibility of tuberculosis has been excluded. Cases are often brought to light amongst old people at home only after a search is made among the contacts of a younger patient who has fallen victim to fresh pulmonary tuberculosis. The grandparent, uncle or aunt is then found to be a flagrant "open" case needing isolation and treatment. Sometimes older citizens utterly refuse to co-operate in X-rays and testing; fortunately most of them are "loners" and tend to keep themselves to themselves.

The reason why tuberculosis is still affecting numbers of old people is not certain. It is possible that the immunity they once had as younger men and women has declined so that they fall victims of a fresh infection; certainly an unexpectedly high proportion of older people react negatively to the Mantoux test. Otherwise they may have had an old infection – as many did of those generations – which remained healed for years, and then broke out again.

Many of the older patients with pulmonary tuberculosis undoubtedly have the bacilli in their sputum, but getting sputum from them for test is remarkably difficult because they swallow it. One may have to resort to swabbing the larynx or testing gastric washings. It may require repeated testings and repeated X-rays before deciding if an old man's pulmonary tuberculosis is quiescent or healed, and that he is safe to mix with people. Treating older people at home is unsatisfactory where, as so often happens, their homes are sub-standard. If they are booked to attend clinics as out-patients they often fail to attend, though regular attendance for months will be required to achieve success; or they are forgetful over taking their drugs – and irregular drug-taking in tuberculosis invites the organism to become insensitive. Supervision of this kind or follow up of patients who have left hospital should be part of the work of a Health Visitor, while the Social Service departments should be responsible for helping in their domestic resettlement. Teaching older men hygienic habits may be difficult, and they do not always see that they have social obligations to other people. Old men who spit will just go on spitting. In-patient hospital treatment is the best solution of the worst of the treatment problems, yet keeping old people for many months in hospital itself leads to well-known difficulties.

COLLAPSE OF THE LUNG

Old people who are frail and not able to cough vigorously may, when lying in bed, get a mucous plug blocking a large bronchus. This causes collapse of a part of the lung. It is most liable to occur when the patient has bronchitis, with thick sputum, especially if he is paralysed and lying on one side, as happens with severe stroke cases. It is just one more reason for patients being turned regularly from side to side or from back to side. The same trouble is liable to result if a weak patient inhales a solid piece of food or a tablet. A patient with a collapsed lung becomes suddenly breathless and ill. If the apparatus and the skilled operator are close at hand, what is needed is aspiration of the plug through a bronchoscope. Slow collapse of part of a lung is the result of a growth in the bronchus, obstructing it, or of an abnormal growth or gland mass pressing on it from its outer side.

LUNG CANCER – AND SMOKING

Lung cancer, which as everyone now knows is often the consequence of the lifelong cigarette smoking habits of the victim, does occur in old people. A few who develop it – but only a minority – were non-smokers. It would be unrealistic with so much evidence now accumulated, to deny the close link between smoking and lung cancer. This opinion is supported by the number of doctors and nurses too who have given up this dangerous habit. Older men (or women) may say that because they have smoked a long time – and come to no harm – it is too late already to alter things, so they think they may as well continue. The evidence is against this argument. If one stops smoking the risk of paying the penalty for past folly steadily gets less, until after ten years it is no greater than for a habitual non-smoker. Besides, smoking is harmful to the heart and seriously aggravates bronchitis, and there is nothing in its favour. It seems a pity that an old person's pleasure and perhaps his or her sole remaining vice is so harmful, but there is no denying it is. There was once a hallowed old rule which was taught to medical students, as follows:– "You should not try to alter the established habits of anyone over forty". We have plenty of evidence now that this "rule" is nonsensical, though it must still be said that we do not always succeed when we try to alter these faulty habits. Health Education still has a long way to go.

Cancer of the lung is a dreadful disease. It is fairly slow in onset, causes cough, pain, often blood in the sputum, wasting, lung collapse, and great distress and depression in its victims. Because of this and because patients are often relatively young and in their prime when afflicted by it – sometimes between fifty and sixty years old – they may nevertheless find themselves in a geriatric ward for terminal care (there being no other place). They are difficult patients to treat and to nurse. Treatment by operation or radiotherapy is tried, but the chances of success are very small, and the older victims – those over seventy or so – do not have the pulmonary capacity to withstand removal of a whole lung, so their fate is virtually certain. Those who have nursed and treated lung cancer cases are utterly convinced of the need for prevention – and that means breaking the smoking habit.

THE ARTERIES

It would be impossible to overstress the importance of artery disease in the medicine of old age. Since the arterial system feeds all organs, disease within it could produce effects anywhere in the body; yet it develops according to distinct patterns, and these the following pages will describe. No one yet knows the causes of arterial diseases: the commonest, arteriosclerosis (or more accurately athero-sclerosis) *might* be due to specific dietary faults; it is in some way thought to be linked with stress, or physical inactivity and lack of regular brisk exercise; obesity and diabetes enter into it; a very important factor is each person's hereditary endowment at birth. The best way therefore to achieve trouble-free old age is to be born of stock with a good "arterial history"!

Many people suppose that if artery disease exists anywhere, then all the patient's arteries are probably involved. Though this can happen, one could just as likely find certain vessels affected while the others were normal. Furthermore, it is quite a mistake to think that every old person is bound to have artery disease. Many post-mortem have been done on very old people whose whole arterial systems are quite healthy.

GIANT CELL ARTERITIS

There are certain diseases of arteries which need not be discussed here, but one is of special significance in geriatrics. This was originally described as *temporal arteritis* because it appeared as if this was inflammation of the arteries of the temples or forehead, and caused a very distressing throbbing or stabbing kind of headache – headache not being a very usual symptom in old people. We now know that this is only one way in which a particular arterial disease shows itself. The microscopical appearance of the diseased vessel gives rise to its new name, *giant cell arteritis*. It is a general disease as well and gives rise to blood chemistry changes and sometimes a little fever. It could perhaps be the reason for various other symptoms, even rheumatism and stroke-like attacks, depending on the portion of the small artery affected; there are disputes about this. In some old people's eyes however, giant cell arteritis has a dramatic effect and causes blindness. The patient says that the blindness "came on as if a blind was being drawn down" – as quickly as that. Naturally, there are other causes of sudden blindness, but giant cell arteritis only lasts a few months and it can be treated with corticosteroid drugs. They must be started at once if the patient's sight is to be saved.

ARTERIOSCLEROSIS

Old arteries become less elastic and more tortuous, and the largest artery of all, the aorta, frequently does so. When they become diseased, arteries develop raised patches of fatty material, called atheromatous plaques, on the inner lining, which partially obstruct the vessel. So arteriosclerosis is better called "atherosclerosis", though we may talk to patients and their relatives about "hardening" of the arteries. The greatest risk is that thrombosis of the blood may take place where the atheroma already exists and a complete blockage may result. Atheromatous vessels may rupture – causing cerebral haemorrhage for example – or in the case of the aorta, blood may burst through between the various coats of the vessel causing a *dissecting aneurysm*, which is a dramatic and dangerous event leading to very severe pain in the chest and a variety of other signs.

Though the cause of atheroma is hotly disputed, there are certainly unmistakable links between it and high blood pressure and diabetes. If these were to be controlled by treatment as soon as they appeared, the risk of artery disease later would be greatly reduced. Atheroma is patchily distributed in the arterial "tree", and it seems to affect large or medium-sized vessels but not very small ones, except perhaps in the eye, where it causes damage to the retina. When a partial blockage occurs the blood supply may be enough for everyday activity but not enough when special demands are being made on an organ supplied by that vessel. So, a patient who walks too quickly may get ischaemic cramp in his calf and start to limp – the so-called intermittent claudication or angina cruris. Other people get angina pectoris when they exert themselves; others may get very transient stroke-like symptoms. If the flow of blood from the heart should happen to fall quickly, which is by no means rare in old age, then any partially obliterated vessel would not let enough blood pass, and symptoms might appear or a thrombosis could take place. This is one of the reasons why geriatric physicians are cautious about artificially lowering the blood pressure in their patients. When artery disease of this kind develops it is sometimes possible for the necessary blood to arrive by a different route, and this alternative circulation expands to bypass the original obstruction, being then called a "collateral circulation".

Blockage of Peripheral Arteries

We have already seen (page 93) the effects of coronary artery blockage and the same process, as it affects cerebral vessels and causes strokes, will be discussed in Chapter 9. Blockage may be by the atheromatous plaque itself, or by clotting (thrombosis) occurring over it. Alternatively there may be a fragment of blood clot broken off from a thrombus and carried down an artery until it lodges in a narrower part and causes total obstruction, a process called embolism. The source of such emboli is usually a clot in the left auricle of the heart in mitral valve disease, especially if the patient has inefficient auricular action because of atrial fibrillation, or from a clot which tends to form over the damaged wall of the left ventricle of the heart after a coronary thrombosis.

Blockage by thrombus or embolus quite often affects the blood supply of the intestine (i.e. the mesenteric vessels) causing abdominal pain and perhaps a surgical crisis. This is quite uncommon in young people but fairly common in the elderly. Much more common is blockage in the vessels of the legs and the arms, though the legs are many more times affected than the arms. The symptoms appear much lower than the point at which the obstruction has taken place. This is a fact which surgeons must always take into account. The symptoms include numbness, "pins and needles", a cold foot or leg (which may be pale or sometimes dusky red), pain on moving about, and painful ulcers of the toes or feet or the lower leg which will not heal. Perhaps one of the worst symptoms is "rest pain"; the patient feels pain in the leg at all times but it is more intense at night, when she may have to hang the foot out of the bed clothes to try to get relief. This ischaemic pain is often so bad that the patient may even ask for the foot to be amputated.

The ultimate misfortune is for gangrene to develop, almost always starting in the toes, but extending up the foot and leg in the worst cases (see below). It is plain to see that arterial obstruction is very serious, it causes most unpleasant symptoms, and it endangers limbs or even life itself. We may not be able to prevent it yet, but we can help to avoid the worst complications by teaching the patient all the rules of good care of the feet, as must be done for diabetes also (see Chapter 10). Warm clothing and warm rooms, too, help to reduce the natural sympathetic nervous constriction in response to the cold, which aggravates arterial obstruction. It is hardly necessary to emphasize that with any patient suffering from or even suspected of a poor circulation extra precautions must be taken to prevent pressure or frictional sores on the heels or the feet. After any splints or plasters are applied care must be taken to watch for sore places or signs that the circulation is impeded. Medical treatment here is not satisfactory, mainly because the drugs which are used to dilate arteries work much more on healthy arteries than diseased ones, so they could redistribute the available blood to just the wrong areas. Anyway, the more powerful of these drugs lower the blood pressure, so this might reduce the flow of available blood. One point of view is that the patient needs what blood pressure he possesses to overcome the obstruction; so reducing high blood pressure by any artificial means is, by that reckoning, nonsensical. Alcohol in the form of whisky or brandy (by mouth!) is probably one of the best general vessel dilators, and it is now often used in treatment. Surgery is often needed in the end. The benefits of arterial graft surgery or the avoidance of diseased parts by insertion of artificial bypasses are generally being brought to older and older patients as time goes on.

Gangrene

Gangrene is so common in old people's limbs that it warrants being discussed separately. It can appear "out of the blue", but is more often seen in a limb known to have a poor blood supply. It is a greatly feared complication of diabetes. It usually affects the toes first, but it can involve patches of skin on the foot alone. So many cases are due to stubbing the foot, ill fitting shoes, or badly treated corns. The dry, black appearance is well known to all people who deal with the elderly; if it becomes infected the tissues will be moist and contain pus. Sometimes it remains unchanged for weeks, and it is not essential for such people to stay under observation in hospital all this time, provided they are being regularly seen at home. Often the affected toes mummify and fall off with healing taking place underneath. In cases where gangrene advances, especially if it is moist and septic, and involves the front part of the foot, amputation becomes necessary. There is a crucial point at which the elderly patient becomes more ill and "toxic", with a rise in pulse rate, and if the chance is not taken then amputation will be too late to save her life. Everyone agrees that a gangrenous part must be kept cool and exposed. Some surgeons insist that no moist dressings must be used, but others like, for example, paraffin and eusol dressings because, they say, dry gangrene of the skin lifts at the edges and allows infection to get in.

If amputation is needed – and no patient likes the idea, least of all an old one – one can very often reassure the patient that she will be able to walk again with an artificial limb. Many thousands of older patients with courage have succeeded in this. The author once had a woman patient who had two legs amputated after the age of ninety-one, and yet she walked again without human aid! Surgeons may have to operate at a higher level in the limb than the patient would like, but a mid-thigh amputation is most satisfactory from the standpoint of having an effective artificial limb. Some patients without the will to succeed with one of these, or who have too many other disabilities, still manage to enjoy life in their wheelchairs. Amputation for gangrene is of course life-saving, but we must respect the wish of a frail, crippled old person who, when given all the facts, finally decides this mutilating treatment is the last indignity and she would rather die. A double amputation is possible in some cases, but it is a disaster and a fearful psychological blow. Everyone must take all possible care not to do anything which increases the risk of this – like letting a pressure sore develop on the remaining heel after the first operation.

Rehabilitation of an old person after an amputation is a difficult art. The stump has to be skilfully bandaged to accept the socket of the artificial limb, and the joint close to the amputation site must be well exercised and kept mobile. The patient's morale may be low because it has been a mutilating operation, and some people would like to give up the struggle. Because of other illnesses, some simply cannot summon the energy for the hard fight back. Nevertheless, it is nonsense to suggest that patients should not be bothered with artificial limbs just because they are old. The wheelchair life should be the last resort, not the first idea in our minds.

BLOOD PRESSURE

Most doctors and nurses have been taught that the blood pressure rises with age. This may, within limits, be natural but it may mean that a general tendency to artery disease, or stress, or overweight, has been raising it. Certainly there are many old people whose blood pressure remains normal as judged even by the standards of, say, middle life. This is no disadvantage to them; indeed it is a positive advantage, for it lessens the risk of many degenerative diseases. Since so many people have some rise above the pressure they had when they were young, but are nevertheless surviving in good health, we must be careful what standards of normality we use for old people as a group. A blood pressure of 160 systolic over 95 diastolic is quite usual. Careful surveys have suggested that realistic upper limits, might be as follows:

For men of 60 to 69   – 195/100
For men of 70 to 79   – 205/104
For men of 80 to 89   – 215/108
For women of 60 to 69– 200/102
For women of 70 to 79– 215/106
For women of 80 to 89– 230/110

Such figures as these would be regarded as seriously abnormal in any younger age group. We must listen to the experience of life insurance companies – that high blood pressure leads to an earlier-than-usual death. Perhaps the elderly we encounter in our work are the survivors of those who did *not* have high blood pressure as middle aged people! The practical fact remains, that many older people seem to survive their somewhat raised pressure remarkably well; the critical period when trouble is most to be expected is in the fifties for men and the sixties for women.

We must not concern ourselves too much with the bare figures. Patients are individuals; we must treat *them* and not their blood pressure figures. Anyway, the blood pressure varies remarkably from day to day or even from hour to hour in some people – even quite old people. Their blood pressure is said to be "labile". A labile blood pressure is usually thought to be a youthful characteristic, but this is not entirely true. Quite often we find the diastolic blood pressure reading as normal, but the systolic is higher than expected. This would be what one would expect if one was pumping a liquid round a rigid set of pipes; so it may indicate simply that old arteries are less elastic than young ones, or more "hardened" (i.e. atherosclerotic).

HIGH BLOOD PRESSURE

Raised blood pressure (hypertension), when it occurs in elderly patients is almost always of the benign or "essential" type. Most other causes of permanently raised blood pressure would have caused the patient's earlier death. Only one of them is still found commonly in geriatric patients; this is chronic pyelonephritis – and it happens that many sufferers from this kidney infection do not have a blood pressure as high as might be expected from experience of younger patients.

No one doubts that high blood pressure can eventually cause heart failure and ischaemic heart disease too, or strokes – particularly cerebral haemorrhage. In a certain number of cases prolonged high blood pressure leads on to gradual intellectual deterioration, and there is a link with arterial disease which explains why some hypertension sufferers develop dementia of the typical arteriosclerotic type (see Chapter 11). Yet it is extraordinary how many patients with an apparently raised blood pressure die from other causes. Many of them are quite unaware of the fact that their blood pressure is in any way abnormal. They quite seldom have the expected symptoms – like throbbing headaches, or hissing in the ears (tinnitus) in time to the heart beat. Some have a tendency to giddiness, to attacks of falling, and some may feel easily exhausted if their heart is under strain. For the rest, they seem to have grown old gradually with their raised blood pressure; they have grown used to it, it is "part of them", and they might feel less well if it were to be reduced.

As a general rule it does nothing but harm to tell old people that their blood pressure is raised above normal. It turns them so easily into frightened invalids, asking "What's the pressure today, Doctor?" at every visit. This is really not a matter which should be allowed to worry them.

When a clearly abnormal blood pressure is discovered, deciding what to do is difficult. Obesity ought to be corrected, for it is often part of the picture. Yet it is of little use saying to older people "Be careful; be moderate in all things": they are not inclined to take such rules very seriously. Nevertheless it would be wise also to limit their salt intake.

Artificially lowering the blood pressure with powerful modern drugs is a different question. The temptation to do so exists when people's hearts are under strain or if one thinks that a stroke might overtake them one day. But there is always the opposite view: that they need their higher blood pressure now to compensate for their partially blocked arteries. Anyway, control and supervision of blood pressure-lowering treatment is a difficult business involving many visits to the surgery or to the hospital. Old people with no symptoms will not put up with it for long. Geriatric physicians are usually very cautious about using anti-hypertensive drugs: they see so many tragedies like strokes from ill-considered lowering of blood pressuure in older patients. The unhappy fact is that it is already too late to alter what is to be. The prevention of high blood pressure (with drugs or any other method) ought to have been started ten or twenty years earlier.

LOW BLOOD PRESSURE

Generally speaking a blood pressure on the low side of normal in an older person is a matter for congratulation. By this is meant a figure of say 110/60. In Chapter 5 the question of fainting attacks from low blood pressure was discussed. This can happen when the patient stands erect (postural hypotension), and some of the causes were mentioned. Apart from this sort of attack, which is disconcerting to the patient and worrying to her relatives, there are much more serious causes of sudden fall of blood pressure, including an internal haemorrhage, cardiac infarction, a severe pulmonary embolism or a fulminating attack of septicaemia. They involve a serious risk of death. Any systolic blood pressure recorded at 100 or below might cause fainting, especially in someone whose usual blood pressure was much higher. It is very surprising how low the systolic blood pressure can be in some old people and yet life can be sustained. However the risks of complications are great; these include total failure of the kidneys to secrete urine – for lack of a sufficient head of pressure – and gross pressure sores because there is not enough pressure to force the blood into the muscle and skin capillaries shut by the weight of the body lying on them.

Any sudden "collapse" or appearance of profound prostration in a geriatric patient is a signal to get the blood pressure taken, though a very "thready" small pulse is a good first clue. It is especially helpful to know what that patient's usual blood pressure was before the collapse. Whatever the cause of the latter, the foot of the bed must be raised at once and the legs firmly bandaged, so that what pressure exists can be utilized in supplying blood to the brain. Treatment then is a matter of highly skilled nursing in hospital and the repeated and controlled use of pressor drugs like Aramine or Levophed with intravenous fluid therapy. Naturally, many patients struck down this way at home do not survive to reach hospital.

The getting of a persistently hypotensive patient back to normal standing and walking will very likely be a slow and tedious process, requiring graded postural tipping exercises (for which a special pivoting chair – the Buxton Chair – is now made), abdominal binders and bandaging of the legs. Some patients never achieve more than reclining in bed, their pressor reflexes having become so deranged, and with it all their self-confidence vanishes. To feel one is always in danger of a fainting attack is a miserable existence. Nevertheless patients with simple postural hypotension often improve after a while.

Chapter 9

PROBLEMS OF MOVEMENT: STROKES AND REHABILITATION

The two previous chapters dealt with conditions which might make it difficult to move easily – the first, because pain and stiffness are the two most important symptoms of joint disease; the second, because any sort of activity is made difficult if one has not the breath to do it. The present chapter is concerned with abnormalities of the muscles, the nervous system and other mechanisms which greatly hinder movement generally, walking, standing and even sitting, because of stiffness or paralysis. At the end comes an account of strokes and rehabilitation after those strokes, which make up so large and so difficult a part of Medicine in old age. The methods of rehabilitation used in stroke cases can be applied, with simple modifications, for assisting back to activity almost all elderly people, whatever their illness has been. This final objective should fill the minds of everyone in geriatric hospitals and of everyone who is fighting this same sort of battle on the home front even after a relatively mild illness.

Before we deal with the several ways in which walking mechanisms go wrong in disease, we should look at the way in which people usually sit, stand and walk about when they are old. Those of us who are younger never give a thought to these activities; anything goes when one is young and athletic. Nevertheless good posture is a thing to acquire and preserve so that it remains as good for the years ahead. Correct habits can preserve good health but bad ones start people on the downward path.

Sitting well

Inevitably older people spend a good deal of time sitting, if only because being constantly active and upright tires them out. Their chairs are perhaps the most important part of their domestic equipment, but how few give any thought to their chairs! Modern, low, sloping-backed chairs with thick upholstery and broad arms are the worst imaginable for old people. They need chairs in which they can sit up well, with their backs straight, hips at 90°, and knees at 90° also – or with at least a chance of getting them to 90°. It is important to keep the back straight even while sitting, and to distribute the weight over the buttocks and the thighs; people who sit slumped down in chairs for long periods may develop sacral pressure sores.

There should be arms on older people's chairs too, because these help them to get in and out; but the arms should be slender at their ends and able to be grasped by hands which may be weak or arthritic. A partly upholstered wooden arm is best. These considerations may explain why some older people like old high-backed, wooden-armed Windsor chairs. We ought at least to be able to match them for convenience by our modern chairs, and to give the sitter more comfort too. The really critical measurement is the height of the seat from the floor, and this depends on the measurement from the sole of the foot to the knee. It is much better to have too high than too low a chair. Many hospital ward chairs are totally unsuitable for older people; they are too low, too sloping backed, and are impossible to get out of (perhaps this is what the Ward Sister secretly wants!; geriatric ward staffs believe differently!).

The providing of suitable chairs for geriatric patients at different stages of their illness is a matter of the very greatest importance. There must be a variety of chairs ranging from firm high chairs with wings and built-in trays and foot rests for the very frail and disabled, to light modern dining-style chairs for those who are convalescent, or usually spend their time fairly actively in dayrooms. The author has had for over twenty years standard dining chairs from the firm of Parker Knoll, a number of which either have two inches, four inches or more added to the length of the legs, these being made to special order but quite cheaply (see Plate 8). Not all people need high-backed wing chairs; the less ill ones will hold a better sitting posture and keep more alert if they have lower backs to their chairs.

Few people understand how to get safely out of a chair. This even has to be taught. Forgetful old people have to have it demonstrated time and time again, and it is wise to teach their relatives the trick too. When getting out of a chair one should bring the feet back underneath it, put one's hands as far forward as possible on to the chair's arms, lean forward till almost overbalancing, and then thrust forwards and upwards with arms and thigh muscles together, pausing, still holding the arms of the chair till all seems well, and then finally stand upright but waiting till one's balance is perfect. Sitting down should always be the reverse process; calves against the seat edge, feeling back for and grasping both chair arms, leaning forward a little, and finally sitting gradually back. Flopping back in a rush is bad – and very damaging to the furniture.

Some nurses and patients' relatives are afraid their old people will fall forward out of high chairs. This is just where the modern British "geriatric chair" in its various versions comes in; its swivelling but fastenable tray-table will lessen the risk (though some patients may manage to slide down underneath even this!). Otherwise it is possible to place the patient in her chair facing towards the side of her bed, so that the risks of falling forward are then much less.

Getting out of chairs is specially difficult when one knee is quite stiff; with *two* stiff or straight-splinted knees the chair seat might have to be made 26 or more inches from the floor, yet even this can be done. There could be no better example of how necessary it is to match furniture to people and their physical problems.

Standing well

The standing posture of an old person can be as erect as anybody else's, but this is not usual. In a man erectness usually suggests a military habit, learnt young and kept up always since (for example, a Chelsea Pensioner's upright appearance) or else a very strong sense of personal pride and character. These are matters of habit, and the good habit can be acquired. Most old people can stand much taller when asked to do so, but they very quickly forget and relapse into their old stooping habit. When they do this the head inclines forward and the neck and the spine bend forward, which tends to constrict the chest, heart and lungs; the arms hang drooping at the sides or are bent (in flexion), while some sagging at the knees tends to make the hips semi-flexed too. This is a awkward position to maintain, because it calls for muscular action all the time. It is made all the worse in people who are afraid of falling and are to be seen stooping right forward holding on to their furniture as they move.

In the fully erect state the body is held up largely by the bones of the legs acting through the pelvis and the erect spinal column, which is like a pile of bony cylinders standing on end, all held together by strong ligaments. The erect posture should mean relatively little muscle effort; flexion must mean steady effort, and fatigue quickly sets in. It is not too fanciful to think that a bad flexed posture is one important factor producing "rheumatism" in later life, because so many muscles, tendons and ligaments are working hard just holding the old person up. Everyone could improve his posture just by standing fully upright on tiptoe two or three times a day, holding his arms by his sides and rotating the palms of the hands forwards and outwards.

Walking

Old people can walk very well, but seldom very fast. They walk more and more deliberately as they get older, as if concentrating on what is anyway a complex activity. Failure to concentrate often does lead to disaster. When old people begin to stand flexed their gait soon suffers and they lean forward, sliding their feet, with arms often not swinging. Arm swinging would help greatly in keeping the balance and it is well worth encouraging. Most old people could take longer paces than they do and lift their feet higher. Some who walk very badly on the flat, can still (surprisingly) walk upstairs quite well. One gets the impression that so much poor walking in people who have no real abnormality is because they have bad habits and do not make much demand on themselves. Nevertheless, we must be careful not to judge them wrongly in the matter, because some have locomotor disease, some painful feet, and some do not possess the good lace-up shoes which they ought to have. Certain people spend all day in their bedroom slippers, which give no support and no firm base for walking.

The gait of fat people is characteristically waddling, trying to distribute the weight safely, but waddling can also indicate a bone disease like osteomalacia. Old people are especially afraid of falling over backwards, so it helps them to push something in front of them, like a stable walking aid (e.g. a Zimmer lightweight aid) (Fig. 8), and this can also help those who are frightened of having a giddy attack. They adopt a leaning forward position instinctively, by holding a stick far out in front of them. People who have lost all confidence, or who have been ill and lying down for a long time, show a very strange gait; they totter forwards with tiny steps and show every sign of terror, or sometimes do the same thing with their feet far ahead of their bodies, leaning back and putting all their weight onto their helpers. This form of walking has a hysterical look about it. It is basically a terrible fear of falling, and it is very difficult to overcome. Sometimes we have to put such patients for periods on to an inclined board to help them get a more normal balance. Some start to walk normally as long as there is someone there to hold them, but revert to their "stuttering" steps as soon as support is withdrawn. Methods of walking beside patients when they are taking their first steps again after illness will be described below.

When old people are learning to walk again they should try to look up, but many of them say they "must look at their feet". This may be true in some cases when they have lost the sense of feeling where their feet are in space – a rare condition. All we can do is to assure them that the way is quite free of obstacles, and give them a target to watch at eye level. Sometimes it pays to ask people to stamp their feet down, and after a while their path can be strewn with pieces of wood over which they have to step. A fear of slippery floors, or what *appear* to them to be slippery floors because of the reflections on them, makes some patients very reluctant to try; they may then do better on carpets or on floors patterned with coloured tiles to split up the appearance of uniform polished surfaces (see page 249).

So many people who need sticks to give them confidence will not use them because they think it will be taken as a sign of great age or decrepitude. This is a bad mistake: they should ignore what other people

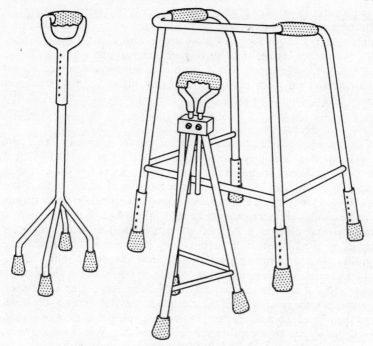

Fig. 8 Walking aids for elderly invalids: a four-footed stick, a tripod ("Warral") stick and a lightweight "Zimmer" walking frame. Note: all are adjustable in height.

might think and use this simple tool, which could make the difference between activity and being confined to a chair. A stick is surely only a badge of seniority, not a hint of having one foot in the grave. All sticks for invalids should be rubber tipped, stout enough to bear their weight, and long enough so that when they are held by the patient's side the elbow is just bent.

Regrettably there will never be enough physiotherapists to help all old people who do not walk. Therefore everyone who can *must* help. This includes nurses, relatives, doctors or social workers, home helps and anyone else who is near the patient. On geriatric ward rounds it is very usual for the doctors to ask to see a patient walking, even though the disease does not happen to be a matter of paralysis or joint disease. Watching a patient walk is a highly important piece of observation because it gives clues to what is wrong, and is a useful part of treatment besides.

Though a good deal which is critical has just been said about the walking habits of elderly patients, we must recognize that large numbers of people still do manage to get about with great courage and ingenuity in spite of serious disabilities and pain. One may even see an old person with crossed, straight legs struggling along with sticks, taking paces of only two inches, rather than staying confined absolutely to a chair or bed. Many very old people would rather slide downstairs on their behinds each morning than not go up to bed every night. Such determination should be an inspiration to all of us.

Care of the Feet

Old feet are often deformed and painful, but for getting about efficiently it is important that they should be neither deformed nor painful. Some surveys of people at home have shown that four out of five have some abnormality of the feet. What a field for prevention of disability this would be. All the money spent on one heart transplant operation could perhaps keep thousands of older patients going a little longer if it were spent on detection and correction of foot abnormalities. The problems are, of course, corns and callosities, hammer toes, bunions and hallux vulgus, or dreadful twisted horn-like nails, which have the picturesque name of onychogryphosis. Sometimes these come from failure of the old person to reach and cut his own nails, because of being too plump or arthritic. Sometimes there is a failure of the chiropody services to reach those who need them most; sometimes there has been simple self-neglect over many years and refusal to accept what help is available. Where self-neglect is present it will without fail show itself clearly in the state of the feet. In this all-important business of keeping moving, regular foot attention is a most crucial matter. Orthopaedic abnormalities should be put right, nails should be cut, and other faults like corns should be dealt with somehow or other, through a chiropody service available to all who need it, every four to eight weeks. With diabetes special risks are involved (see page 156). Diabetic patients should *never* attempt to cut their own nails or corns, they should wear good stout shoes with no "snags" inside, and be careful to avoid any injury however slight to the feet. They should wash them frequently in warm water, dry them, and powder them carefully. These are good rules for any aged, or not-so-aged feet whose owners want them to be healthy for lifelong use.

Neurological Diagnosis

Trying to make a precise diagnosis of the diseases of the nervous system which cause trouble to older patients and to assess their physical capabilities, can be most difficult. The doctor's examination has to be very exact; it requires a great deal of co-operation from the person being examined, and that is not always forthcoming, especially when the patient is muddled or deaf, or thinks the tests are nonsensical anyway. All nurses know how some elderly people cry out as soon as their limbs are touched; does this mean they really have pain? Some tense their muscles involuntarily as soon as anyone tries to bend their legs; does this mean that they have increased muscle tone? Some cannot apparently exert any strength; but can one be sure they are really trying to show it? Some say that their limbs are "useless" at the same time as they move them about doing things for themselves! There are many pitfalls in diagnosis, therefore, and doctors will be grateful for all the help and careful observation that nurses and others can provide, especially since their well-tried diagnostic tests give so many false answers when applied to old people.

SOME SPECIAL DISABILITIES

Quadriplegia

This is a very serious condition consisting of paralysis of all four limbs and often sensory losses at a high level too. It may mean the patient has no appreciation of pain, heat or cold, or even of discomfort over most of the body. In young people such severe paralysis could be the result of a fall or a motor accident. In the elderly it would more likely be due to some abnormality like a tumour in the vertebrae of the neck, or to widespread destruction of those vertebrae and their intervertebral disks from a degenerative disease (cervical spondylosis). Two severe strokes one on each side of the body might produce the same general effect, but there would be other tell-tale signs; there are a variety of rarer diseases too. The outlook for a quadriplegic patient at any age is grave, while the older patient with quadriplegia, whatever the cause, is at special risk from pneumonia and from pressure sores. She might not be able to move any part of the body to relieve pain caused by pressure, or she might not even be able to feel pain if there was sensory loss, so the pressure effects would be occurring without her knowledge. Bladder and bowel control might be lost also. Quadriplegia is a stiff test of nursing skill, but some patients in this state are devotedly nursed for long periods in geriatric wards, everyone else having admitted therapeutic defeat.

Paraplegia

This is similar to quadriplegia but less extensive and much more common; it means paralysis of the body below a certain segmental level; most often both legs are paralysed but the trunk and the rest of the body escape. There may be loss of sensation also, and in many cases it is possible to discover accurately where the trouble lies. Its causes are similar to those of quadriplegia – an injury, or pressure on the spinal cord by a secondary tumour from the spinal bones, and many other things besides. Yet not all paraplegia is hopeless in old age, for occasionally a small benign spinal tumour arises, and can be removed if it is recognized promptly; then the patient recovers altogether. Some cases are caused by arterial disease or other serious abnormalities within the skull which happen to affect the power of both legs together, in which case sensation from the lower half of the body may not be affected at all. The intricacies of diagnosis are very great. What is vital for nurses and others to know is first, what paraplegia is – for it must be recognized at once if there is to be any hope of relief for it by surgery; secondly, what effects it has which require special observation and nursing skill. There is no possible justice in labelling a patient with paralysis from the waist down as being a case of "senile paraplegia"; The paraplegia must have a clear-cut cause if anyone will trouble to search it out. Nevertheless patients with paraplegia do arrive in geriatric hospitals with no proper diagnosis having been made, even after months of home care – by which time it will be too late, and the diagnosis might never be made. From the nursing standpoint this is also a great test of skill. Some patients have severe and painful spasms of the legs which either shoot out straight or start suddenly and uncontrollably bending up at the hips and knees, and these spasms are aggravated by unskilful handling. The bladder may become "automatic", emptying without warning as soon as it has become full. If there is sensory loss the risk of pressure sores is very great indeed, and attention to the back and heels and turning of the patient from side to side might be needed *every hour*, day and night. Nevertheless some paraplegic patients, even very elderly ones, survive and manage to live in wheelchairs though needing a great deal of personal attention. Never was there greater need for bed cradles, Lennard pads under the heels, bladder and bowel attention, and all the other paraphernalia of good nursing care, for a paraplegic, of all people, runs most risk of all the usual hazards of immobility. There is often a case for using a mechanical patient-hoist to make bathing easier; the same device provided at home makes it possible for the patient to be managed, and moved about from bed to chair or to commode by one intelligent but untrained "nurse". We should not forget also that very profound psychological effect which loss of all strength and sensation from half of the body, with bladder disturbances, must have on any patient. Most elderly patients who understand what is going on think that paraplegia is a cancerous illness – and in many cases, unfortunately, they are right.

Hemiplegia

Hemiplegia (or hemiparesis, as milder cases are described) is a paralysis down one side of the body. It is sometimes, but by no means always, linked with loss of feeling (hemianaesthesia) down the same side, with visual loss and other changes. It is usually the result of a catastrophe in a cerebral blood vessel. This is the most usual effect of a stroke, which will be analysed in detail later in this chapter.

Ataxia

Walking and all muscular movements are made remarkably difficult if they cannot be properly controlled, even though the strength to perform them still exists. Normally the control mechanism is exceedingly accurate. Ataxia is in essence a failure of co-ordination, but it has many possible forms and causes. When the disease process is situated at the back of the brain in the cerebellum, there may be gross uncontrolled movements, with tremors and speech difficulties, so that for example the patient, though trying hard to walk, is so unsteady that she has to be held up by two helpers. Weakness in stroke illnesses is difficult enough to overcome; when this weakness is linked with ataxia it is a great deal harder for all concerned, including the patient.

Involuntary Movements

(a) Tremor

Fine shaking movements are common in old people, but they have a great variety of causes, and recognizing the differences is not easy. Fine tremor of the hands in cases of over-activity of the thyroid gland has been mentioned elsewhere (page 155). First in importance after that there are the tremors with which some people are born, and about which they will know already. Secondly, there is the so-called "senile" tremor, which is fine and rapid and involves the hands and sometimes the arms, the head, neck and face quite often, in people of a great age. Probably the head-noddings and incessant jaw-champings one sees in some very old people are similar, but these are sometimes called "habit spasms". These movements, and the repetitive gruntings which some people indulge in are upsetting to the other patients and try the patience of nurses. A special tremor, the "pill rolling" shake of Parkinsonism, will be described at the end of this chapter. There remain other kinds of tremors brought on by years of alcoholic excess, and sometimes by excess of tea and coffee drinking.

(b) Chorea

Certain types of special twitching movements are important to recognize. These are involuntary and seem to have no positive purpose; they are coarse and cannot strictly be called tremors. The head or hands and arms fly about in random movements and are never kept still. Chorea is seen in children with acute rheumatism. In older people chorea is usually a late-appearing hereditary disease (Huntington's Chorea) of which we have most of us seen examples – when older people are walking about, grimacing and flinging their arms about and perhaps embarrassing the passers-by. There is in old age a form of this so-called "senile" chorea which looks the same, but is not carried in families. Such patients with gross movements usually end up in hospitals or mental hospitals for their own safety.

One other special variety with the movements on one side only, linked with certain strokes and called "hemiballismus", responds dramatically to the drug Dartalan.

PAINFUL DISABILITIES

(a) *Shingles*

Herpes zoster (shingles) is not strictly a disorder which causes difficulty with moving about, but is a real disability nevertheless. An infection of the nerve roots with a virus, it is remarkably common amongst late-middle-aged and old people, and makes them quite ill. It first causes intense pain; this is followed by a severe blistered rash which takes days or weeks to disappear, the rash being distributed in a sharply marked band over the territory of the nerve root which is affected. In the elderly the head and face, including an eye, is often affected, and the pain is intense. Worse still, the pain or acute tenderness when the skin is touched may persist for many months or even years after the rash has gone. This causes the old person to be in great misery, and depressed almost to the point of suicide. Treatment of this pain is notoriously difficult.

There is a close link between herpes zoster and childhood chickenpox, so grandchildren are often liable to transfer the virus to their grandparents. If they develop chickenpox, therefore, it might be best to keep them away from contact with older people. When an old person's eye is affected by shingles, expert ophthalmic advice is urgently needed.

(b) *Trigeminal Neuralgia*

This excessively painful condition is almost unknown under the age of fifty. It is a condition causing severe "lightning" flashes of pain in parts of the face supplied by the fifth facial nerve – that is, in the forehead, cheeks, nose and mouth. Attacks are brought on by cold winds, movement, eating, touching the "trigger" area, shaving etc., and the poor patient is in real dread of firing off an attack. She may even be frightened to wash her face or even chew lest it should start the pain off. This is a difficult condition to treat, but the drug carbamazepine (Tegretol) is often helpful. Otherwise, a most delicate operative injection of the particular nerve root as it leaves the skull behind the face has to be tried, and repeated every two years or so when its effect wears off. The pain is so distressing that even a frail old lady, unable to get relief any other way, may beg for this special injection to be done.

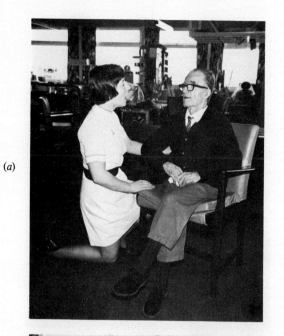

(a)

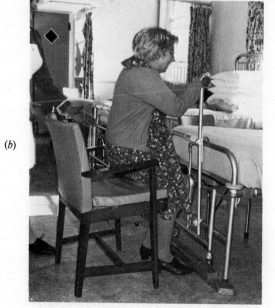

(b)

1(a) The correct way to approach an elderly patient
1(b) Early stage of rehabilitation: "end-of-bed"
       drill, using the T-bar

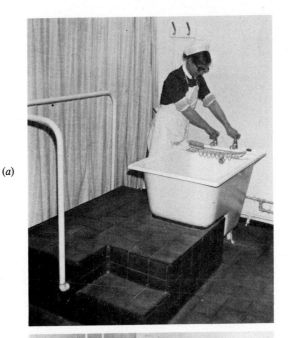

(a)

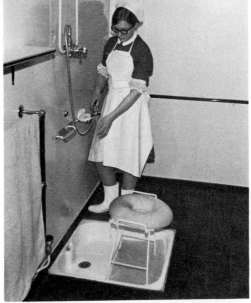

(b)

2(a) Preparing a sitting type bath specially built-in
Note: normal working height for nurses
2(b)   Preparing to shower a patient

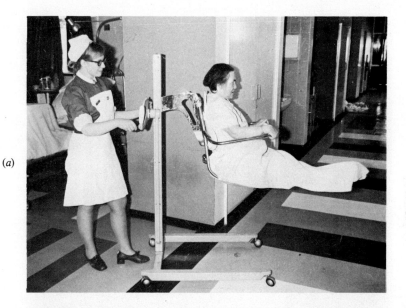

(a)

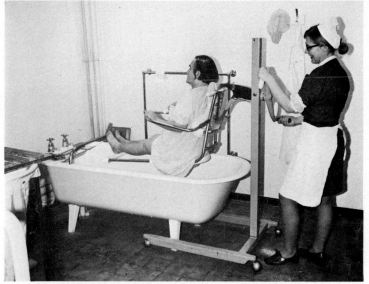

(b)

3(a) Use of the "Ambulift"—on the way to the bath
3(b) Use of the "Ambulift"—in and out of the bath

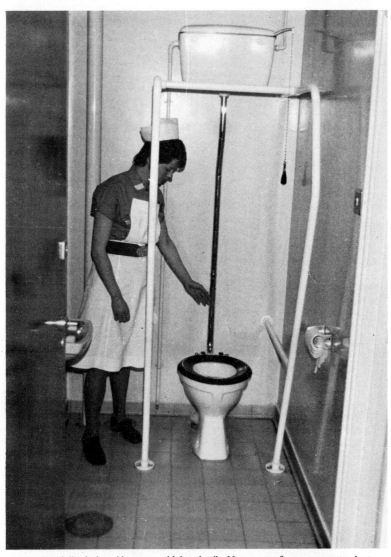

4 Specially designed lavatory with hand rails. Note: room for nurse or attendant
to help

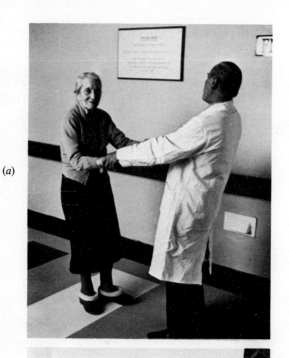

(a)

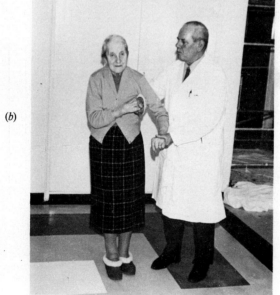

(b)

5(a) Walking with a frail old person—incorrect method
5(b) Walking with a frail old person—a good method

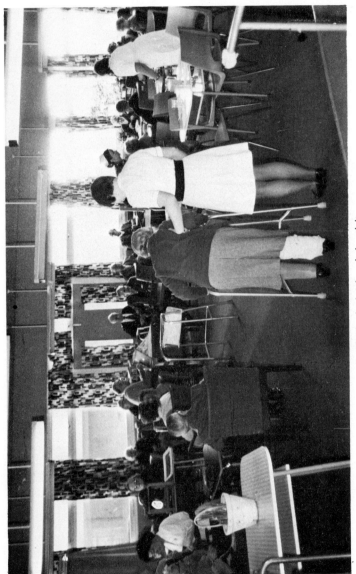

5 Geriatric day hospital activity

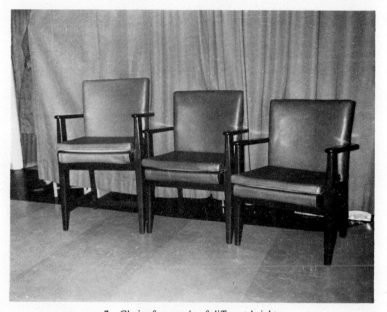

7 Chairs for people of different heights

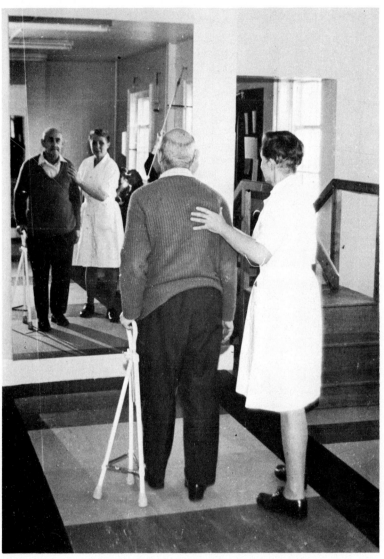

8   Walking training after stroke: value of a mirror

(c) *Headache*

Though in younger people this is common, older people are not commonly headache sufferers, and a fresh type of headache must be carefully investigated. Certainly it is not always true, as some people say, that migraine sufferers improve and have fewer attacks as they grow older. "New" severe headaches could mean a cerebral tumour, or suggest that a stroke might be in the offing. When after a stroke has happened the patient admits she was first seized with a severe headache or vomiting, it is good evidence that this was a cerebral haemorrhage.

Headache could be a symptom of depression needing treatment, or of renal failure (uraemia), or intoxication with bromide, etc. Most important of all, a persistent headache in the forehead or temples raises the possibility of giant cell arteritis (see page 102) for which corticosteroid drugs are certainly required, for they are highly effective.

SPECIAL NERVOUS SYSTEM ABNORMALITIES

Before we can turn to the largest group of physically disabling conditions, the strokes, we should consider a group of diseases with some points in common, and all of which cause difficulty in getting about. Two at least might be improved by early detection and treatment. They have in common some suggestion of "neuritis". "Neuritis" does not mean the same thing to patients as to doctors and nurses. To patients it often just means "pain" or "rheumatism" especially in the neck or arms. To doctors and nurses neuritis should mean a diseased condition of the nerve trunks going out from the skull or spinal column to the periphery, and giving signs of sensory losses or loss of muscle power, or both. "Polyneuritis" simply means that these signs are attacking a wide variety of the peripheral nerves.

(a) *Subacute Degeneration of the Cord*

This is a nervous system disorder caused by the same abnormality which leads to anaemia of the Addisonian or "pernicious" kind – with large red blood cells circulating because cells of the proper size do not mature as they should. Also because of a lack of Vitamin B_{12} there is a degeneration of certain pathways in the sides and back of the spinal cord, and of the nerve trunks themselves. This first causes tingling of the hands or feet and then gradual reduction of power and various kinds of sensation, whilst vibration sense and the sense of position is lost, and the patient has a staggering, unsteady gait. If this were allowed to proceed unchecked, the result might be a total flaccid paralysis of the legs with anaesthesia (rather like paraplegia), which could not then be put right by the standard treatment, i.e. large and regular doses of Vitamin B_{12}. The tinglings (paraesthesiae) of the hands and feet are valuable warning signs, and should suggest the need of a neurological examination and a blood count. The severity of the anaemia is not a good guide to whether or not subacute combined degeneration might develop – for some patients develop it before the anaemia even appears. Subacute combined degeneration is quite common in old age because pernicious anaemia is common too.

(b) *Diabetic Neuropathy*
Diabetes itself will be discussed in Chapter 10. It does not always come to our notice in the standard ways, with thirst, loss of weight, passage of urine frequently, or as eye problems or gangrene. Quite a proportion of cases in the elderly have signs of "neuritis" first, that is, numbness or tingling, cramps, loss of feeling for a pinprick, or tenderness in the calves and even weakness and foot-drop. It is not easy to make the distinction between this and the other forms of "neuritis" (neuropathy) being described in this section – and arterial disease produces some of these symptoms too. The important thing is that we should be suspicious of diabetes in any old person with these symptoms, and should at once test the urine for glucose.

(c) *Carcinomatous Neuromyopathy*
It is becoming clearer that certain nerve-muscle disorders which lead to weakness of groups of muscles, or wasting, or losses of sensation, are associated with the presence of cancer. Sometimes these nerve symptoms appear before the cancer has been detected, and they have to be taken as a warning sign.

(d) *Cervical Spondylosis*
The cervical spinal vertebrae often show changes of degeneration in people from middle age onwards. In X-rays there are very often some signs of degeneration and extra bone growth (osteophytes) even when no symptoms have appeared; so we have to be cautious in diagnosing a disease which might never appear outwardly. The discs between the vertebrae also degenerate, and between them these irritate and compress the nerves as they leave the spinal cord to pass down the arms. The tendency of older people to let their heads droop forwards may bring on the condition all the faster. It would be interesting to know how many old regular soldiers develop it!

In the afflicted patient there may be pain and tingling in the arms, hands and fingers, and signs of muscle wasting and weakness in the hands and arms. Pressure on the higher regions of the spinal cord may occur in the worst cases, so that effects are felt right down to the legs. Occasionally a patient may be so crippled with the combined arm and leg signs of this very distressing condition that she is virtually quadriplegic, totally crippled, and in need of total nursing care. The treatment may be rest in bed for a while, but immobilization of the neck with a plastic or plaster collar or a metal brace may stop the condition getting worse. Flexing of the neck forward is to be avoided at any cost, and the idea of treatment is to hold it back, with support, if need be, under the chin. Unfortunately older people take even less kindly to these conspicuous and restricting collars than younger people do. We should do all we can to encourage older people to use them because the later results of cervical spondylosis which progresses are so serious. Some neck splints made of firm paper, sponge rubber or foam-padded polythene plastic are not unbearably uncomfortable.

STROKES

The technical name given to a stroke illness is a "cerebral vascular accident". Presumably "stroke" is a word which refers to the suddenness of the start of the illness. We talk of many things being done "at a stroke". Suddenness is in fact the usual characteristic of this kind of illness; the disaster may be quick and severe, and although things look bad at the start, recovery will often take place, rapidly in the first stages perhaps, but more slowly later. In the most severe cases, of course, no recovery takes place. The word "stroke" itself is very disturbing to older people – "I haven't had a *stroke*, have I doctor?". Certainly this is a serious matter and not to be made light of. "Seizure" is another word commonly used, since for some people this carries a suggestion of not being quite so severe. The author usually tells the patient as soon as she can understand, in language like this, which aims to lessen the anxiety and immediately starts the patient looking forward: "Yes, you have had a bit of a stroke, and now we must set about getting you better; are you willing to help us?". There is always a great deal for us to do to help the patient, except in the severest cases when he or she is struck down and never regains consciousness, dying in a few minutes, hours or days. In such severe cases everyone can get a grain of comfort from being told that in the event of survival the disability would almost certainly be complete, and the patient's life an empty existence, perhaps even without power of thought or speech; even the most devoted of relatives might not wish survival for them on those terms.

Strokes are increasing in number every year, but so are the numbers of older people (see Chapter 1). Every year there are over two new strokes for every one thousand of the total population; this means in Great Britain between 100,000 and 120,000 new strokes every year. There are besides large numbers of people who have only partly recovered and still need a great deal of personal help in hospital or at home. It would not be an over-estimate to say that a total of 250,000 people in this country at any one time are requiring treatment or support because of stroke illnesses. This gives some idea of the size of the problem.

Strokes, with few exceptions, are caused by cerebral vascular disease. The first of these exceptions can conveniently be dealt with at once: it is a subdural haemorrhage, that is a haemorrhage outside the brain substance but within the skull.

Subdural haemorrhage would not in many doctors' opinions count as a stroke at all. It is due to a collection of blood clots under the dura mater, one of the coverings of the brain, but not bleeding into its substance. It results usually, but not invariably, from a head injury. The clot enlarges by further bleeding, causes pressure, and may indeed lead to paralysis rather like a stroke, but with signs of increasing pressure inside the skull (as one would expect also from a tumour). This is a relatively common happening in old people, and it is vital that it should be noticed, because quite simple surgery can cure it and save a life. Most characteristically the patient is at times quite alert and at times drowsy or in coma with unequal pupils. If this sequence of events was to be discovered in a patient, especially if he had had a blow on the head recently, it would be highly important to report it, for the surgical treatment is not difficult – but it must be prompt.

Cerebral Embolism

The other cause of strokes which cannot strictly be blamed on any abnormalities of the cerebral arteries is cerebral embolism. Here a fragment broken off a clot in the left atrium (auricle), or a vegetation from a valve, or a clot over a damaged internal area of the left ventricle, is suddenly driven into a cerebral vessel by blood flow, and lodges at a point depending upon its size. The effect of this is a very sudden stroke-like attack, which from that moment on needs to be treated just like any other stroke illness, except that steps may have to be taken with anti-clotting drugs to prevent it happening a second or third time. A large cerebral embolism could cause instant death, but this is not usual.

Almost all other stroke illnesses, then, are caused by arterial diseases or abnormalities. Rupture of a congenital small aneurysm sometimes causes a subarachnoid haemorrhage, but this is much more often a disease of younger people. The strokes we are discussing are essentially catastrophies which happen to people over the age of fifty.

There no need to discuss here the detailed lay-out of the cerebral blood vessels. One point however is of special importance – the four main arteries supplying the brain, the internal carotid arteries and the vertebral arteries, are all connected together by a circle of vessels at the base of the brain (the Circle of Willis). In theory then, a blockage of one of the four main vessels would not be too serious as blood could get round the circle the other way. This indeed is what happens in many cases; if it were not so the number of severe strokes would be much greater. Unfortunately the arteries of the Circle might be diseased in old age or perhaps were never properly developed at birth. Or perhaps one channel might already be blocked by disease, and the stroke would occur after a second main artery, previously using the Circle of Willis, had become blocked. Usually it is rather a pointless exercise to spend time debating which precise artery is blocked. A stroke, after all, is a stroke. We need to know at that point what *disability* there is, so that we can start at once on the slow job of overcoming it. Even the precise reason for the damage is only important to the rehabilitation team if it alters the line of treatment, or the speed at which treatment goes, or the outlook for the patient in the long run.

THE TYPES OF STROKE DISABILITY

It will perhaps be helpful, before discussing the causes and treatment of strokes in more detail, to concentrate on the types of disability caused by strokes. The pattern depends much on the simple anatomical fact that all the main motor and sensory nerves of the body cross from one side of the brain to the other before they enter the top of the spinal cord. Therefore damage in the left half of the brain (hemisphere) produces most of its effects on the right side of the body, and vice versa.

Hemiplegia
Hemiplegia is the commonest disorder. It is a paralysis down one side of the body, usually arm and leg together. The lower half of the face muscle may be affected too. The upper face muscles and the trunk muscles are usually not much affected because they are controlled by both halves of the brain. *Hemiparesis* is the term for a milder paralysis of the same sort.

Monoplegia
Monoplegia is a paralysis of an arm or a leg singly, as one small branch of an artery may be blocked.

Hemianaesthesia
Hemianaesthesia is loss of sensation of various sorts down one half of the body, but it is less serious than loss of muscle power, and usually passes off more quickly. With a straightforward stroke hemianaesthesia normally occurs on the same side as the paralysis; less than one in ten of strokes has this sensory disturbance.

Hemianopia

Hemianopia is loss of half of the visual field of both eyes. In strokes it is the same half of field of both eyes and is on the same side as any loss of power or sensation. This disability is of particular importance to nurses and therapists, because the patient is unable to see anyone approaching or trying to interest him in anything if she does it from his blind side, whilst he may be very startled by someone unexpectedly appearing in front of him from that side. As a rule his central field of vision, the part used in reading, writing and handwork is, fortunately, preserved.

Ataxia

Ataxia or inco-ordination of movements has been mentioned already in this chapter (page 117). It is relatively uncommon to find in stroke cases, but when it does occur there are extra difficulties in rehabilitation.

Dysarthria

Dysarthria is a common disturbance of speech not confined entirely to stroke cases. It consists of slurring of the words, but their meaning is usually clear enough to us. In severe strokes involving both sides it may be so severe as to make communications very difficult. Old people very often have slovenly speech, strong dialects, or are minus all their teeth; so they may seem to be dysarthric when they are not really so!

Aphasia

Aphasia is a most complicated group of speech disorders, rarer than dysarthria, where basically there is a failure in the use of the words we all employ as symbols to communicate names of things and ideas to each other. These difficulties are characteristic of certain strokes or other sorts of destruction of brain tissue. There are two main types. First there is *motor* aphasia: here the patient cannot put his thoughts into recognizable words. At worst he has no words to use and is silent though longing to speak; or he might just have "yes" or "no" – often used at the wrong times; or there might be one or two words which are used for everything; or he might use nonsense words, expecting us to be able to understand them; or he might do well except for putting names to people and things, which he finds difficult (nominal aphasia). All this is exceedingly frustrating to a patient, who may get angry and red in the face at the apparent stupidity of everybody else in not understanding what he is saying. He may not even realize that his nonsensical words are nonsense to us. Uncomprehending relatives often think this is a sign of mental derangement, and they have to be told just what is the unfortunate patient's problem. Many aphasic patients are quite capable of understanding what is said to them and it is a common (and humiliating) mistake to speak about them in their presence assuming they do not understand. The other principal form of aphasia is *sensory* aphasia, when the patient cannot understand the meaning of the words we use to him. This raises immediate problems of communication between nurse and patient, and therapist and patient. Teaching and rehabilitating are then much more difficult. Something can be done by gesture, and pointing to different items of food (to offer him a choice), and demonstrating what one wishes him to do, but trying to convey abstract ideas or business matters will probably be beyond us. Disturbances of reading and writing words often takes place at the same time. Many people have mixed forms of aphasia – which just adds to our difficulties of interpretation.

Aphasia is a very great handicap, but teaching by deliberate use of simple words and pictures, like teaching a child to read and talk, is possible in many cases. This is the real work of speech therapists, and most valuable it is. Even so, a great deal can be done under expert guidance by nurses and intelligent friends and relatives with some time to give to this most rewarding part of rehabilitation. A patient who has recovered from the rest of her stroke but is left with motor aphasia may be quite incapable of doing her shopping; but patients who cannot utter words but can read them could be given lists of helpful phrases and the names of objects, so they can point them out to people trying to help them.

Dysphagia

Some stroke patients have a disturbance of their swallowing so that they are in great danger of choking and inhaling food or drink. This is terrifying to them, as often they would realize only too well what the risk is. When there is doubt about safety in swallowing, it is best to pass a naso-gastric tube. Often safe natural swallowing returns quickly, but sometimes a tube has to be left in place for long periods, and sometimes permanently (see page 257).

Emotionalism

Emotionalism is a very common difficulty for patients who have suffered strokes. They tend to be emotional and weep when people talk to them or try to help. A few do the reverse and burst out laughing. This is, in fact, part of the illness. Though some of the emotionally disturbed people seem to be deeply depressed at the blow which has fallen on them, the probability is that the normal "brakes" which we all apply to our basic emotions ("keeping a stiff upper lip") were released when the brain was damaged, so weeping is the result. Some patients' relatives suppose from these floods of tears that they are doing wrong, or that the nurses are ill treating the patient. Thus, this emotionalism has to be explained to them as something which we must expect in most stroke patients.

Pseudobulbar Palsy

In people at the age of fifty to sixty one stroke is possible, and unfortunate enough; older patients with cerebral vascular disease might have two or more strokes and still survive. If these various events occurred on different sides of the body, the picture is unusually pathetic. There may be signs of the double hemiplegia, on top of which there is fixity of the expression, difficulty with moving the tongue, very dysarthric speech, and swallowing problems, profound emotionalism. Every time the patient is spoken to he bursts into tears. This picture of so-called "pseudo-bulbar palsy" is common in geriatric wards, and rehabilitation from it is difficult.

Flaccidity

At the start of most strokes the paralysed arm and leg is totally powerless and floppy or "flaccid", lacking all the usual muscle "tone". If held up and released it falls loosely back on to the bed. In most cases this stage gradually changes to one of spasticity.

Spasticity

Spasticity after a stroke is a state (usually a later stage) when the limb after having regained a little power, perhaps, is obviously stiff, and resistance is felt as one tries to move each joint. It is due to an excess of muscle tone. Severe spasticity is a great hindrance to recovery, especially when there is only a little return of power.

THE EVOLUTION OF STROKES

In the managing of strokes it is convenient to think of them in three ways, according to the manner in which they behave in the early stages. First comes the *completed stroke*: here the beginning is a sudden and urgent catastrophe, as was described at the start of this whole description of strokes (page 121); the damage is done unmistakably, and will get no worse provided the patient does not have another stroke on top of the first. Secondly, there is the *stroke-in-evolution*: here there may be loss of speech or use of an arm, and a few hours later further signs like paralysis of a leg appear, until finally the whole picture is complete, usually within a day or two.

The third type is the *"little stroke"*: a minor stroke appears and disappears again in a few hours or even a few minutes. These are known technically as transient ischaemic attacks (T.I.A.s). They may be frequent, each lasting a short time. Some are caused by sudden alterations in blood pressure and flow when the cerebral circulation is only just enough for the brain's usual needs. The balance of the cerebral circulation is very delicate indeed in such people and almost anything can upset it. Anaesthetics certainly can. Such attacks could be warnings of worse strokes to come, and for this reason anti-coagulant drugs are sometimes used to try to forestall them.

WHEN IS A STROKE NOT A STROKE?

In certain patients the illness starts as if it were a stroke, but does not develop quite as expected. There may be numbers of little events over a long period, like T.I.A.s, but each leaving the patient a little more disabled; or the stroke disability does not go step-wise, but shows a steady slow deterioration when the opposite might have been expected. Perhaps later, uncharacteristically in a stroke, signs of a rise in the pressure of the cerebro-spinal fluid develops, such as headache and vomiting and visible changes in the fundus of the eye as shown by an ophthalmoscope. Then the suspicion dawns that the patient has a tumour or other cause of a rise of pressure within the skull. These are classed as 'space-occupying lesions'. Some tumours are primary (e.g. an astrocytoma or glioblastoma), and some are secondary to a primary cancer of the lung, breast or elsewhere.

Now there are available tests to help with this diagnostic problem. First an electro-encephalogram (E.E.G.), which could show changes in electrical patterns of the brain, especially if the test is repeated. Next is an echo-encephalogram, which can show if the centre line of the brain has been pushed to one side or the other – and this may be detected in an X-ray of the skull also. Thirdly, radioactive isotopes, when injected into the blood, may be taken up in different quantities by normal or abnormal parts of the brain substance, and show up on special recorders or X-rays, suggesting a tumour perhaps. This is the brain scan, "gamma scan" or brain scintogram. Even more recently, there has appeared Computerised Axial Tomography – the so-called C.A.T. scan, or E.M.I. scan, after the British firm which invented the apparatus. Done in an elaborate machine, this test is only available in larger centres as yet, but it can give accurate pictures of the lay-out of the soft tissue of the brain and its ventricles and other spaces, and show up tumours and other abnormalities without any operative procedure.

Though some of these new tests are complex, and the cost of the apparatus is high, they have the great virtue of being painless, not frightening even to old people, and they are safe – far safer than any other previous methods. It is perfectly reasonable to subject older patients to these tests if there are reasons for doubt, for example, about the diagnosis of a stroke. One must have an accurate diagnosis in order to plan future tactics and to be able to tell the relatives what to expect. Besides, some cerebral tumours like meningiomas, and almost all subdural haemorrhages (see above) can be operated on successfully, even in older people. It seems likely that more and more people will be having these scanning tests in future. The C.A.T. scanner can be used equally to explore other parts of the body "from the outside".

THE CAUSES OF STROKES

(1) *Cerebral Haemorrhage*

When there is severe disease in a part of the cerebral artery, and especially if the patient's blood pressure is high, the vessel may rupture and blood will pour out, doing great damage to the brain substance. The result is often a very dangerous stroke starting off with violent headache and vomiting, and the patient falls unconscious with stertorous breathing, head and eyes turned to one side, and one cheek "blowing". The neck is often stiff, and down one side of the body there is total flaccid paralysis. Instant death takes place in the worst of these cases. In some of the others in whom death is delayed a few days there may be high temperature, and in some the temperature falls well below normal (hypothermia).

The nursing treatment is simply that for any patient in coma. The outlook for such patients is very grave, and many never regain consciousness. If they do, the disabilities which result are likely to be very great, and recovery even of walking capacity is doubtful. This is a "completed stroke" with a vengeance. Further haemorrhage can take place into the original area affected, so these patients must be kept in bed and as little disturbed as possible consistent with giving them the basic nursing care which is so vital. Such patients are very vulnerable indeed to all the worst complications (see pp 46–54). Occasionally neuro-surgeons open the skull to try to remove the blood clot from within the brain, but the hope of recovery is still very remote. This is not often attempted in geriatric patients.

(2) *Cerebral Embolism*

Cerebral embolism has already been mentioned. It comes on just as suddenly as a haemorrhage but is often less severe, the brain tissue being damaged by loss of blood supply rather than by being torn apart. There is usually a clear-cut cause for the formation of the blood clot and later the embolus, like atrial fibrillation or recent signs of cardiac infarction. This too is a "completed stroke", but activity can be allowed as soon as the stage of coma is past, and not all such patients are unconscious at the start. One of the problems of cerebral embolism is the risk that it will be repeated.

(3) *Cerebral Thrombosis*

Cerebral thrombosis may be a milder stroke with a "gentler", slower onset without loss of consciousness. Cerebral thrombosis can come on at any time of day, but it is common for the patient to wake up, start to get out of bed, and fall down because the leg has lost its strength; or she may be sitting at the tea table and drop her cup as the hand loses its strength. A monoplegia is quite common. Occasionally there may be hemianopia or aphasia with no other signs of a stroke at all.

Many cases of cerebral thrombosis develop as strokes-in-evolution, a little at a time, over some hours. There is artery disease (atheroma) at a crucial point in the cerebral arteries, and clotting takes place at that point, perhaps due to slowing of the blood flow or lowering of the pressure. This is one reason why geriatric physicians are doubtful of the practice of trying to lower high blood pressure by powerful drugs in old people who might have – indeed probably will have – artery disease. A certain proportion, though a small one, of examples of hemiplegia come from a thrombosis in the carotid vessels in the neck, i.e. outside the skull. It is then possible to operate on this area of the diseased artery to try to restore a good blood flow when, for example, the Circle of Willis was only just maintaining a small flow. Some carotid obstructions or threatened obstructions are operated on with the object of preventing a stroke later.

A patient with cerebral thrombosis has a relatively good outlook for recovery, even when a full hemiplegia develops. Paralysed legs often recover better than arms, so one frequently finds at the end of weeks of treatment that the patient can walk without help but has only one effective arm. Patients with cerebral thrombosis seldom lose consciousness, or only do so for a short while. As no haemorrhage is taking place there is no need to keep the patient quiet and in bed. Hence it is the author's policy to have these patients starting to sit out of bed the very next day, for there is no sense in wasting precious rehabilitation time.

One cannot always be sure which process has been the cause of the stroke. If the doctor does a lumbar puncture and blood appears in the cerebrospinal fluid, haemorrhage is almost certain; if no blood appears it may be a thrombosis or embolism, but it still could be a small haemorrhage without blood appearing; the diagnosis is a matter for delicate judgement. In this the doctor is guided by what precisely happened in the early stages, and even the days just before the crisis, when there might have been little episodes of confusion or speech difficulty and signs which might suggest transient ischaemic attacks, but which soon reveal their true colours in a stroke illness which does not disappear again so quickly as a T.I.A. This is not how a cerebral haemorrhage or embolus would begin. Any nurse or social worker who can get the story of the case from the friends and relatives, and records it faithfully, will therefore do a valuable service – for so often the patient himself can communicate nothing.

THE OUTLOOK FOR STROKE PATIENTS

It is not an easy matter to predict what will happen. Severe cases with haemorrhage and coma seldom recover, and most of those patients who reach hospital come into the milder group, who at least survive the critical first few hours. Patients with completed strokes from a cerebral thrombosis do best. The recovery is fast in some, and in some it is slow; no one can predict at first how much damage has been done. Younger stroke patients and those with the strong will to fight back obviously do better than the rest. It is impossible to give a realistic outlook in under one month, and even after three months from the start some very remarkable recoveries take place. However, once the patient has got through the first fortnight safely, he is not likely to die of that stroke attack. Of people who survive long enough to start active rehabilitation in a good geriatric department, about two out of three recover enough to be independent in walking, but not all of them will have the use of their affected arm and hand, and about one in four remains a severely disabled invalid. In addition there are many recoveries which take place from mild strokes (or T.I.A.s) where there was no need for admission to hospital because the attack was mild and the home circumstances were especially favourable. Bad signs are listlessness, the development of a pressure sore, and the appearance of periodic breathing (Cheyne-Stokes respiration). A good sign is an alert eye and a patient longing to help himself right from the start. If anyone after a stroke is at any stage able to lift his affected leg straight up from the bed, there is a strong possibility he will in due course be able to walk after a fashion. Persistent mental confusion, often the result of the brain damage but possibly present before, is a bad sign, since it makes rehabilitation particularly difficult. One thing is certain – rehabilitation of most stroke cases is likely to be a long business, requiring care, determination and a great deal of encouragement from everybody concerned. It is wrong to call off the attempt too soon; some patients still make progress after six, nine or twelve months' treatment.

THE TREATMENT OF STROKES

Drugs have little place in the treatment of a stroke which has already developed. Pain has to be relieved sometimes, and drugs to relieve muscle spasticity have a place, though they are not usually found to be very effective. There is a dispute about the use of anti-clotting agents to attempt to *prevent* certain strokes – i.e. to prevent them being repeated – and only a minority of doctors think that using drugs against high blood pressure to influence the risk of strokes (see page 107) is of any use by the time the time the patient is old.

In essence, then, the treatment of the stroke is by active measures aimed at getting the affected limbs working again in a positive manner, using the patient's own brain-nerve-muscle systems as far as they can be used. This means physiotherapy, linked with speech and occupational therapy. Furthermore the same techniques will lend themselves with only slight modification to the rehabilitation of any elderly patient from almost any other disease, whether it be someone who is frail and has "gone off her feet" after recovering from an attack of pneumonia, or a patient crippled with arthritis. There is a tendency for elderly patients and even some of their relatives to imagine the treatment, for strokes, etc. consists of *being* treated: that is, they imagine themselves sitting under lamps and electrical apparatus and having their limbs moved or massaged, but taking no active part themselves. This is incorrect. Lamps and electrical gear will do nothing more than relieve pain. Passive movements of limbs are a very poor substitute for the patient's own active movements, when she can make them. We have to convince patients that their progress very largely depends on their own efforts, taught, guided, and encouraged by ourselves. There are some patients who are treated for long periods and make no visible progress; as long as they are "having physiotherapy" they believe that this is progress. It is a hard but necessary decision sometimes to stop treatment – after a long enough interval to be sure that progress has stopped – because the needs of other patients are greater and not enough physiotherapists are available.

We must all school ourselves not to help any patient to do anything which she can do reasonably for herself. If we do help we hinder progress. This is a particularly hard discipline for nurses to accept, brought up as they are in the tradition of service to other people in adversity. It is almost an instinct to go to help someone out of a chair, but if that person *can* do it, she *should* do it, and it will be easier for her the next time.

There is often a conflict as between home and hospital for treatment for strokes. The patient may desire the comfort and familiarity of home; the relatives may be torn between compassion and knowing they cannot do all that is needed. The doctor and the Home Nurse perhaps are torn between the two. Yet there cannot be much doubt that for treatment of a fairly severe stroke a well-equipped active geriatric rehabilitation department has more to offer than a well organized private house. It has, after all, skilled nurses day and night, therapists and therapy departments, various equipment and aids, a bright optimistic atmosphere and, above all, space for the active training which is needed.

Rehabilitation is team work. The team comprises the doctors, the patients themselves, the therapists, the entire nursing staff from the Nursing Officer downwards, and friends and relatives also; and at various stages the Social Worker's contribution is vital – maintaining communications with the outside world, solving financial and legal problems, preparing for the homecoming and persuading authorities to provide the home care and adaptation which may be necessary if recovery is not quite perfect – as it so often is not. All these people must be aiming at the common objective – the greatest independence of the patient and the earliest return to as nearly normal a life as possible. Everybody must rely on everybody else's special skills, and there must be free consultation frequently. There is never enough of the special skill needed: this being so, it is often necessary for the nurses to assist in walking patients about, or for physiotherapists to help lift particularly heavy patients back to bed after treatment. What applies to the nurses and others should apply equally to the doctors and everyone else who has the welfare of the patient at heart. Teams need leaders, but there is no time in geriatric rehabilitation for demarcation disputes!

This is not the place for a fully detailed account of the principles of rehabilitation and treatment for strokes. What we do now is not necessarily new; much of it was thought of in the fifth century A.D., but it was mostly lost sight of until about the middle nineteen thirties! Nevertheless, some of the main principles and the particular parts of stroke treatment which will particularly interest nurses and social workers will be discussed.

In the first days after the stroke, following the dangerous stage with coma and with swallowing difficulties, the patient may have to be nursed in bed for some hours or some days and every night, according to the circumstances. The special risks are pressure sores, pneumonia and contractures. All necessary precautions must be taken to supply plenty of fluids and to control incontinence, which will be of the "cerebral type" (see page 52): it may require habit-training, or at worst a self-retaining catheter in the first stages.

The patient must, whenever in bed, be sitting up with a cradle in position, her legs straight, her feet supported at a right angle, with a wooden support or sandbag, and with "tubipad" heel protectors and a Lennard pad to keep the heels clear of the bed. The affected arm is kept away from the side (to try to prevent a "frozen" shoulder), with the weak arm supported on a pile of pillows with the elbow slightly bent, and the wrist and fingers straight out on the pillows, or splinted out at night if they are tending to contract. All this, with regular turning and attention to the back, and perhaps the use of a "ripple bed", should ensure that complications do not arise and the paralysed limbs do not get into incorrect positions.

Some paralysed legs contract up especially at night and need to be splinted straight. The plight of a patient with a neglected, flexed, contracted leg tucked up permanently under her buttocks is pathetic to see, as she can neither lie straight nor sit in any chair.

As soon as possible the physiotherapist should move the limbs through a full range of movement, on both sides, affected and normal, to maintain joint mobility and preserve normal muscle tone. These passive moments are important and can be taught to and practised by nurses, husbands and wives, friends and everyone else interested, so that they can be done repeatedly during the day. They can be to some extent taught to the patient herself, to be practised while she sits in a chair, using the sound hand, for example, to manipulate the weak hand and arm. By this time the patient needs to be sitting out of bed for considerable parts of the day, dressed in her own clothes and if possible in a day room well away from the beds. Beds, night attire and all the sickroom and ward paraphernalia make anyone feel an invalid, but we must try to make her feel as normal as possible.

There follows from this a stage, supervised by the physiotherapists, where every flicker of returning movement is used actively, by devising exercises where the therapists resist pushing or pulling arm movements and kicking or leg raising movements which the patient is attempting to make. Pulling of weights on pulleys, punching of suspended punch balls, and exercises in suspension all help in this first attempt to use the patient's own returning powers. Suspension means the effect of gravity is counteracted, the limb is held up from an overhead frame with ropes, slings and springs, so that small muscle power can produce large ranges of movement. By special suspension techniques, which only help some people, it is possible to make muscle groups work harder and harder by working against more and more powerful springs. Home Nurses, with the help of relatives who are handy men, can often set up simple suspension exercises for patients to do, by attaching pulleys and hooks to ring bolts in the ceiling.

Nurses and orderlies should help to supervise and encourage patients in all these activities because their attention and determination so easily flags. Everyone must recognize the fight back is long and hard.

At the same time speech and occupational therapists are at work overcoming aphasia and dysarthric signs, and giving the patient something positive to do. At first occupational therapy may have to be confined to using only the good arm, but as some activity starts to reappear in the other hand and arm, effort has to be concentrated on encouragement of its activities, however small they may be at first. The weak hand in particular should be working at squeezing a soft rubber ball, a roll of plastic foam, or a piece of so-called "plastic putty". Only at a later stage, supposing hand-arm recovery is proved to be unlikely, should occupational therapy be concentrated on making it possible for the patient to live, dress, cook and manage generally with the remaining normal hand.

At an early stage of course the patient should be fully dressed in his own clothes and good shoes. He can do end-of-bed drills by bracing his feet against a board and pulling himself up and down from a chair by using the bed rail or a specially raised "T-bar" (see Plate 2). This is one of the first steps to independence and is vitally important for morale.

Even more important are the first steps in walking after trunk and leg extension exercises on the bed. The therapist walks beside her patient bracing the uncertain knee, and coaxing the whole leg forward. At this stage it may be necessary to be using splints for the wrist and for the leg to hold it straight and stable, and a caliper with a back-stop and other devices to counteract the foot drop which is so commonly a part of this illness, but is made so much worse by neglect of providing foot support and of a cradle in the bed right from the start.

Nurses need to know the practical details of how calipers (Fig. 9) and splints help patients, and how they should be put on, for they are an essential part of the patients' day by day equipment.

Most physiotherapy departments organize classwork for stroke patients so that they can benefit from competition, perform group exercises, play indoor ball games and indulge in other activities which encourage particular muscle movements in a cheerful, competitive team spirit. Simple they may appear, but they have positive value (see Plate 9).

By this time occupational therapy should have progressed to making definite objects, giving the patient a sense of creative activity, and concentrating on techniques of dressing, toilet, cooking, despite disabilities which are often only too obvious. The patient should be being taught how to get out of bed safely, out of chairs (see page 203), off and on to the lavatory, and off the floor supposing she were unfortunate enough to fall down. Having been taught how to tackle such problems before they arise gives great confidence. At all points the nursing staff should be involved in these activities, encouraging, congratulating, showing sympathy but optimism equally, and seeing that the sorts of activity which patients are taught are continued in the ward and bathroom and at the wash basin after stroke-therapy hours.

The patient should by now, unless grossly aphasic, be able to communicate and even to write a little, even though it may have to be with the wrong hand. She is put through the range of normal daily activities and has her performance recorded preparatory to her return home. Certain aids, sticks and gadgets may be necessary. There is a great variety of such aids for eating, cleaning teeth, pulling on clothes, stockings and shoes, lifting, cutting bread, reaching for distant objects, and for generally making independent life possible for people whose recovery may only be partial. It would pay all nurses, social workers and doctors to get to know what possibilities there are of this kind.

This is one of the stages at which the Social Worker and other Local Authority staff should be most involved. They should see the patient, discuss his capabilities with the medical, nursing and therapy staff, see what his remaining needs are, and try to get the home adapted as required and the gadgets that the patient needs to continue a semi-active life at home. These adaptations may have to include a second handrail to a staircase, a

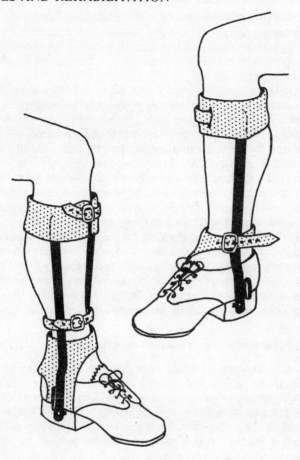

Fig. 9 Calipers to help patients with foot-drop. Note: the backstops and T-straps.

ramp up in place of steps, elimination of hazards, grab handles in strategic places, and others, depending upon individual circumstances. All these could be provided under present legislation, but many rehabilitation departments are still frustrated at the long delays in getting these requirements provided. It is useless for a Social Worker from outside to interview the patient but not consult the various health professional staff; patients often cannot communicate, they may be muddled, and they may give a pessimistic account of their capabilities because they fear the problems ahead, and after several weeks or months in hospital look on that as security to be hung on to. It is our collective duty then to help the patient over that last difficult hurdle.

In certain circumstances the offer of a place in a Residential Home is gladly accepted, as it offers some regular and reliable help, and an absence of certain chores like preparing meals. Nevertheless the ideal solution is for a patient to go home to be in a family, or even alone with aids, and *wanting to do so*.

Some patients (naturally, the less robust, the older ones, the most afflicted) do not achieve enough independence to leave hospital; even so, they need certain aids and ungrudging assistance, and things to do with their limited abilities, and a personal wheel chair perhaps, and cheerful surroundings, and a sense that people are still interested in them even though their illness did not allow them quite to come up to our best hopes for them. It helps them tremendously if they can still be cared for by members of the same medical, nursing and social work team rather than being sent away, cast off, failures in their own eyes, to be cared for by strangers who never knew how hard they tried.

By contrast there is great rejoicing by the team when a severely handicapped patient, by dint of her own hard work and theirs, finally takes the homeward road. They like to follow her progress in a follow-up clinic, and they will repeat the whole rehabilitation process if need be, supposing there is a second stroke or any other illness takes her off her feet. A bond has been forged which will only be broken later by death.

SPECIAL PROBLEMS IN THE TREATING OF STROKES

Careful observation of a large number of elderly stroke patients by Professor G. F. Adams and his colleagues in Belfast, as well as other people in other places, have shown us how often the best efforts of doctors and nurses in treatment produce results which are not as good as anyone might have expected from the first examination of the case. Sometimes it happens that a patient "does not seem to be trying very hard". It is difficult to communicate with him; his attention wanders; he keeps on making the same kind of mistake time and time again. Analysis of this kind of problem now suggests that it is we ourselves who may be making the mistakes, by not understanding just why that particular patient has this difficulty, why he fails to make progress. First, however, there are more obvious causes of delay or frustration in treatment. These may be the very great frailty and the very great age of the patient. Trying to rehabilitate a stroke patient in her nineties is a formidable proposition even if hers was only a mild stroke. Next, she might be deaf and unable to understand, and not able to take to a hearing aid. Blindness would be even more of a problem. Next, the patient's heart condition might not keep up with the extra expenditure of energy – for struggling to do things with limbs that are inefficient is physically exhausting. Next, there may be the mental confusion, or aphasia, or emotionalism which have been described before. It is hard to get anywhere teaching a hemiplegic patient to walk if half the time he is in floods of tears. Incontinence of urine may be present, and this seriously upsets things in a rehabilitation department; it also upsets relatives, and they have to be reassured that this is part of the illness and not just the patient's wilful neglect of proper behaviour. *Hemiplegic oedema* is another difficulty. In this condition it is noticeable that the hand and arm and sometimes the leg of the side affected becomes swollen with fluid like the swelling of a thrombosed deep vein. Limbs like these are then heavier and more clumsy, and less able to bend – just at a time when the need is for them to be lighter and supple because they have less power than normal. We do not fully understand why this should happen, or how to get rid of the excess fluid.

Mental Barriers

Finally there are a number of mental barriers to progress in certain strokes. Sometimes it is *poor comprehension* which may be mixed up with aphasia; the patient can perform actions which are shown to him, but does not fully understand when instructions are given by word of mouth. Other patients have such short memories that they forget one day's lesson by the next. Far more difficult to understand are the cases where the patient is not aware of his body as the rest of us are. This is known as *disturbance of body image* (see Fig. 10). He may entirely neglect the one half of his body; even if asked to draw a clock face he would leave out half the numbers! A fairly common difficulty, especially seen in cases of left hemiplegia or hemiparesis is *sensory inattention* on the same side of the body. One tests for it as follows: the patient has her eyes closed, and first one touches one hand or leg while she identifies which side. Then one touches the opposite side, and again the patient is able to identify which side, always provided there is not any anaesthesia (see page 123). However, when she is touched on both sides simultaneously she will be found to identify the touch as being on one side only (usually the right), the other being ignored completely. Patients with this strange disability are especially difficult to rehabilitate, because they are just not able to concentrate enough attention on improving the activity of the affected side.

In some cases the patient absolutely denies there is anything wrong with the paralysed side when everybody else can see that it is paralysed. This is not a pose; it is some kind of thought disturbance and is part of the stroke illness. Sometimes too there is a state called apraxia where the patient has the power to move certain muscles, but no power to make them do particular actions. Thus, if you ask him to put out his tongue to order he cannot; yet you see him lick his lips a few moments later! This kind of thing is common, and it must never be assumed that a stroke patient is "playing up". Some patients once they have started a movement go on repeating it even when given a different instruction; this, as it is with repetition of speech, is known as *perseveration*. Then there is the patient whose reaction to a stroke is one of total despair, frustration and rage that this should have befallen him. It results sometimes in total unwillingness in every respect.

It must be plain from all these possible impediments that stroke rehabilitation is often a slow, difficult process which takes a good deal out of the staff and a good deal out of the patients too. When one of them does not react as well as expected, it must not be a matter of scolding him but of getting medical advice about the impediments to his progress.

PARKINSONISM

Next to arthritis and strokes, Parkinsonism probably poses more problems of moving about than any other disease of the locomotor system. This disease takes its name from Dr James Parkinson who first described it in London in 1817. He called it then "the shaking palsy", having noted its two main characteristics.

There are now thought to be three main types, one due to encephalitis lethargica (sleeping sickness) earlier in life, another to cerebral atherosis, and a third type for which we know no real cause as yet. It is not helpful to describe them separately now. A few mild cases develop after taking certain drugs like chlorpromazine (Largactil) but the symptoms disappear if the drug is stopped.

Parkinsonism is a malady, then, of later life. The disease is a disturbance – perhaps a chemical disturbance – in the basal ganglia deep in the brain between the cerebral hemispheres. The characteristics are a tremor coupled with rigidity, but some cases have more of one, and some more of the other. Typically the tremor begins to affect one hand with repeated movements as if the patient were "rolling pills", the fingers oscillating rhythmically at three to five movements a second. It may affect the whole hand, or arm, or the leg of the same side, or the opposite arm and leg, and can in the worst cases affect the head, tongue and lips. Often the patient dribbles saliva from half closed lips. Trying to move the limbs affected gives a curious noiseless clicking sensation, and the muscles seem rigid and hard to move. This is in fact called "cog-wheel rigidity"; it is the rigidity which impedes the patient's activities, but it is often the tremor which she dislikes most because it is so conspicuous. With the rigidity goes some muscular weakness, and difficulty with fine movements. Often the face is unmoving, expressionless, looking like a dismal mask, the voice becomes small and monotonous, so no play of emotion is seen. If the patient can walk, her steps are tiny and fast as if she is leaning forward with her feet trying to keep up with her body, arms bent across

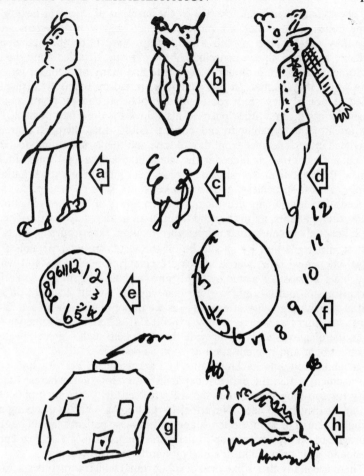

Fig. 10 Drawings done by patients with strokes.
    (After Isaacs, B., (1971), Modern Geriatrics Vol 1, pp. 398–400)
      Request: "Draw a man"
(a) Patient with minimal brain damage
(b) Patient with right hemiplegia and aphasia
(c) Patient with severe brain damage
(d) Patient with left hemiplegia and neglect of the left half of space.
    Request: "Draw a clock"
(e) Minimal brain damage
(f) Left hemiplegia: note "escape" and reversal of figures.
    Request: "Draw a house"
(g) Minimal brain damage
(h) Left hemiplegia with visual agnosia (the patient could not understand the parts
    were incorrectly related).

her chest, and head bent forward in the position of "general flexion". Some patients, once they are moving, literally run with tiny steps and they may not be able to stop without help. Very often the patient is perfectly alert and all too conscious of the pathetic, disabled state she is in. Some patients are profoundly depressed and many of them get into a state where they cannot get any activities started by themselves (this is called akinesia); they seem rooted to the spot, but can get going again once they are given a little "push". This akinesia is the worst obstacle to our attempts to rehabilitate the patient. Often, too, there is a great difference in performance from day to day, and this is something outside the patient's control, as indeed is the whole illness. The final state of advanced Parkinsonism is very sad: a rigid, bent individual with agitating tremor, almost speechless, and with flexed limbs with contractures, and in need of every nursing attention, yet often aware of her own affliction. Many such patients, naturally, find themselves in long-stay wards of geriatric hospitals because their proper care requires expert nursing skills.

It is important that we should be on the watch in older patients for those who move little, whose voices are colourless and slow, and who may have a ghost of a tremor from time to time. This might be early Parkinsonism, and it might well explain why the patient does not do so well in regaining activity after illness as we might hope, or why she fails to run her house as we might have expected. It is helpful for someone to make the diagnosis early, to provide the extra help such a person needs, and treatment and rehabilitation as soon as possible.

Rehabilitation has its limitations in Parkinsonism: activity and encouragement within the patient's capability are important, whereas inactivity for too long means that she will get "set fast". Yet such patients cannot be driven too hard. Nevertheless the tremor is not as disabling as it might seem. The author often suggests that these patients should be encouraged to do the washing up in the ward kitchen; this gives them confidence in their own abilities, and they hardly ever drop a plate!

There are many drugs like benzhexol (Artane) which sometimes help a little; the very number of the drugs used suggests how relatively ineffective they were. In the author's experience benzhexol is an unsuitable drug for most older patients for it is not very effective though it often makes the patients confused. Of these many older drugs, orphenadrine (Disipal) is perhaps safer than most. Some twenty years ago a surgical operation on the affected brain centres by elaborate techniques to destroy an overactive area by means of an electric coagulating current or a small alcohol injection helped a great many patients, especially those with pronounced tremor. These operations have been performed too in some fairly old patients in their seventies with good results, though they did not always control the disease for very long.

In the last ten years or so we have seen the arrival of two new types of drugs, amantidine and levodopa (L-Dopa). These have greatly changed the outlook for Parkinsonian patients and some almost miraculous cures have taken place – provided the patient continues with the drug. Unfortunately these drugs, especially L-Dopa, have many unpleasant or dangerous side effects such as vomiting, twitching and fall of blood pressure, and they are not often proving miraculous in the cases of very elderly patients. Levodopa is one and carbidopa is the other constituent of the compound drug Sinemet, now widely used. The combination appears to be more effective and usually less liable to unwanted side-effects than levodopa by itself. A newer – and most expensive – drug bromocriptine, has lately emerged, but its special advantages (if any) are still being assessed. Pharmacologists seem still to have a long way to go, unfortunately, before producing the ideal drug for this distressing disease. Yet the cause is biochemical, and success should be within our grasp. The story of a case of Parkinsonism so far is often also the story of drugs causing as many problems as they solve; whereas the illness is still, in geriatric work, a major problem of how to keep a sensible, often very willing, but very immobile patient "on the move". The underlying rigidity and akinesia are the stumbling blocks. It must be said, too, that some older Parkinsonian sufferers develop a characteristic rigidity of outlook and gradual mental deterioration, and are not the easiest of patients to nurse and treat. It is dangerous to stop drug treatment of this disease abruptly, because patients go into coma. Drugs can and should be reduced gradually.

Chapter 10

THE BLOOD, KIDNEYS AND ENDOCRINE GLANDS

Age does not have much effect on the tissue which forms blood and which has to go on replacing it so regularly throughout life because the cells deteriorate and break up. Red blood cells themselves have a life of only two to four weeks. The active, red bone marrow which produces them extends down the length of many bones in young children, but it later retreats from the long bones into the bones of the chest and vertebrae, and perhaps the very tips of the long bones in adult life, and there it continues its work. Under the microscope the blood of old people looks the same as young blood. Anaemia is not a feature of old age as such; yet in spite of this fact, anaemia is often found in older people. When found, it needs to be treated. Indeed, anaemia is one good indication of ill health waiting to be discovered. The normal haemoglobin level is always lower for women than men, at all ages. Normal levels even in old age can be taken as 13.5 to 14.2 gms per 100 ml for men, and 12.3 to 13.4 gms per 100 ml for women. Surveys of old people at home have shown that more than one in every twenty, perhaps even one in ten, has a haemoglobin level below those figures. There is much to be said, therefore, for regular routine blood testing of older people so that these signs could be detected earlier and disabling disease prevented.

ANAEMIA

For practical purposes anaemia can be said to be present in geriatric patients if the haemoglobin is less than 11.9 gms per 100 ml. Amongst those admitted to geriatric hospitals, who after all are usually not the most healthy of old people, up to 40% may be found with some degree of anaemia. Anaemia is often associated with infections; thus a long-standing kidney infection (pyelonephritis for example) may result in persistent anaemia, and an acute infection of any kind may suddenly cause the haemoglobin to drop by one or two grams per cent. To keep abreast of these changes blood counts need to be done more frequently in old invalids than young ones.

The effect of anaemia is to produce weakness, palpitations and breathlessness, but the last is often absent in people who are inactive (see page 40). There may be giddiness, particularly on standing up, and swelling of the ankles. The effect of anaemia may be to produce angina pectoris or congestive heart failure, or even mental confusion when it is very severe. The proof of the pudding is in the eating; if curing the anaemia cures these other symptoms, anaemia was the cause.

One looks for anaemia particularly in the skin of the face and the beds of the nails, but especially in the mucosal surfaces of the mouth and lower eyelids. Many mistakes can be made if one only looks at the skin of the face, for some people have only a small number of capillaries per square millimetre. They look anaemic though they may not be so. Others have many capillaries, or spend a good deal of time out of doors in all weathers and look ruddy-complexioned and therefore not anaemic – though they may in fact be so. Judging anaemia by these clinical means is never accurate, and the only reliable method is a blood count, in doing which all the special indices are calculated so that the type as well as the severity of the anaemia may be settled. Some anaemic patients have a yellowish tint to their skin, almost like jaundice; others have smooth tongues; other have ridged or spoon-shaped fingernails (koilonychia). In the investigations it may be necessary to look for bleeding in the motions (fresh or occult blood), test the acidity of the gastric juice, and perhaps take a sample of the marrow with a marrow biopsy needle. The latter is an unpleasant investigation to undergo, but even in old age it is sometimes unavoidable. It is never justifiable for a patient to be treated for anaemia without a full diagnosis of its cause. In some emergency cases treatment has to be started without the complete diagnosis, but at least the basic type of the anaemia should be known.

A severe anaemia found (or suspected) in a patient at home may be an indication of serious malnutrition, simply because people who eat too little, or not enough of the "protective" foods, may be very short of iron. Usually anaemia comes on quite slowly; there is so little change from day to day that the people who are always with the patient fail to appreciate the problem when it is quite obvious to the visiting stranger. Sometimes even in hospitals a severe anaemia is eventually detected in a long-stay patient, though, to their embarrassment, the staff failed to notice it gradually developing! Anaemia may appear so slowly that the victim becomes accustomed to its gradual effects and fails to report any symptoms. People like this may believe that it is "just old age creeping on". Only when specifically asked do they admit to weakness or breathlessness. The power of adaptability of the aged human being to a very low haemoglobin level is quite astonishing. Adaptation of this kind is not possible when the anaemia develops quickly, as it would with sudd bleeding. Then the patient may suddenly faint or pass rapidly into h failure. A point worthy of special mention is that old people who are severely anaemic are especially sensitive to sedative drugs and hypnotics in which case an otherwise normal dose could be lethal.

Modern methods of diagnosing anaemia (using "absolute" values as calculated from a full blood count) distinguish between those with red cells which are normal in diameter, and those which are too large, or too small; similarly, the cells may each contain a standard quantity of red pigment, too little, or too much. Thus in the common anaemia of iron deficiency, the usual picture is of red cells which are too small in size and each contains too little haemoglobin (microcytic, hypochromic anaemia). In Pernicious or Addisonian Anaemia the cells are variable in size, may be too large and are packed with excessive haemoglobin (anisocytosis, macrocytosis and hyperchromia).

CAUSES OF ANAEMIA IN OLD AGE

In the simplest terms the causes are (1) loss of blood, (2) failure to form sufficient normal red cells, (3) increased destruction of red cells. The latter, the so-called "haemolytic" anaemia, is too rare to concern us further.

Blood Loss
(a) *Rapid Loss*
Loss of blood may be sudden, as from a haemorrhage from the stomach or bowel, or even a severe nose bleed. The effects would be the well-known effects of any bleeding, though old people stand severe blood loss less well than other people. A transfusion may be needed, and quickly, but transfusions always carry the risk of cardiac complications because of the extra fluid added to the circulation. Without transfusion, and following upon it, the lost blood has to be made up by bone marrow activity, so iron and a good protein-rich diet will be needed.

(b) *Slow Loss*
This can arise from a large number of causes; a hiatus hernia or oesophagitis which bleeds (see page 71), chronic gastric or duodenal ulcer or gastric cancer, colitis, diverticulitis, or cancer of the large bowel, even haemorrhoids. At least female geriatric patients are not suffering from the anaemia of abnormal menstruation which is common in younger women.

Several investigators have suggested that old people bleed from the alimentary tract more easily than young people. Certainly if one looks carefully enough for hidden (occult) blood in the motions, one finds it often. Several groups of drugs are notorious for causing gastric bleeding, which may be slow and regular as long as the drugs are being taken.

They include aspirin and phenylbutazone (Butazolidin) and other drugs which are used in treating rheumatoid arthritis. With this disease there is a tendency to develop anaemia for other reasons as well. Anaemia from slow blood loss always requires extra iron to be provided (see below).

Failure to Form Normal Red Cells

The explanation of these various common anaemias is a deficiency of some vital substance or "building material" like iron or vitamins. Alternatively, there may be inefficient absorption of these building materials as might happen, for example, after a gastrectomy. Again, though the building materials are available, the marrow may be unable to put them to use.

(a) Iron Deficiency

Bleeding causes loss of red cells, and the iron they contain is lost also. It therefore leads to iron deficiency when the reserve stocks have been exhausted. Again, iron may be lacking from the diet. The reason is usually faulty dietary habits. To this extent this anaemia would be preventable if it were possible, from the economic and habit standpoints, to get an older patient to change her dietary ways. The main sources of iron are meat, especially kidney and liver, egg yolk, fruit and green vegetables. Cereals, bread and milk can in a complex way hinder the absorption of such iron as there is in the diet. Thus, we can easily see then why some old people have this dietary kind of anaemia!

The treatment of iron deficiency is, first, the treatment of its cause – bleeding or dietary faults. To restore the haemoglobin level iron itself is needed; this may mean taking iron tablets daily for many weeks or months, because only a small proportion of the iron can be absorbed through the wall of the gut. Ferrous sulphate is the cheapest drug, but other iron salts may be needed to avoid gastrointestinal upsets. Oral treatment sometimes fails. Then it is usual to try injections of iron-dextran complex either repeatedly into muscles (which causes brown staining) or intravenously in a dose carefully calculated to supply the deficiency and replace the reserves for the future. This so-called "total dose infusion" is gaining in popularity, because iron by mouth is so disappointing in its results, and older patients cannot be relied on to continue regular tablets three times a day for long enough. There was a suggestion that intramuscular iron might lead to cancer after a long interval, but for elderly patients this slight risk seems a reasonable one to take for dealing with a difficult therapeutic problem. In a few cases iron treatment does not seem to get under way with the anaemia until a preliminary blood transfusion has been given to set the patient off with a "flying start".

(b) *Pernicious Anaemia (Addisonian Anaemia)*

This type of anaemia was called "pernicious" because, before the discovery of its cause, it responded to nothing, and its effects were serious and eventually lethal – pernicious indeed! It is essentially a failure of the marrow to produce enough normal-sized and normal-shaped cells, because of a lack of Vitamin B_{12} or folic acid. In this case red cells start to be formed in the marrow but fail to mature; this gives the cells of the marrow of these patients a particular appearance under the microscope (hence it is called a "megaloblastic" anaemia). The cells which do reach the blood stream are unusually large (macrocytosis). It is a rare disease in young people but it is progressively more common the older one's patients are. The oldest patient of the author's who developed pernicious anaemia for the first time was ninety-six years old. Half the patients who develop this condition are over sixty at the time.

There is a number of complex factors which may be involved in anaemia of this type; thus it may appear sometimes after gastric operations, in the state of mal-absorption, in diverticulosis and other abnormalities of the gut, and because of taking certain drugs like Epanutin, certain barbiturates and nitrofurantoin – which many older patients are taking. The story is complex, but basically the Vitamin B_{12} which is usually available in the diet should combine with a substance normally found in the stomach wall (the "intrinsic factor") before it can be properly absorbed. In some older people, then, the stomach fails to produce the intrinsic factor and it happens also to be incapable of producing hydrochloric acid, which is a helpful factor in diagnosis. In the other forms of this type of anaemia failure of the absorption of the Vitamin B_{12} is usually the problem, even though the intrinsic factor is available.

The anaemia develops slowly and takes on a characteristic clinical pattern with a smooth glossy tongue and a yellowish skin tint. There may be mental changes too. Some patients develop tingling of their hands and feet as a preliminary to a form of paralysis known as "sub-acute combined degeneration", the spinal cord being affected (see Chapter 9). It may be for these symptoms, not the anaemia, that the patient first consults her doctor. At the time of making the diagnosis most patients have only two-fifths of the normal number of red blood cells, and some have only one-fifth. This indicates how insidious the anaemia is.

It is most important that the diagnosis is made accurately before treatment begins; cancer of the stomach, which also causes there to be no acid in the gastric juice, has to be ruled out. If treatment is started before the confirmation of the diagnosis it may be impossible to be sure, and the patient then may continue having injections for the rest of her life without anyone being certain they were really required.

The treatment of this kind of anaemia is injection of Vitamin B_{12} (Cytamen) at intervals, and never ceasing. For maintenance when the blood count has returned to normal, injections fortnightly or monthly are needed. The newer drug Vitamin B_{12} (Neocytamen) requires doses at only every two or three months; but using this newer drug means that the older patient will be seen less often, so there is less check on her general health. A number of elderly patients on treatment for pernicious anaemia do well at first and then get no further; this is because in the rush to make new cells they have used up their small iron stores and are now needing extra iron before they can fully recover.

Anaemia due to lack of folic acid is very like pernicious anaemia. It is occasionally a straightforward dietary deficiency, or is part of the picture of malabsorption.

Hypoplastic Anaemia

One much rarer form of anaemia is found in geriatric patients but is of special interest. The true cause is not known, but the bone marrow, in spite of having all the substances needed, is inactive and does not produce cells as quickly as it should. This is sometimes called "senile hypoplastic anaemia"; it can only be surely diagnosed after a bone marrow examination, and the only treatment is repeated blood transfusions at intervals, depending on the blood counts. No one likes giving regular blood transfusions indefinitely but this policy, expensive and unending as it is, is nevertheless justifiable in these cases to preserve reasonable health and happiness. (The same policy might *not* be justifiable if adopted to try to keep an elderly patient going who was known to be slowly losing blood because of an inoperable cancer.)

*   *   *

It has been hinted that blood transfusion is risky in old people because of the chance of overburdening the heart with the extra bulk of fluid. Nevertheless it has to be done sometimes. It is usual to transfuse "packed cells" prepared in the laboratory rather than whole blood, because of the smaller bulk; usually a dose of a diuretic drug is given at the same time to rid the body of the unwanted fluid, thus forestalling heart failure. Some doctors, seeing how bad the results are, believe it is never justifiable to transfuse a patient with pernicious anaemia. The author believes this rule must be broken sometimes in desperate cases.

OTHER BLOOD DISORDERS

Anaemia may be associated with infections like pneumonia or urinary infection, and with rheumatoid arthritis, as has been mentioned. There are other special forms too – like the anaemias of chronic renal disease, scurvy, protein deficiency, and subnormal thyroid activity (myxoedema). Whenever in geriatric work an anaemia does not respond as we expect it to, we should consider these other possibilities.

A condition in which too many blood cells are produced (*polycythaemia*) is common in old age, and the cause is not known though some patients have kidney diseases. The patient is noticeable for having a very red face and suffused eyes. It is important because there is a greater tendency for clotting – with all that implies at an age, when diseased blood vessels are so common – and it can be treated by X-ray therapy or a radio-active phosphorus injection.

Leukaemia is not only a disease of children and young adults. The two more chronic types – chronic myeloid and chronic lymphatic leukaemia are not so rare in older people. They usually take a slow course, needing drug treatment and occasional transfusions of blood over a period. Lymph glands are enlarged and can be felt – this is unusual in old age, except in this kind of disease or secondary to cancer. Certainly, lymph gland enlargement is unusual in infections. Very rapid gland enlargement can be seen in some rarer tumours of the lymph glands themselves.

Multiple myelomatosis is a disease of middle and old age; it is common, but no treatment is effective and it is unfortunately slowly lethal. Deposits of special "myeloma" cells are found in the bone marrow and in many other places, and there may be pain in the affected bones.

KIDNEY AND BLADDER DISEASES

In Chapter 2 the changes which take place in the kidneys with age were briefly described. Steady loss of function year by year takes place without any external signs appearing. The tendency is shown by the fact that the urine cannot be concentrated as well as it can in young people. The detailed determination of kidney function is a very precise scientific exercise; for the present purposes we need consider only the simpler, practical points.

Normally the kidneys produce most urine by day, and almost "close down" at night. In certain old people the process becomes reversed – which might help to explain the excessive incontinence of some of them at night! Normally the first morning specimen is the most concentrated. If the specific gravity (S.G.) of this specimen is above, say, 1015, then for an old person we would say the kidney power is reasonable. If the S. G. never rises above, say, 1009 to 1012, then severe kidney disease is quite probable. This is a very important consideration indeed, when as the result of an estimation of the blood urea level, there is talk of *uraemia*. The upper limit for the blood urea (i.e. the level of blood waste nitrogen products) is 9.9 mmol/litre (equal to 60 mg per 100 ml) in later life, which is half as high again as would be allowable in youngle. The two most usual causes of a high blood urea are (a) kidney disease, and (b) lack of fluid (dehydration). The latter is treatable just by giving the requisite fluid; the former may be very difficult to overcome. So a specific gravity figure of 1009 to 1012 suggests kidney disease itself, especially if it is combined with a high blood urea reading, but a higher S.G. figure suggests some form of cause is responsible outside the kidney. Such causes should be deprivation of fluid, diarrhoea, vomiting, a heart attack, traumatic shock or burns.

CHRONIC KIDNEY FAILURE

This is a serious condition at best, but in an old person it is even more grave, especially since the elaborate modern treatments of organ transplants, artificial kidneys peritoneal dialysis, etc. can so seldom be offered to them for economic and practical reasons. The possible causes of kidney failure are many: any kind of long-standing kidney disease itself, including nephritis from earlier disease, the effect of kidney stones, some cases of gout and high blood pressure, myelomatosis (see above), back-pressure from bladder diseases including cancer, and from prostatic disease. The patient passes large quantities of very pale, dilute urine and still cannot excrete all the waste products; this eventually gives rise to symptoms such as hiccup, diarrhoea and vomiting, itching, twitching, pallor of an earthy colour, deep sighing breathing and finally coma. In young people there is always high blood pressure, and albumen is found in the urine; in old age this may not be the case. It is a most distressing end, but not so very often seen in geriatric work. In the nature of things most people with chronic renal failure do not live to be old. At this stage of uraemia the best anyone can do is to give the patient plenty of fluid and alkalis, treat any urinary infection, and treat the immediate symptoms. Truly uraemic patients who are old will not survive for long. Nursing these patients in the terminal stages is difficult and distressing work, because the symptoms, particularly the hiccup and vomiting, are so hard to relieve; a stomach wash may be helpful; towards the end heavy sedation may be the only possible course.

Unhappy experiences have taught the author the inadvisability of drastically cutting down the quantity of protein in the diet of elderly patients with uraemia. In younger people this is the standard treatment, but in the elderly it may cause the sudden appearance of huge pressure sores, and the patient is far worse off than she would be on a normal diet.

BLOOD IN THE URINE

Blood appearing in the urine (haematuria) – an alarming happening at any time – can be the result of any disease of the kidneys, bladder, prostate gland or any other part of the tract, or even because of some blood diseases. Stones and cancers are common enough in the bladder or kidneys. From the practical standpoint the commonest causes are either a very severe infection of the bladder (haemorrhagic cystitis), bladder cancer or trauma from a catheter. Finding the cause of haematuria is a precise technique, but it requires the use of a cystoscope and usually an anaesthetic, so such an investigation of the kidney tract is not often taken so far in a frail old person. Bleeding due to infection quickly subsides when the infection is treated.

INFECTION OF THE URINARY TRACT

Invasion of the urinary tract by bacteria is one of the most common misfortunes of older people. For anatomical reasons it seems to be more a scourge of women than of men. Over 50% of the patients in long-stay geriatric wards may have infected urine. Some researchers have found the risk is even higher than that. Infection tends to recur time and time again. Personal hygiene may be involved in its cause, but by no means is this always so. The patient's mental state is obviously very important here. People who drink very little are probably more liable to have an infection than those who drink well, and women seem to be the worse offenders when it comes to not drinking much.

Incontinence is more often the cause of infection than the result of it, and faecal incontinence is particularly to blame. Catheterization is also a well-known cause, though modern plastic catheters have a better reputation than the older rubber or gum-elastic catheters in this respect. Infections pass up the urethra and become established in the bladder. Apart from symptoms of frequency, and urgency, and pain in passing urine, which are all highly suggestive, proper proof is needed from a laboratory culture of a *clean* urine specimen which has been examined and cultured as soon as taken. It should not be necessary in most cases to take a catheter specimen, though the Alexa bag system is efficient and easy. A few bacteria or a few pus cells mean very little, but many pus cells or a large bacterial count (more than 100,000 per ml) spell out infection, and the sensitivity of the bacteria to various antibiotics must be discovered for treatment to be properly prescribed.

Bladder infection (cystitis) is what most of us mean when we talk of a urinary infection. It happens particularly if the bladder cannot be fully emptied or has pouches (diverticula). Stagnation of urine is the thing to avoid, and drinking plenty undoubtedly helps to avoid this. Sometimes there are no symptoms or infection; sometimes the urine looks normal but cultures positively; sometimes it looks and smells like pure pus, and sometimes there is blood in it (see above).

When chronic recurrent cystitis has developed it may cause the bladder wall to go into spasms and thicken and contract, so that eventually it will only hold 50–100 ml of urine; then the patient has great frequency, passing urine perhaps every thirty minutes, accompanied by much pain. We now know, though it is a fairly recent discovery, that repeated bladder infections permit bacteria to travel back up the ureters and infect the kidneys (see below). Treatment, apart from insisting on plenty of fluids, consists of using one of the many urinary antiseptic drugs like sulphonamides, nitrofurantoin (Furadantin), hexamine mandalate (Mandelamine), nalidixic acid (Negram) or antibiotics. Each course has to be short and sharp, or the bacteria will become insensitive. Bladder washing with a mild antiseptic solution has to be done if there is much pus and debris, and it should relieve the patient's pain and urgency.

Kidney infection (pyelonephritis) is very often caused, as has been said, by bacteria passing up the ureter from the bladder. When the infection is acute, at any age, there is fever, pain in the loins and perhaps a rigor – it is one of the few causes of a rigor in old age. The chronic state is exceedingly common, and may be found at post-mortem examination when it was in no way suspected. Clearly it is quite a frequent cause of death, and for this reason particularly it must be detected early and treated. So must the bladder infections which are so often to blame. Yet it is not easy to be sure of the presence of chronic pyelonephritis; one cannot even be sure of finding an infected urine specimen at any one moment. The illness itself can be very vague, with a little pain and fever, or none at all. When patients finally show kidney failure with no warning in old age this is very likely to be the cause. The treatment is as it is for any urinary infection, but long courses of drugs may be needed, changing the drugs frequently in the hope that the bacteria will not become insensitive to all drugs. A kidney affected singly might have to be removed to avoid other complications. Loss of one kidney in an old person is not necessarily a total disaster; if the other is healthy there may be enough kidney capability left for life to go on quite well.

Occasionally a kidney which has an obstruction to its outlet is distended like a useless, sealed off bag of fluid (hydronephrosis), or of pus (pyonephrosis) if it was infected. The latter is one of the causes of severe "hidden" infection from which old people can die.

RETENTION OF URINE

All nurses know how often this occurs in older people, and how seldom the patients themselves complain of any pain or discomfort which would draw attention to the condition. The only answer is to acquire the habit of putting a warm hand on the lower abdomen of patients very frequently as they lie in bed, just to be sure there is no tell-tale cystic swelling rising out of the pelvis. In the hospital ward this avoids the embarrassment of the doctor discovering it first! There are a great many possible causes, including prostatic disease, the use of diuretics in men, a pelvic tumour or a long-forgotten pessary in women, and dementia and gross faecal impaction in either sex. In unconscious or paraplegic patients and those who have lately had strokes or are recovering from recent operations, it is a particular hazard. Seeing evidence of urinary incontinence on the clothes or bedding is no proof that the urine can flow freely, for retention-with-overflow can occur, especially with men. Then the bladder remains distended, the pressure within forces a little urine incontinently out, but the bladder remains overfull. In this kind of retention the bladder need not be tender when pressed on. Nevertheless it is a serious state requiring hospital treatment.

Removable causes like impacted faeces must be got rid of first. Next there are the time-honoured "tricks" of helping the patient to stand up and pass urine, or setting the taps running as a psychological inducement. An injection of carbachol is sometimes used especially if the patient is a woman and is not too frail or ill. Usually, however, catheterization with the usual strict aseptic precautions has to be used, and if there is any risk of recurrence the catheter, a self-retaining type, can be left in place a few hours or days, after which a trial without it is made. Some patients who are old and "bad surgical risks" – very old men with prostatic disease for example – may have to "lead the catheter life" permanently when repeated attacks of retention show that they need it. Provided one can be certain that the retention has only been present a few hours, all the urine can be released at once from a distended bladder; but if it might have been present for a long time, gradual "decompression", 100 to 200 ml at a time, is necessary to avoid serious complications like haemorrhage.

DISEASE OF THE PROSTATE GLAND

It is so often the case that old men have prostatic trouble that it counts as one of the facts of life. At the start they experience a little difficulty with the act of passing water, which is slow to start and uncomfortable, and the flow is small. Even so, many men do not report their symptoms; perhaps they think it is "just natural", as so many of their friends are likewise troubled. Unrelieved prostatic disease leads to incomplete emptying of the bladder, to infection, and to the risk of back-pressure on, and even infection of, the kidneys.

Benign Prostatic Enlargement

Most cases of prostatic disease are benign; we do not know why the gland becomes so large in the base of the bladder; even this might not cause trouble but for the fact that the urethra passes through the gland

and the channel is made narrower, so that it might even be obstructed. Besides the usual symptoms of a delayed and reduced flow of urine, there may be haematuria or true "dribbling" incontinence, with retention or retention-with-overflow as the ultimate difficulty to be expected.

The treatment of this disorder is surgical; it is certainly possible to perform a prostatectomy with reasonable safety in very old men who are otherwise fit. Many such operations have been successfully carried out in men in their nineties. The question is whether or not the patient is likely to become continent afterwards, because an operation is little help otherwise; in deciding this question a good deal depends on his having a "go-ahead" outlook and clear mental processes. Many old men do not have operations, and therefore have to have permanent self-retaining catheters and leg-bag urinals, etc., or have to remain in hospital indefinitely because they get into such an unhygienic muddle if they are on their own, or because they only have female relations to help them – for this is more than the latter can stomach. For the same sorts of reason, patients of this kind are not very welcome in Residential Homes. Matters are all the worse when mental confusion complicates the picture.

Malignant Prostatic Disease

This is the most common form of cancer in elderly men. It is often present in very old men without producing any significant symptoms, and men may live as long as ten years from the first date of the diagnosis being made, with steady but slow deterioration. The growth is usually confined to the gland itself for the first two or three years, perhaps causing difficulty in passing urine, but very often not. It may then extend to the bladder itself or the nearby organs in the pelvis. More commonly perhaps, secondary spread takes place to the bones, or to the liver, lungs or bone marrow. In the latter it gives rise to anaemia as the blood-forming tissue is displaced. Secondary deposits in the bones, mostly the spine and pelvic bones, cause pain, especially in the back and legs, and the old person gradually – very gradually indeed in some cases – becomes weaker, thinner and paler.

This form of cancer can be held relatively at bay for months or years by hormone therapy; that is, by giving large doses of oestrogenic female sex hormones like stilboestrol or chlorotrianisene (TACE).

ENDOCRINE DISEASES

The ductless (endocrine) glands, or glands of internal secretion, were once thought to be the key to the ageing process. People, knowing in particular that the pituitary gland is reckoned to be the "leader of the endocrine orchestra", took the view that ageing was a matter of pituitary failure. Certainly in very rare cases pituitary failure makes a patient look prematurely old, but there is much more to the matter than that. There is no justification for giving glandular extracts indiscriminately to try to ward off old age, and "rejuvenation" experiments with gonadal extracts have all been failures. Giving extract of thyroid for example, "just in case it might be deficient" would be a dangerous practice. Anyway, giving a gland extract often has the affect of reducing the gland's own output.

Relative under-activity, or in one case over-activity, of these glands nevertheless causes a number of characteristic states of disease which have special features when they affect older people. Most of these are treatable diseases. There are tumours of endocrine glands which produce certain strange and dramatic effects, but these do not appear in geriatric patients often enough to require special description here.

FAILURE OF THE ADRENAL CORTEX

This disorder (otherwise known as Addison's Disease) can be caused by tuberculous disease in both glands or by cancerous deposits in both. The latter is the more likely cause now, but the condition really is not common in old age. The picture is of a patient with a deeply pigmented skin and mouth lining, with very low blood pressure, and with a disturbance of blood salt chemistry. However a very brown-coloured skin and low blood pressure are common anyway in old people, so this disease is more often suspected than finally confirmed. Both adrenal glands have sometimes been removed surgically as a delaying treatment in carcinoma of the breast (particularly), when secondary deposits have already occurred. After that is done corticosteroids then have to be given for the rest of the patient's life.

OVERACTIVITY OF THE THYROID GLAND

This disease, hyperthyroidism (or thyrotoxicosis), shows itself in younger patients by the well-known signs of a goitre, staring eyes (exophthalmos), and signs of general body overactivity, with rapid movements, high pulse rate, fine tremor, persistent diarrhoea sometimes, good appetite but loss of weight, or a generally excitable or nervous temperament. All this happens, too, in some older patients, but quite often the disease is hidden; so there may be no noticeable goitre and the eyes look normal; yet the pulse may be rapid and irregular with atrial fibrillation (see page 88) or unexplained heart failure, and these may in fact be the main or even the only signs whatever of thyroid disease. Other older patients are strangely depressed, frustrated or apathetic – and are usually thin and ill-looking too. On a cool night, with a patient who has no fever or heart failure and is sleeping, the pulse rate should be below eighty; if it is above, the thyroid might be overactive and needing appropriate treatment. The detection of thyroid overactivity is not easy because many other geriatric patients are thin, somewhat nervous and agitated, and have tremors – though the tremor is not usually the fine finger and hand tremor of the thyrotoxic type. The particular importance of detecting the disease early is that further cardiac damage and heart failure could be forestalled. Provided it is suspected, making this diagnosis is a fairly accurate matter, involving complex methods measuring the excretion or thyroid gland absorption of radio-active iodine compounds or more recently by estimation of the thyroxine (T_4) or tri-iodothyronine (T_3) in the blood. Treatment is by an antithyroid drug like carbimazole (Neomercazole) or a therapeutic dose of radio-iodine (I^{131}). Surgery was much used, but is seldom suggested now for elderly patients.

UNDERACTIVITY OF THE THYROID GLAND

This is a common ailment of older people, and some of its clinical signs do closely suggest signs of the ageing process itself – the loss of hair, slowness in movement and speech, and thickening of the features. However there are differences. This disease (hypothyroidism) is usually a malady of later life; its cause is uncertain as yet and it may be related to several different disorders. Failure of the gland is not just simple "wearing out", nor is it an effect of the ageing process itself. We discover sometimes that a patient has the neck scar of an operation earlier in life, so this would be a case of overactivity of the gland rather too energetically treated, which resulted in underactivity later in life.

The hypothyroid patient slows up, that is, moves slowly, thinks slowly and talks slowly, and may even go into coma or into a highly dangerous state with low temperature though this is one of the less common causes of hypothermia (see page 59). Particularly in the elderly the voice changes: it is slow, very deep, the words are hard to decipher, and it is, as some say, "clotted" in the way it is produced. This is a particularly telling sign in old people. So is the texture of the skin, which has deposits in it under layers (myxoedema) giving an extra fullness and puffiness round the eyes with a characteristic look. The pulse is usually slow, and the heart may go into failure and will not recover with the usual treatment until the thyroid deficiency is also treated. The patient meanwhile is lethargic, dislikes cold, gains weight, has leg cramps, notices increasing constipation and sweats very little. Anaemia may develop too. It is as if the clock was running down.

This illness is so slow in coming on that, like a slowly developing anaemia, the people near the patient do not notice the subtle changes, but a stranger sees at once that there is something wrong. Some research workers believe that it takes three to five years for hypothyroidism to develop fully. Meanwhile such a patient is usually pleasant and easy-going and all her friends tolerate her slowness, and just think she is growing old rather faster than she might. Once again, electro-cardiographic changes are typical, and laboratory investigations are complex but give fairly precise answers. There could hardly be a more important diagnosis to make, since an under-active thyroid changes the whole way of life and activity of the patient, whereas treatment restores it all to normal.

Treatment used to consist of giving thyroid extract itself. This was slow to start its action, taking at least two weeks to give noticeable effects. A more modern drug, successful for old people, is thyroxine, which acts more quickly, but not too quickly. Many people believe a period of hospital care is needed for elderly patients with this disease, because in starting treatment the state of the heart is usually precarious, and overdosage with thyroid drugs could do harm.

Hypothyroid patients are very sensitive to some drugs like sedatives and morphine; the risk of hypothermia in cold weather is always present; the patients are rather liable to arterial diseases, and if they do not continue taking their treatment indefinitely they will surely relapse. This means that this insidious disease must be taken seriously, and patients under treatment must be seen by a doctor or nurse or health visitor regularly.

DIABETES

Diabetes mellitus in old age poses us some pretty problems. It is common, and will become more common as the population grows steadily older. It is not necessarily so serious a matter in itself as younger people's diabetes is, but its complications are many, serious and insidious; it is not easy to treat if (as so often happens) the elderly sufferer cannot be bothered with dieting carefully, does not care for injections, or is forgetful about the tablets which she might have to take regularly as an alternative, and cannot check the treatment by testing her own urine.

Artery disease, that is, an increased risk of the usual kinds of degenerative arterial disease, is the complication most to be feared. In old age this seems to be more the disease than the complication! The question of how much diabetes exists in the community and how much it could be detected will be discussed in Chapter 14. The cause of the condition is a change in the islet cells of the pancreas, so that insufficient insulin is available, the blood sugar level is usually above normal, sugar appears in the urine, and other biochemical faults become apparent, which lead to the state of ketosis. This short book is not the place for a discussion of the underlying cause. Two simple facts can be mentioned nevertheless. First there is a strong family tendency in diabetes; secondly, obesity is a factor in its causation, for indeed half the elderly sufferers are overweight; their insensitivity to insulin will correct itself again if they can lose weight; but if they cannot they have a very much higher mortality rate than thin diabetics.

In young people it is well known that diabetes starts with thirst, loss of weight, and frequent passing of urine. So it can be with the diabetes of old age; but very often the patients have no symptoms at all, or they come on so slowly that they are hardly noticed. Often the first signs of diabetes are detected at a routine urine examination. If all patients attending afresh at clinics and surgeries routinely had a urine examination, we should detect many more early cases and perhaps be able to prevent many complications. Special symptoms to note and inquire about are irritation of the skin, anus or vulva, cramp, and loss of vision.

Besides the arterial disease which has already been mentioned and which so often leads to coronary thrombosis or ischaemic heart disease, strokes, or gangrene of the feet, there are other troubles, namely, neuritis (neuropathy), kidney disease, changes in the retina (diabetic retinitis) and cataracts. The latter are theoretically speaking no different from other or "senile" cataracts, but in diabetes they come on earlier and much more commonly than they otherwise would. The well-known complication of diabetic coma is much rarer in older people, when all the difficulties of control are considered, but severe diabetics who contract an infection are always at risk. Hypoglycaemic reactions certainly do take place in older patients from too energetic treatment or (more often) from the patient's failure to eat enough to "cover" the treatment she has had. In older people this is a special hazard because patients in the midst of these "reactions" quite commonly develop strokes or cardiac infarctions. This risk is so real that most geriatric physicians prefer not to control treatment too rigorously, preferring to let their older patients show a little sugar in their urine rather than having it always sugar-free. Control is made all the more difficult because many older people have a high "threshold" for sugar passing into the urine; that is, such patients show no sugar in the urine though they may have excess sugar in the blood – which is what really counts. In the standard test (glucose tolerance test) fairly strict limits of what is normal or not can be set for young patients; when older people are under investigation the standards have to be relaxed, otherwise nearly all of them might be classified as diabetics – which would not be realistic. However, any random blood sugar test over the level of about 11.0 mmol/l is highly suspicious even in older people (though some have higher peaks than this), but usually the blood sugar level quickly falls to normal again.

The treatment of diabetes was made much easier when various new forms of insulin appeared, and since tablets of various controlling drugs were found to be effective by mouth. In the matter of diet there are always difficulties for old people. Apart from the domestic problems they have to face diet-wise, most of them do not understand Calorie values or the composition of various foodstuffs, and carefully weighing a diet would be quite out of the question. Many of them cannot see the need for strictness of diet in a disease which, at first anyway, has so few symptoms. Few people, least of all the elderly, will willingly restrict themselves for the sake of the good it might do them later on! Fortunately we can afford to let old people be a little more free in what they eat than younger ones who have a more "brittle" diabetes. Anyway if we did not allow more freedom they would take the liberty themselves! It is best to demonstrate a series of correct-sized meals and then try to insist the patient specifically avoids certain carbohydrates like sweets, sweetened drinks, biscuits, cakes and puddings.

It really is essential that obese diabetic patients should reduce weight, and the aim might then be a diet of 1,000 calories a day, or less, with 80 gms of carbohydrate. For people of normal weight, leading sedentary lives, a diet of 1,200 calories with 100 gms of carbohydrate should be sufficient, but those who are a little more active might need 1,400 calories with 140 gms of carbohydrate – and in each case the protein and fat would be adjusted to suit. These allowances ought to be apportioned sensibly through the day, but if twice-daily insulin was being used, particular care would be needed. About one-third of the cases of diabetes in old age can be controlled by diet alone, always assuming the patients' co-operation is sufficient.

These days, with the relatively mild diabetes of the elderly, and with so many alternative treatments available, soluble insulin is not often needed alone, except in the control of unstable states, or just prior to operations. If insulin is needed, a mixture of soluble insulin and protamine zinc insulin will suit some people, but many are better treated with one morning dose of insulin zinc suspension (lente insulin) – provided the patient does not need more than a total of about 40 units, and is not very obese.

In hospital there are no problems about insulin administration; nor should there be in Residential Homes if a member of the staff is a trained nurse. It does often present very great problems of management in private houses. Few old people manage to master insulin dosage and injection unsupervised, unless they have done so for years already. Some meanwhile have developed tremors, or arthritis of the hands, or paralysis, or loss of confidence, all of which might make this delicate but essential operation impossible for them to perform. When eyesight is bad – as it so often is from cataract or retinitis – they cannot see the numbers on the syringe or cannot be sure the syringe is not half full of air. Naturally, many elderly diabetics are helped in their treatment by their relatives.

Nevertheless some must rely on a regular morning injection from a Home Nurse. The problems of the poor nurse who has two or three rather helpless elderly diabetics at different places in a far-flung territory can be imagined.

The use of oral tablets of tolbutamide (Rastinon), chlorpropamide (Diabinese), phenformin (Dibotin) and the newer varieties has quite changed the picture for geriatric diabetes, for they have removed many – but not quite all – of the problems of using insulin itself. These oral agents are not suitable, of course, for dealing with diabetes complicated by infection, gangrene, gross obesity, pre-coma, before operations, or where there is liver or kidney disease as well. Tablets do not remove the need for reasonable care with the diet, and they can cause hypoglycaemic attacks if dietary care is not exercised; some of them cause skin rashes. As with all such treatment, especially where taking liberties leads so easily to serious complications, the patient's willingness to swallow tablets regularly, and the fact that she must have a good memory, are crucial. For a lonely, unstable diabetic, or a demented one, or one who just will not trouble to learn and abide by the simple rules, long-term hospital care may regrettably be the only solution. Notwithstanding, the management of elderly diabetes is not the problem it once was, and should not usually cause anxiety except in the situations mentioned above. We must continue to hope that good control of as many elderly diabetics as possible will help to reduce the fearful toll which the complications of diabetes still takes.

Older diabetics need regular supervision and urine testing. Attendance at diabetic clinics is the ideal system. There is every justification for running special clinics for them in small towns or in country geriatric hospitals which they can easily reach. They must all be expressly warned of the necessity of good foot care (see page 114), and of the folly of attempting to do their own chiropody or even cutting their own toenails. They must be made aware of what to do in the event of illness, and those on insulin or drugs must be warned of the need to take sugar promptly if a hypoglycaemic attack (a "reaction") threatens; and they must of course be told precisely what the early symptoms of such a reaction might be if they have never experienced one.

The warning symptoms include light-headedness, changes in eyesight sometimes, clamminess and sweating, and behaviour as if they are a little intoxicated.

OSTEOPOROSIS

This is an abnormality of ageing bones which can reasonably be discussed at this point even if it is not basically a disorder of the endocrine glands. It is so common in old age that it is usually called "senile" osteoporosis. This does not however explain its real cause; in fact the cause is still a matter for argument. The only fairly certain thing is that it is not just "old age". Some research workers claim it is due to insufficient protein substance in the bone structure; others more recently have believed that it is a dietary deficiency of calcium in people whose kidneys also happen not to be good at conserving the body's calcium; most recently it has been suggested that it is closely allied to osteomalacia, which is due to Vitamin D deficiency in the diet of older people (see Chapter 6). This type of deficiency was reported from Scotland, London and elsewhere. Perhaps there is an element of all three causes in the various cases of osteoporosis.

The main lines of treatment are (a) anabolic steroids, to build up bone structure; (b) a good diet with milk and bread, (c) extra calcium tablets; (d) Vitamin D. The use of these drugs reflects these various theories. Sometimes all three are given to one patient.

Once osteoporosis has developed, treatment has to go on for a very long time for the bones to approach their normal state again, and the X-rays may not show improvement after many months. The symptoms of osteoporosis are pain in the bones and bending of the back, so that the patient loses a good deal of her height. The disease is especially common in women; many of the sharply bent backs of old women have this as their cause. They seem suddenly to have been dwarfed by the bone disease, and characteristically have a deep crease across the upper abdomen as they sit in bed all hunched up. Pain may be due to some of the vertebrae having collapsed; this is compression fracture, the bodies of the vertebrae being like wedges instead of cylinders. Though painful this seldom leads to neurological complications.

The diagnosis is made by X-rays when the bones look "ghost-like", and thin, and they may have sustained fractures. This is because so much calcium has been lost over a very long period. We must also remember that osteoporosis also occurs in bones which are not able to do their normal job, because of a patient's long immobilization in bed, because of joint disease (especially rheumatoid arthritis), and in paralysis of muscles near the bones in question. Even more importantly, corticosteroid drugs given over a period cause a steady drain of calcium from the bones, so that osteoporosis occurs. One has seen such a patient have both her femurs fractured just by being gently lifted into bed by two careful nurses (and the feelings of the unfortunate nurses can be imagined). This is just one of the reasons why steroids have to be used very carefully and for restricted periods for geriatric patients; treatment as outlined above often relieves back pain dramatically, but that is only the start of the business. Many old people need special corsets or spinal supports to prevent further angulation of their backs, but some do not take kindly to this cumbersome gear and have to be constantly encouraged; or their expensive support might be found discarded and hanging in the coal-shed! It is a mistake, in spite of the risk of fractures, to forbid an old person with fragile osteoporotic bones to move about. Great care is certainly needed, but old bones will never strengthen and regain their calcium unless they are put to their proper use – the bearing of weight.

Chapter 11

MENTAL UNRELIABILITY

The mind changes as the man grows older. We have seen already in Chapter 2 that this mostly shows as a conservative outlook, a tendency to be pessimistic rather than the other way, to be rather turned inwards, bound by routines – sometimes necessary for keeping on the right domestic rails – and to be less able to absorb new notions and interests. Some slight loss of memory is fairly characteristic, especially loss of memory for recent happenings; but neither this nor any of the other tendencies are true in all cases; in this, as much as in any other things in ageing, individuals vary greatly. Even if peculiarities do appear, they need cause no one much distress. We shrug these things off as part of growing old; young and thoughtless people may poke fun at the absent-minded and the "square", and that is as far as it normally goes (but our turn will come soon enough!).

However, when symptoms of mental change become too prominent they cause more distress than almost any other symptoms. We are accustomed to think of our friends and relatives as distinct personalities with predictable behaviour, and any alteration of these patterns comes almost as more of a shock than a physical incapacity, which seems more understandable. Most sensitive, thinking people have a horror of "going out of their mind" and of becoming a burden to others because of it. Yet many people have a feeling that gradual mental failure is in some way inevitable in old age – one of its special penalties – which is not true. In reality it is not easy to draw a clear line between what is normal and what is abnormal in mental trends. Something abnormal may start to take place on top of a perfectly natural decline in speed and intellectual capacity. Then the normal shades imperceptibly into the abnormal. As well as this, we must take due account of eccentric behaviour in people who have always been that way inclined, and of the process whereby older people develop exaggerations of their earlier behaviour – like the careful, thrifty person who becomes a hoarder of everything imaginable. How far though is this mental disorder?

In a practical sense, the kind of behaviour which is abnormal enough to require special action may be determined by how much public opinion

162

will tolerate. Numbers of gently pixilated old people are kept going at home by tolerant friends and neighbours; but there are others, especially the more disagreeable ones, who overstep the mark. Then the neighbourhood, even the police sometimes, demand action from someone – and usually that "someone" has to be the doctor, the nurse or the social worker.

This chapter has the heading "mental unreliability" because it is time everyone moved away from the old idea that geriatric mental changes are always inevitable, irreversible and unmistakably due to brain disease. Sometimes – very often indeed – they are only evidence of other illness. The aged brain with no abnormality of its own is perhaps being starved of enough blood, or poisoned by bacterial toxins, and even by the drugs used in treatment of physical diseases. Unreliable the brain certainly is then, but it is not necessarily diseased.

There seems little doubt that the amount of mental abnormality in older people is increasing, but of course there are more and more of them, and the proportion of really old people grows steadily higher (see Chapter 1). For example, the total number of patients over 65 in mental hospitals in East Anglia went up between 1959 and 1969 from 1,635 to 1,827, despite the fact that the total number of in-patients of all ages in those hospitals fell by about 12%. The number of long-stay elderly patients in all mental hospitals is rising and causing special problems. Besides, large numbers of old people with some mental abnormality are being looked after in the long-stay wards of geriatric departments, while about 10% of the elderly who are being looked after at home have some degree of dementia (see below), and another 12% have other mental abnormalities like depression. This taken altogether amounts to a great load of care to be provided. If the friends and relatives of the ones at home refused to do their bit, with the help of domiciliary workers, the other services would be utterly overwhelmed.

It is sad to think that until recently such pessimism existed about mental disorders in old age that many doctors did not see the need to make a detailed diagnosis from the symptoms and classify the type of disease involved. All good treatment and all advances in knowledge follow on accurate understanding and classification of disease. In former days, then, the doctors' summing up of the patient was usually confined to words like "demented", "arteriosclerotic" or (worse still) "just senile".

SOME DESCRIPTIVE TERMS

In the process of discussing and reporting cases as between doctors and health and social workers generally, using correct terms is most helpful in conveying clear meanings.

The meanings of words like "*agitation*" and "*depression*" are clear to us all; so is *"aggression"*. Some of the others which are in common use to describe mental disorder are as follows: (a) *Delusion*: an idea in the mind which has no basis in fact ("they are trying to poison me", etc.); (b) *Hallucination*: an impression of something heard or seen or smelt which is not there in fact ("I hear voices talking to me . . ."; "I can see men under the bed", etc.); (c) *Retardation*: abnormally slow thought and speech; (d) *Mutism*: making no utterance, though capable of speech; (e) *Nihilism*: believing that nothing will come of anything, and bodily functions have all ceased working, etc.; (f) *Perseveration*: repeatedly doing or talking about the same thing; (g) *Confabulation*: telling untruths to cover up gaps in one's memory or understanding, hoping that will somehow satisfy the questioner (a classical example: Q. "Where are you now?" A. "Here!" or "In bed, of course!"; Q. "Which year is it?" A. "I never bother with that sort of thing!"); (h) *Disorientation*: failure to know where one is, or what the day, date and time is, or who one's nearest and dearest are. Disorientation can therefore be noted in place, in time or in personal relationships. There are many other technical terms, but these are some which are most often used.

Some other descriptions are less precise, but we nevertheless still use them. *Confusion* is one; this is a general state of muddle and disorientation, with mistaken ideas; it may mean a failure to manage simple things like handling cash. Confusion is a useful word (if not a scientific one) to describe the fact that an old patient is not able to reason clearly. This is very often the case when ill old people suddenly find themselves in strange surroundings like a hospital ward. Their basic personalities are often quite intact. Having used the word confusion, we can then by further observation of the patient's state describe things more accurately. The word confusion is often preceded by such telling adjectives as "pleasant", "gentle", "mild" or "agitated". It is certainly best to restrict the use of confusion to changes which have just lately taken place and which might not be permanent.

Dementia is more than confusion. It implies severe mental failure combining disorientation, intellectual losses – so that simple calculations, for example, are not possible – and eventually alterations in general behaviour, with destruction of the patient's normal personality (see below).

It is helpful to think of the common mental disorders in old people within a definite scheme or classification, even though two states can occur together and there are often some points of overlap. A simple classification is as follows:–

(a) Acute confusional states.
(b) Disorders of the emotions.
(c) Late paraphrenia.
(d) Organic psychoses (certain types of dementia).

Naturally there are other diseases not included, but they are rare, like syphilitic General Paralysis of the Insane, which is a state of dementia too.

This kind of disorder may not be acute in the sense of being very rapid and dramatic, but it is acute in the sense of being unexpected and related to some incident. Attacks like this have been called "toxic-infective confusional states", because these are two of the common reasons. When a patient who was yesterday and previously mentally normal, but today has become suddenly confused, this is a most valuable pointer to a physical illness – indeed, one of the most valuable and most common signs of all. It is much more common, for example, than a rise of body temperature. Perhaps the patient is deluded or hallucinated, has clouded consciousness, is restless or wakeful, even noisy and resisting people who want to help him; alternatively, perhaps he is quiet and bemused. Either way, the likelihood is that it is due to a chest or bladder infection, a boil, kidney failure (uraemia), heart failure, a painless heart attack, unstable diabetes, a stroke, or any other fresh illness; alternatively it might be due to drugs – some of the sleeping preparations like barbiturates (especially pentobarbitone – Nembutal), drugs to treat Parkinsonism, and many more besides. Other reasons might be anaesthetics, broken bones, even a full bladder or impacted faeces in the rectum. Almost any disease can cause a state of confusion in older patients. It is the link between the sudden change of mental performance and the use of the drugs, or the onset of the infective illness, for example, which is so unmistakable if one goes into cases fully enough. Naturally it is difficult to be sure of the facts if the patient is alone, and is found to be in this state but unable to give a proper account of what happened. In all mental upsets, the account given by those near to the patient is of the greatest importance. It is so often the Home Nurse or the Social Worker who is the only one in a position to get this information and note it down. It would be fair to say that almost any significant bodily disturbance is likely to cause confusion in certain old people. In the case of bacterial poisons, or drugs even when used in standard doses, the confusional state is not hard to explain, for it is an intoxication. In the case of other illnesses a change in metabolism or the distribution or availability of the blood might take nourishment to other organs which would have gone to the brain; cardiac infarction or strokes are particular cases in point, and they do indeed frequently cause bouts of confusion.

The combination of physical disease *plus* confusion is more serious than the same disease would be if the sufferer were clear in mind. A careful diagnosis *must* first be made and then the illness treated energetically. It could happen that the admission of the patient to the wrong place could prejudice his chances. Such cases usually need the full facilities of a general hospital with a laboratory. Active geriatric departments with good assessment wards are usually very willing to accept acute confusional states speedily – even as emergencies.

Patients who recover from the primary physical illness are likely to recover their mental balance also. Some do not do so because the brain damage (e.g. after a stroke) was too great, or because the illness had already started as a slowly progressive mental disorder which was brought out into the open by acute confusion at the start of a physical illness: this was the last straw, and they were left demented.

The risk of acute confusion should be a deterrent to families (and nurses too, sometimes) who always press the doctor for something to make the patient sleep or just to keep him quiet. It ought *not* to be a routine matter to prescribe sedatives and hypnotics for old patients just in case they might need them. Frequently, mentally disturbed patients are admitted to geriatric wards for investigation, yet they recover as soon as all their medication, especially their sedation, is stopped. In some cases of confusion sedatives are used to give everyone a little peace, but more confusion results, and even more sedatives are given for that. It turns into a vicious circle, especially if barbiturate drugs were chosen.

People usually do not all look kindly on confused patients. In particular those who work in acute medical and surgical wards find a noisy old person unwelcome, and so, understandably, do other patients who are trying to rest. But we for our part must understand that there is no wickedness in the confusion; the patient is ill, not aware of what trouble he is causing, and is most seriously in need of understanding, help and treatment. A single, quiet side ward is a help, but the patient must not just be left to his own devices. He needs reassurance and explanations repeatedly, and gently shaded lighting without long frightening shadows, people with sympathetic and familiar faces who have time to talk gently to him so he can reorientate himself. There really should be in every general hospital a small quiet "acute confusion" ward set aside for treatment of this common condition, staffed by experienced, calm nurses who take special pride in their skill.

It is strange that an old person who becomes muddled in an illness may get herself described as "a dreadfully confused old lady", whereas when referring to a bright young man who is ill with a high temperature people will say "poor fellow, he is delirious". The trouble is the same, but the feeling about it is rather different!

DISORDERS OF THE EMOTIONS

To talk of disorders of the emotions usually indicate that a patient is either quite unreasonably elated, ebullient, talkative and irrepressible, or that she is in the depths of depression. Some patients' moods swing quickly from one state to the other, though this tendency is much more common in younger adults. An excitable, over-active, talkative patient, flitting about, never sticking to the point, is so unlike most elderly people that such a patient is easily picked out as suffering from "*mania*" or "*hypomania*" (the latter being a less severe form, usually found in older people). At least such a person will enliven a group and will either stimulate or annoy everyone else.

DEPRESSION

Much the most common emotional disorder is depression. This depression is more profound than the usual minor pessimism of so many older people. It is an abnormal state requiring a speedy diagnosis and treatment. For this mental disorder treatment is certainly available: it is given either as electroconvulsion therapy (E.C.T.) or as antidepressant drugs, which are a recent innovation and extremely effective in many cases. E.C.T. is thought by some to be rather drastic for old people, even though there is no actual convulsion when present day techniques are used.

Apart from the upset caused to everyone near the patient by her misery, nihilism, and thankless attitude, and her apparent distress, depression carries a serious risk of suicide. Older, inactive geriatric patients might not carry out a threat of suicide, but younger old people can, and do. Some of them talk a great deal about the futility of going on living, without really meaning they wish to end it all. With depressed patients however this must not be taken as an empty threat and nurses and social workers need to be on the alert.

Sometimes depression is the natural outcome of bereavement, enforced retirement, loneliness, loss of status, or poverty. The first should pass with time; the others Society could prevent or alleviate. Most depression in old age, nevertheless, comes from within the patient, having no obvious external cause. Sometimes there is an earlier story of repeated attacks, or members of the family have had the same trouble. It may be a biochemical disorder. Both varieties can be helped by treatment.

The difficulty of separating true depression from the normal pessimistic state of old people has been discussed already. In addition we find that a number of geriatric patients with stroke-like illnesses are apt to weep and to look the very picture of misery, whatever is said to them, and however much one tries to help or comfort them. They burst into tears (or occasionally laughter – tears and laughter being very close). This is excessive emotionalism, and just part of that kind of illness; it probably has little to do with depression. Nevertheless, truly depressed patients do weep frequently, they complain of "fears" and sleeplessness, they have guilty feelings and delusions of being "ruined", they have poor appetites and are obsessed with their bodily functions, which they say do not work. Extreme hypochondriasis and neurotic obsession with illness is sometimes a mask for depression, or an early sign. In spite of all this, most depressed patients are well orientated and capable of normal mental attitudes otherwise, and they do try to keep up personal appearances. However, in advanced cases great apathy and slowness of thought and activity appear, and the patient just sits hopelessly mute, refusing to do her housework, to dress, to walk or even to eat. It is a pathetic state and the cause of immense frustration to everyone else. Yet if it is diagnosed wrongly as "senility" or "dementia" the chance of a cure will be missed. It seems likely that many cases do exist undetected in the community. Various surveys have suggested that from 8 to 30% of old people at home suffer from emotional disturbance, of which depression is the most common by far. This is a real challenge to detection, and a fruitful field for Health Visitors' work.

Severe cases of depression need treatment in mental hospitals, and it may be necessary to admit them there against their own inclination by using the Mental Health Act. It is useless to try to talk a depressive out of her symptoms by suggesting she should "pull herself together": she needs rest, encouragement, good food, occupational therapy and electroconvulsion therapy or drugs. In agitated depression some tranquillizer will be required like chlorpromazine (Largactil), promazine (Sparine), or one of the many others now available. The most recent advance is to find drugs which "lift" the patient's mood, like imipramine (Tofranil). There are many others of the same kind. These drugs can be given as syrups, which are often easier than tablets to administer to disturbed patients. Depressive states tend to recur, and patients need to be kept under regular review.

LATE PARAPHRENIA

This interesting but not very common mental illness is often looked on as a type of schizophrenia found in later life. In this group are found those strange patients who are shrewd and intelligent in most things but develop a compelling delusion or series of delusions, coupled sometimes with hallucinations. Deafness or blindness would have the effect of aggravating paraphrenia. These people believe they are being persecuted or "influenced" by rays or other unlikely things; they work out a whole tissue of improbable explanations for this and their own reactions to the belief. These are called "systematized" delusions, and the patients themselves are often paranoid and aggressive. Most of these unfortunate people shut themselves away, barricading their doors, blacking out their windows and discouraging callers. They are the "old witches"; their houses are the ones children hurry past; their neighbours (if they do not understand this is an illness) are mortally offended by their behaviour and by the insults they hurl from their doorways. Some are uneasily tolerated for years; some get into such a mess that action finally has to be taken, when the state of their houses almost beggars description. Unfortunately, treatment seems to have little effect on this disorder.

ORGANIC PSYCHOSES OF LATER LIFE

This group comprises the largest proportion of the true mental disease of older patients. These are the "dementing illnesses", progressive as a rule, and at present virtually incurable. They are unsatisfactory both because the numbers of patients are so large, and the domestic disruption they cause can be so great. The two main varieties are so-called "*senile*" *dementia* (psychosis), and *arteriosclerotic dementia* (psychosis). Some cases show features of both. They are not so very different in duration or final outcome. The "senile" type is slowly and steadily progressive. The other type is progressive but by steps, and the patient often, in the earliest stages anyway, is aware of his shortcomings and is determined to show himself at his best, especially while strangers (or a visiting specialist) are present, but becomes just as abnormal as ever an hour or so later. People who live with them know of these marked swings of behaviour and often are obliged to say to those of us who have called, "Well, you have only seen him on a good day!". Arteriosclerotic dementia is associated with artery disease and sometimes with high blood pressure; there are often tell-tale signs in the nervous system, such as those of an earlier mild stroke.

Dementia is a state of severe intellectual loss, coupled with personality change, leading to more and more abnormal behaviour. Of course a severe stroke could reduce a patient to dementia overnight from gross brain damage. In the present context however, dementia is almost always a slow process, taking weeks, months or years to develop. To start with, memory is lost, but patchily; the patient may mislay things and accuse others of stealing them, or go out and get lost in her own home town. There is increasing restlessness and disorientation, especially towards evening, poor sleep and a habit of getting up and dressing at all hours of the night. The patient can manage less and less of her own domestic and money affairs; then she may begin not to know her friends or relations; she talks less sense, and shows perseveration. The voice tends to become harsher and her emotions are blunted so that later she does not show any consideration for the feelings of others, becomes slovenly and deteriorates in her personal habits and cleanliness. Eventually the patient is incoherent, demanding, incontinent, and even has dirty habits and anti-social behaviour; her whole personality has disintegrated, and she is just the shell of her former self. This is a deeply distressing picture for her family to see. The same trends result from the arteriosclerotic process but the losses are more patchy and vary from moment to moment; there is intellectual loss, but the personality perhaps survives a little longer. Many of the latter patients die eventually of some other complication of arterial disease like a stroke or a heart attack.

The very essence of the diagnosis of either of these kinds of dementia is that it has been quite a slow, relentless story of downhill progress. It is an unforgivable error of geriatric work to make such a diagnosis hastily, without the right evidence. Some patients arrive quite unknown to anybody, but with every appearance of great confusion, and they might be thought to be demented. The proper assessment of this kind of patient must be delayed until someone can find a sensible relative or neighbour to describe how this patient has been during the preceding few weeks.

Patients who are victims of senile dementia itself may survive quite a long time in a protected environment, provided that they are well fed and kept from lying in bed. Neither of these groups are easy patients to nurse, and those who look after them do not have the satisfaction of seeing them get better, nor yet get much thanks for the care they give. There is nevertheless some special satisfaction in seeing that these sadly handicapped patients are up and dressed attractively in their own clothes, habit trained, and treated with consideration and good humour. They may be shells of their former selves, but they are not to blame, and they gave of their best, no doubt, when they were able. The community owes an immeasurable debt to the nurses who devote themselves to the care of elderly demented patients. The type of care which can be given to such unfortunate people is said to be a measure of the civilization of a country. The present trend, instead of herding these patients into long-stay wards forever, is to encourage them to be cared for in the community either in private houses or in specially equipped Welfare Homes set up for those who are mentally unreliable. Mild dementia can be managed well in a Home if the staff are skilled and sympathetic, and if there are enough of them to give adequate supervision. There must be people on duty at night.

In a private house it requires a person of remarkable patience and good humour to face giving care for any length of time. Being tied to someone whom one dare not leave, who cannot talk sense, and who wanders behind at one's apron strings, whose continence is uncertain and who disturbs one's rest, is altogether too much of a task for many people.

At least, that is what many husbands, wives and daughters decide, and who can blame them? It *can* be achieved by devoted relatives if plenty of help is available – like Home Helps, occasional "sitters", Day Hospital attendances and intermittent or "booked" holiday care in hospital. There is no doubt that if the patient's home and family is a good sympathetic one, home is the place where he fares best, treading his own well-known paths, given a regular regime which does not overtax him, and kind supervision from an understanding relative or housekeeper. But by contrast one can think of hundreds of homes where this never would work out, especially if there is overcrowding and young children are there; then, admission usually becomes unavoidable. Nevertheless we must at least explore the avenues of domiciliary care more widely if the problem of dementia in old age is to be faced realistically, because such patients already absorb a large and increasing share of the available Hospital and Local Authority resources. The problem is much more one of management than treatment. Drugs are only useful to help control the worst of the patient's restlessness, but demented people do benefit from regular occupational therapy chosen carefully to be within their capabilities, and they respond to being approached as much as possible like normal adults. This attitude does win good responses from many of these patients.

We have no real means of preventing dementia yet, but it seems that those who try hard to go on exercising their intellectual powers for as long as possible have the best chance of keeping the advances of the disease in check.

The financial and legal affairs of demented patients and those who are mentally ill often have to be put into the hands of the Court of Protection, an official body, under the direct control of the Lord Chancellor, which can protect their interests and do for them the things which their mental state makes them incompetent to do in the eyes of the Law. Even a properly executed Power of Attorney is no longer valid if the person who has granted it cannot any longer understand what is being done. The Court of Protection can be brought into the matter through a solicitor at the request of relatives; the Director of Social Services can take the first step himself if need be, and the doctor in the case can also do so if he believes his patient's interests require it.

BRAIN FAILURE AND MENTAL TESTING

In recent times medical workers have begun to talk of "brain failure", using the parallel of heart failure, which has many causes but a fairly usual and easily recognisable clinical pattern. Brain failure simply means inability to perform the sorts of mental tasks which previously could be managed easily enough. In layman's language, this is "confusion". There is some sense in this new concept, because brain failure (like heart failure) could be reversible, and likewise it has several different causes. It could be sudden, i.e. "acute" brain failure. Alternatively, it could be slow, becoming gradually worse and finally irreversible, but still showing the pattern of forgetfulness, intellectual losses, and deterioration in habits and personality.

It is common practice now in geriatric departments to give the patient a simple set of questions which would test his memory and capacity for knowing things (cognitive functions), totalling up the score of correct answers (see Appendix 2). This is called "mental test scoring", and various scoring systems have been devised. Used sensibly, it is a good means of assessing capabilities. If repeated later after treatment, it could measure improvement or failure to improve. Such a system cannot of course be used with patients who are unable to communicate because of deafness or special difficulties, or with those who refuse to co-operate.

FACTORS IN THE CAUSATION OF MENTAL ILLNESSES

Some severe but rare mental illness is hereditary, and heredity perhaps comes into the picture at other points, because the children of mentally abnormal parents have a greater than average risk of being afflicted themselves. We have already seen that physical diseases upset the older patient's mental behaviour. Anything which cuts an individual off from other people is likely to increase the risk of mental illhealth. It seems likely that lonely people, lacking the chance to use their faculties on other people, become more mentally vulnerable. So do those with uncorrected deafness or bad eyesight. Age itself is of course a highly significant factor, to the extent that the greater the age, the greater the chance of mental unreliability for one reason or another. Yet poor social conditions are probably not so important, provided there is no loneliness. The reverse is more likely – mental deterioration itself leads to unsatisfactory social conditions and eventually to a squalid house. Malnutrition is suspected by some people to lead to mental breakdown (see Chapter 6), but the evidence is by no menas clear.

We are left, then, with possible psychological factors like bereavement, or retirement without enough to do, or changes of address. Breakdown sometimes does follow these. There are besides certain changes in the culture of our Society which mean that the elderly do not share in the general economic advancement, they lose their former positions of authority in the family, and some become insecure, starved of affection and lacking any real incentive or sense of purpose. This can even happen in a Welfare Home where everything is done to a set routine, and the residents have hardly any obligations or need to assist other people. It could be that the bitterness and frustration of all this leads to deterioration in mentality and in behaviour, but such things are hard to prove. We know for a fact in hospital work that if reasonable demands are made on old people they respond to them; but if they are allowed to become just passive receivers of help, they respond less well in every way. At worst they "regress" to the infantile state – wet, dirty and helpless.

ATTITUDES TO MENTAL UNRELIABILITY

(a) *The Relatives' Attitudes*

Some unintelligent or unimaginative friends and relatives first think a mentally deteriorated old person is doing what she does "on purpose" or "out of devilment". Tolerance and sympathy have often gone out of the window. Later perhaps, when the abnormality is quite obvious, they often think it is "just old age". Very few "lay" people understand at present that this is a disease, and fewer still know that mental unreliability is, as likely as not, a pointer to physical disease as distinct from brain disease. The public has become better educated than to think that mentally ill people are "mad" and dangerous to everyone else, although the old idea died hard. Yet a proper understanding is not yet universal, and many basically kind people are worried and perplexed by the change in people they used to know as rational and reliable. They feel they cannot "cope" with them from then on; so, they say, "something must be done". The reverse side of this coin is that many patients who are mentally unreliable, even deranged, are being patiently cared for with the family doctor's help, and their cases never become known to the authorities, the Social Services or the Hospital. In other cases there is a sad conflict between the younger generation's wish to be free of the burden, and their conscience, which says they should do their duty by their parents or keep the promises about caring for them which they have made earlier – rather unwisely as it may have turned out. A few people, acting defensively, refusing to face facts, want to have their relatives admitted to "a proper hospital" (i.e. not a mental hospital), being unwilling to agree that the illness could possibly be a disorder of the mind ("How *can* you suggest she is mental!"), when it is staring everyone else in the face. The liberalizing of our mental hospitals and the methods of entering and leaving them will gradually result in the public acceptance that mental illness is not so very different from physical disease, that it is not necessarily the end of the road for an elderly person, and that there is no disgrace in suffering from mental disorder or having a case of that kind in one's family. This will all take time. Nevertheless the distress caused by permanent mental unreliability will probably always be great for sensitive husbands or wives, sons or daughters, because they knew the sufferer's capabilities and unique personality in the past, and now it has changed and gone, though the body remains.

(b) *The Attitudes of Hospitals*

Changes are on the way. The large mental hospitals were remote, and largely "custodial" in outlook. Some of their acute psychiatric work is being carried out in the general hospitals, and there is a general bringing together of activities, so that eventually longer-stay mental care even for older patients may also become part of the activities of a district general hospital or at least of smaller Community Hospitals, and all nurses and doctors will understand that older mental patients, just as much as any others, are deserving of care and need as normal a life as can be provided. It is time that all doctors, all nurses and all social workers put out of their minds the whole concept of "old dements", just as modern geriatrics is, we hope, ridding people of the idea of "old chronics".

Old people with mental disturbances, when the cause is not quite clear, can be admitted and observed there by a psychiatrist and a geriatric physician working closely together. Separate so-called psycho-geriatric assessment wards are hardly needed if there is a good geriatric assessment ward which allows people with some mental symptoms to be admitted. There have been opinions expressed that geriatric departments should take charge of all long-stay elderly patients wherever they may be – in geriatric or mental hospitals. This is not practicable. Geriatric departments already have large numbers of patients and they are mostly scattered, whereas there are many more psychiatrists than there are geriatric physicians. This large problem therefore has to be shared by all parties, including Local Authorities' Social Services Departments, each doing what it can best do for certain kinds of patient. This sharing policy must also include home and voluntary community care, and in this the hospitals can assist too by providing good out-patient and day hospital arrangements, admissions to cover family crises, and prompt specialist advice in consultation with the family doctor at the patient's own home.

In days not so far distant the patient's cry so often was, "Oh, don't send me away!"; she knew that the journey to the old workhouse hospital or the "lunatic asylum" was a one way trip. There are many alternatives now; things are not, or need not be, as they used to be.

(c) *The Patient's Attitude*

It is hard to be sure what the patients themselves think of their mental disorders. Those who have depression surely cannot be happy, but those who are hypomanic and overactive are usually cheerful and friendly to everyone. Yet in many conditions, including early dementia, the victims have some insight into their failings, and may be considerably upset. At a later stage all insight will probably be lost. Then who can say what these patients' feelings are? Sadness? Indifference? Bewilderment? It seems likely that many demented patients, living in worlds of their own, are not particularly unhappy, provided that they are sympathetically handled by cheerul people, who go along with their failures, provide them with creature comforts, and help them to preserve their dignity with attractive clothes, hair-dressing, and simple interests within their limited capabilities. The real sadness about irreversible mental disorder is experienced by the patients' relatives, who remember how they used to be in former times. Many people, afraid they will end their days mentally afflicted and desperate, express these fears by wishing for voluntary euthanasia to be legally sanctioned. One can sympathise with this apprehension, but it is not necessarily always well-founded. There might be worse fates than to be demented in sympathetic surroundings.

ADMISSION TO MENTAL HOSPITAL

Most admissions of mentally ill people to hospital for observation and treatment, provided that the patient is not unwilling, are arranged informally, just as they are to other hospitals. Compulsory admission may be necessary in certain circumstances – in the interests of the patient's own health and safety or for the protection of others – even though the patient himself is not willing. This is provided for by the Mental Health Act of 1959. Such an admission is usually arranged under Section 25 of that Act, and the patient can be detained for not more than twenty-eight days, when other action has to be taken if need be, or the patient allowed to go. Most such admissions are to mental hospitals, naturally, but there is nothing to prevent the patient being detained for the same reasons in a general hospital under the same Act. It is necessary to have an application made by the nearest relative or a mental welfare officer who is a social worker, and two doctors must see the patient, one a psychiatrist and the other a doctor specially approved under the Act, though the second doctor need not be a psychiatrist. The Mental Health Act of 1959 preceded the recent reorganisation of the Social Services Departments. The designation, under the Act, of "mental welfare officer" is at present taken to mean simply a social worker. However there has lately (1978) been a review of the Mental Health Act, in which it is suggested that a social worker who undertakes duties under the Act should possess special knowledge and experience of mental problems, and should be called an Approved Social Worker – approved perhaps by the local social services authorities. Legislation on this point will probably follow.

There are also other ways of detaining mentally ill patients in really urgent circumstances, that is, under Sections 29 or 30 of the Act, if the above procedure would take too long. Then the detention can only be for three days. The aim of the Mental Health Act and its various sections is of course to safeguard the interests and rights of patients, also to see that other people do not come to harm, and that any doctors, nurses or social workers involved are safeguarded against accusations of improperly detaining patients. Patients who are not formally detained in these ways are free to leave, but if they have been formally admitted under these various Sections it is proper to inform the police if they attempt to leave. Notwithstanding, there is now a much freer and easier atmosphere about mental hospitals and mental treatment than ever there used to be. Locked doors are unusual, and the general public is becoming much better informed about mental illness. There should now be very little stigma attached to accepting mental hospital treatment, but old attitudes still die hard.

Chapter 12

SURGICAL QUESTIONS:
PROBLEMS OF CANCER

There was a tendency in times past for surgeons to be conservative in their treatment of older patients. Major operation was thought inadvisable except where a real emergency had occurred and surgery was the only answer. Even now we do not advise operations for trivial conditions, and seldom simply for "cosmetic" purposes alone. Nevertheless there have been notable advances in anaesthetics, in surgical technique, and especially in the pre-operative preparation of patients and their postoperative care. The hazards are therefore much less serious than they were. Now it often happens that a new operation is devised and used for younger and resilient patients successfully, after which its use is extended to help people of older generations.

Surgical questions in old age are a matter of balancing risks. Yet the general public and our geriatric patients themselves are often firmly convinced that surgery can have a very doubtful chance of success indeed, and that operations are always likely to be dangerous "at that age". No one can attempt to operate on a patient without his or her consent, and no one should try to put pressure on a patient to accept a line of treatment to which he is utterly opposed. One of the purposes of this short chapter is to help those who are in regular and close contact with older people at home or in hospital to understand what surgery can or cannot do, and to help them to answer the questions of worried patients and their families. In fact about 7% of people who enter geriatric wards benefit from surgical treatment.

It goes without saying that it is best to arrive at retirement in the best of health, and there might be circumstances in which surgical correction of a fault would be better done in middle life when the problems are least, to avoid having to have something done much later and perhaps more hurriedly. Examples of this might be an abnormality of the feet, a hernia, or even severe osteoarthrosis of one hip. In this respect what a younger patient needs is some courage and foresight, an appreciation of what the disability will mean to him in his later life, and of course good professional advice.

177

Surgical aims for older people may not be quite the same as for people in the prime of life; nor for that matter are the aims of rehabilitation. For the young person a total cure is what is wanted, so that he or she can appear as normal and inconspicuous as possible. For the older patient the object is to restore to him as much capability and comfort as is possible in the circumstances, but the result may be far from perfection; it is not to be despised for that. Surgeons who have this broad and humane outlook confer boundless benefits on old people; those (and there are some) who are perfectionists and look upon an aged body as already past benefiting from their skill, are not much help to the elderly. It is usually fair to say that anyone who performs an operation but does not take the patient forward afterwards to the highest point of activity she can reach *by rehabilitation* has not achieved a great deal. If that patient has to be handed over a little later to some other department (usually the geriatric department) to be cared for indefinitely, this does not seem like a great therapeutic success. An artificial hip replacement operation in a demented patient who has not the wits to co-operate in the rehabilitation afterwards really is rather a waste of effort and money, not to mention expensive apparatus. An amputation for gangrene may save life, but that is not the end of the matter; the patient needs to be got onto an artificial limb if humanly possible; and if not, at least she should have a personal wheel chair and every other aid available to make her less dependent on her family or nurses. Geriatric departments can advise before and after operations in cases like these, but they are not often able to undertake rehabilitation of *all* surgical patients who happen to be above a certain age. So an obligation remains for surgical teams to see their patients through, and for nurses in surgical units to help older people to be active again and to avoid preventable complications – especially pressure sores.

We have already seen that fractures and surgical wounds heal well even in very old people, given the right circumstances – which means asepsis, a good blood supply, and a basically well nourished body. Anaesthetics themselves these days involve much smaller risks than they did even twenty years ago. Elderly bodies do not react well to blood loss or lowered blood pressure, so operations need to be as speedy as they can safely be done, and the operating technique needs to be first class. It is in the post-operative stage that the elderly person is most at risk, being inactive, rather vulnerable to chest infection, and liable to all the other hazards of the bedfast state (see Chapter 5), to which the only answer is as rapid a return to the upright position as possible. The risks of dying on the operating table are not very great in any patient who has been carefully prepared, though this catastrophe does happen occasionally when the urgency of the case left no time for proper assessment and preparation. In skilled hands planned surgery of old people carries an operative and immediate post-operative death rate of 2 to 3%, which may be felt a reasonably acceptable risk, considering the circumstances.

The problems caused by multiple disabilities occurring in one and the same patient have already been described, but one further repetition of this point is justified here in respect of surgery. All the patient's disabilities must be listed and considered, in case one, being overlooked, alters the outlook for the surgical disability. Early Parkinsonism, which often passes unnoticed, might for example cause any form of postoperative rehabilitation to fail; so might ischaemic heart disease because rehabilitation calls for a good deal of personal effort.

When considering a non-urgent operation the doctors should be taking into account the average expectation of life of such a patient apart from the surgical disease. Taking an extreme example, not much would be gained by removing a cancer of the breast which was not ulcerating or painful in a woman of 96, for her normal expectation of life at that time might be only a year or so more. All the same, average figures for any group *are* only averages, and must not be too strictly applied in individual cases.

In well conducted geriatric departments working in close touch with surgeons, then, age will count least in decisions to operate or not to operate. The chance of relieving distress will count high; so will the chance of making the patient active after immobility, and an assessment of the patient's general health, his "hold on life", alertness and will to recover, are all of great importance. How relatively simple the same question would be in a young adult person!

It has to be appreciated too that at any age the results of emergency surgical work are less good than if the operation can be planned ahead, and done "cold" – as surgeons are apt to say. In emergencies with geriatric patients the death rate is doubled at least. The sooner a firm decision is taken the better; the opportunity must be seized as it occurs; so we should beware especially of too much of the "wait and see" mentality when surgery is in the offing.

The Patient's Viewpoint

It is no surprise that older patients are very cautious about surgery. When they were young the risks were much higher and many of the operations which we think of as simple these days did not even exist. They cannot judge the chances, and need us to tell them. Even if at first they reject the idea out of hand, many of the thoughtful ones will reconsider the question, provided they feel that they are given the facts honestly. They have a right to know how bad the operative risks are. In urgent circumstances it is fair to say, "The risks are so and so, but if the operation is *not* done, the likelihood is such and such." This does not frighten them – it gives them the facts upon which to make decisions. They must also be told what to expect after the operation, and it is not fair to understate the case. Suppose, for example, a patient has gangrene of a toe, is told she will have a "little operation", and then wakes up to find the whole leg amputated – imagine her feelings. The post-operative plan has to be known by everyone concerned, including the nurses, and the patient most of all. Thus it could be said, "We may be obliged to remove your bad leg, but we want to get you quickly on to an artificial leg; are you willing to try it?".

When the necessary facts have been given, the patient must decide if she is mentally able to do so; if not, a relative may be asked to speak for her. It is *not* a matter which a relative ought to decide, no matter how important he may be, if the patient is capable of giving her own opinion – for it is the patient's, not the relative's life or limb which may be at stake. A patient must not be put under pressure to decide in favour of surgery, and she must be given time enough to think.

Reasons for Operations

We can briefly list some classes of operations which help geriatric patients. Firstly, those done for real emergencies where immediate lifesaving is the object – like an operation for a perforated stomach ulcer. Secondly, an operation to save life, but one which could be delayed and a good moment chosen – for example, slowly advancing gangrene. Thirdly, an operation which might cure the condition but which might not, and time alone would show; the plan would depend on what was found like, for example, a suspected cancer within the abdomen. Fourthly, an operation which could not cure, but which would help with a severe symptom, for example, cutting a nerve root to relieve pain in cancer, or limited removal of an ulcerating cancer of the breast. Fifthly, an operation designed to make a patient more mobile, speed up recovery, or reduce the risk of complications – like a tenotomy for contracture. Sixthly, planned operations to make a patient more comfortable, for example to remove a large hernia or uterine prolapse.

A difficult situation arises sometimes when there is a simple operation which could get rid of a disability and allow the patient concerned to be active or perhaps even leave hospital – but she will not give consent to it. No one can force her to have the operation against her will, nor even force her co-operation in physiotherapy and rehabilitation. Yet there is surely a moral factor in this; we might ask ourselves if anyone has the right to go on using services or even a hospital bed when a small manoeuvre carrying a negligible risk would make it all unnecessary. The question of a small operation to help straighten a contracted leg followed by physiotherapy and a good likelihood of success is just a case in point. Persuasion and careful explanation of the smallness of the risk and the discomfort are needed, and the doctors will require the help of the nurses and relatives in this too. Sometimes, when it is so clearly a moral issue, the Hospital Chaplain can be brought in to help solve this medical yet moral matter; the Parable of the Talents might be a good start to the discussion.

MEDICAL AND NURSING CARE BEFORE OPERATION

Two things have to be decided at an early stage; the patient's fitness for whatever is being contemplated, and the chance of success, bearing in mind the patient's mental clarity and resilience. Next it is necessary for a full examination and investigation to be done, keeping a particular watch for the unexpected where the patient has no other symptom whatever. Because of this, it is usual to have a haemoglobin estimation, a blood count, testing of the urine particularly for sugar, a chest X-ray and an electrocardiograph, because these can all be very revealing. It is only reasonable that all hazards which can be known about in advance should be brought to light before the surgeon and anaesthetist are asked to give opinions: it is they who will have the patient's life in their hands. Every possible attempt should be made to see that the patient is at the peak of condition before going to the operating theatre. So often she is in a poor state of nutrition, and a few days of "feeding up" may be days very well spent. Transfusion of blood or correction of a state of dehydration are vital in some cases. Intravenous fluids can be started if the oral route is not possible to use. If the patient suffers from diabetes, this must be stabilized, if necessary on a routine of soluble insulin and a fixed diet, or a glucose-equivalent fluid diet. It is even a good plan to get the patient accustomed in advance to breathing and other sorts of exercises which she would be required to do to become active again after the operation. Even a hearing aid supplied in advance of a cataract operation might make the rehabilitation stages easier. These are all counsels of perfection. All too often there is no time for more than basic pre-operative preliminaries, and the shorter the time available the smaller the chance of a good outcome.

POST-OPERATIVE CARE

What must be done for a younger patient after operation also must be done for an older, but even stricter attention than usual to nursing detail is needed, and a closer watch must be kept for specific complications, for the older patient has smaller reserves of strength and is not so active in bed. Just as soon afterwards as the anaesthetist will allow, the patient must sit up and begin to do breathing exercises. Just as soon as the surgeon allows, she must sit out of bed and even start to stand. One orthopaedic surgeon operating on elderly hip joints has the patients sitting out on the first day afterwards and starting to take a few steps on the second! This is the sort of approach which geriatric physicians will applaud, provided that it does the patient no harm – and apparently it does not. Most careful watch must be kept for post-operative lung collapse or pneumonia, and for retention of urine. Pressure sores sometimes develop even as a result of a long session on the operating table itself, and during the first few hours and days in bed they are a very great hazard indeed. Therefore nursing vigilance, with regular turning (the real antidote), should be reinforced by using ripple mattresses (see page 206); heels need special attention at this time.

A watch needs to be kept by medical and nursing staff for any fall of blood pressure, any sign of heart failure or change in the type of the pulse (because rhythm changes are so common at this stage) and for a deep vein thrombosis. Elastic bandages can help to reduce this last risk, but getting the patient up or at least arranging for leg exercises in bed are much the best answer. Problems arise over what sort of drugs to give in the hours and days after an operation. It may be traditional to give morphine to relieve pain and restlessness, but morphine is dangerous because it increases the chance of complications of all kinds, and frail patients are very sensitive to it. All sedation is a risk to older patients after operation, and yet they are so liable to be noisy and confused and disturbing to other people. Compromises have to be made, and it is obviously best if such a patient can have a single side room as close as possible to the nurses' station for a few days.

Rehabilitation will be needed, to some extent at least, in almost every case. An operation is a major setback in any old person's life, and it will sap his confidence. Supervision in walking will be needed for sure, even though the operation is small and nothing to do with the legs. Yet it is still common to hear of patients like this being sent back to their homes without ever having been got walking in the hospital; they are lifted out of the ambulance at home, go straight to bed, and stay there, often with disastrous results! Some of them have to be readmitted as geriatric patients, which is surely going about things the wrong way round.

THE SCOPE OF SURGERY IN GERIATRICS

1. *Gynaecology*
Apart from dealing with cases of cancer of the uterus and ovarian cysts, surgeons are often asked to help patients with a mild cystocoele and with "stress incontinence" – that is, trickling incontinence which only comes on with coughing or abdominal straining. A complete prolapse of the uterus is greatly distressing to an old woman, and common enough too. Elaborate repair operations are not often feasible, but there are simple procedures like the le Fort's type of operation which can give complete relief, and earn the patient's profound gratitude.

2. Abdominal Surgery

Almost any known catastrophe in the abdomen could strike an old person and it has to be dealt with on its merits, emergency operations being quite common and all the more serious for being necessary in old frail people instead of robust young people. Some are unusually common, like a perforation of diverticulitis, twisting of the bowel (volvulus) or a blockage of a mesenteric artery by an embolus. What is more, the usual classical signs of perforation of the stomach from ulcer, or acute appendicitis, or strangulation of a hernia may not be present, and the diagnosis can easily be missed. This means it is most important to take all complaints of abdominal pain seriously and get a medical or surgical opinion in good time.

These things apart, there are many abdominal operations which can be planned ahead and carried through with safety and success. These include operations for gastric ulcers, for pyloric obstruction, removal of the gall bladder for repeated attacks of infection or stones, and even operations for slow-growing tumours of the colon or rectum. Colostomy is a feasible operation for a slow obstruction, or to help in the treatment of diverticulitis; all the same, old people have a great dislike, naturally, for being left with this unpleasant and unnatural opening, and some of them never learn to control or dress it with modern colostomy appliances: so they have to remain in hospital indefinitely.

One very helpful small operation is that of inserting a silver wire into the wall of the rectum to prevent a prolapse that "comes down" repeatedly. The distress which this symptom causes to a frail and very elderly lady – the most likely sort of victim – is not hard to imagine. Such an operation has often entirely cured a woman in her middle nineties when she would otherwise have had to stay in hospital and perhaps even in bed, because sitting up caused the prolapse always to be "down".

3. Orthopaedic Surgery

This has great possibilities in the sense of correcting deformity, relieving pain and improving the patient's chances of walking. Successful replacement of diseased hip joints has been done for 25 years or more, and now artificial replacements of knee joints are becoming feasible; they are likely to be suggested for more older people who are crippled by a type of osteoarthrosis which causes great deformity, pain and limitation of activity. Broken hip joints – so common an injury especially in elderly women, for reasons given at various points in this book – can either be "fixed" with nails and plates, or replaced entirely so that the patient can be got walking again in a fraction of the time it took formerly. The old days of full-scale hospital nursing care extending over many weeks for old people strung up with a network of suspension and traction apparatus for broken legs and at risk of innumerable lethal complications, should be nearly over, except in special cases.

Other helpful orthopaedic operations include corrections of foot faults of all kinds, help for patients whose limbs are crippled and distorted from rheumatoid arthritis, and cutting of contractures and tendons (tenotomies) to correct footdrop, for example, to allow permanently bent legs to be straightened, and to overcome gross spasticity so that a fresh start in walking can be made with the help of physiotherapists. There is hardly any limit to the good which can be done by an active team consisting of an orthopaedic surgeon and geriatric physician working together, with keen nurses and therapists. Nor must we forget the large number of patients who have suffered the great misfortune of an amputation and yet are walking again without help, thanks to a good artificial limb and plenty of encouragement. Even *double* amputation need not be a total disaster, though most of such patients have to be content with a double short rocker pylon. The author once had a splendid woman patient who, after her two legs were successively amputated at the age of 91 and 92, was taught to walk again on two full length shaped artificial limbs, with no one supporting her. Here was courage if ever there was.

4. *Neurosurgery*

Geriatric patients are no more immune than any others to tumours and other abnormalities within the skull or spinal column which need surgical treatment. Some of these tumours are *not* malignant, and many of them require detailed investigation because of this, though we must not forget how often it is that cancers elsewhere develop secondary deposits, e.g. from the lung or breast, ultimately in the brain. Other important areas in which neurosurgeons help geriatric departments and their patients are the treatment of the severe pain of trigeminal neuralgia, the investigation, treatment and cure of subdural blood clots (which without surgical removal grow larger and may prove fatal) and the surgical treatment of Parkinson's Disease by what are called stereotactic methods (see page 140). This has become less common now that new drugs have become available.

5. *Genito-urinary Surgery*

Even in quite old people it is possible, indeed essential, to remove a kidney which has been destroyed by stones or is full of pus, or suspected of being cancerous. After all, it may have ceased to be an effective kidney some time ago, so the remaining kidney is presumably keeping pace with the extra load, and its capacity is quite easy to test. Surgery is possible too for bladder abnormalities and cancer. Otherwise it is the prostate gland which offers the surgeon a fruitful field for action. It is easy to see, therefore, that a large part of this branch of surgery *is* the surgery of geriatric patients.

6. Surgery of the Blood Vessels

Here is a part of surgical work which is making great strides forward, and opportunities are opening out for older people because in them, above all, artery disease is widespread. It is possible now to replace parts of diseased aortas with dacron or similar artificial grafts without too great a risk, and larger arteries like those of the leg can have grafts or bypass operations. Certain sorts of strokes or stroke-like tendencies, or cases of narrowing of the neck vessels with atheroma which *might* lead to strokes, can be treated similarly, though naturally if the artery disease is within the skull itself it is not accessible to the vascular surgeon's methods. The techniques of X-raying diseased arteries are advancing rapidly, and this makes it possible to show very clearly where the obstruction is, and whether it might be overcome. Some arterial obstructions, especially if they are just in one place, can be removed by opening the vessel and "coring it out", as one might core out an apple. There is increasing hope for older people from all these advances, but it would be still better if we could learn to prevent artery disease altogether.

7. Plastic Surgery

No doubt certain elderly people consult plastic surgeons to have themselves operated on to give them an outward appearance of youth. Apart from this use of surgery, there are many other ways in which plastic surgeons will save lives and correct gross deformities – by treating serious burns, removing skin tumours, correcting extruding eyelids (ectropion) and removing obvious disfiguring or painful blemishes like sebaceous cysts of the scalp or large fatty tumours under the skin (lipomata). We need plastic surgeons' help too, in treating some leg ulcers which never look like healing by any other means, or providing covering skin grafts for large pressure areas which have unfortunately developed but failed to heal. One must hope that calls of this nature on plastic surgeons will grow less and less in time.

8. Pain Relief

Recent research into pain pathways in the nervous system and the setting up of pain clinics has resulted in a number of effective procedures for relieving intractable pain, especially in people whose illnesses are not dangerous and not considered likely to be fatal. Some older patients can benefit from these advances, and the possibility should be kept in mind. In times past surgeons sometimes cut pain-conducting tracts in the spinal cord. Now it is quite common for injections of alcohol or other drugs to be made into the spinal cord or the sympathetic nerve chain so as to give immediate, and hopefully permanent, pain relief. These techniques are often studied and perfected by anaesthetists.

CANCER

Cancer is not the worst problem in geriatric work, but it is large enough to cause us deep concern, and common enough for almost all elderly people to fear it and to imagine, perhaps, that this is the cause of their symptoms. We would be well advised to think of this ever-present fear, and if we are sure that cancer is *not* the cause, then we should say so quite plainly.

Growths account for, or are associated with, about 15% of all old people's deaths, and more than half of all cancer deaths take place after the age of 65. In many organs the chance of cancer rises steadily with age – for example the skin, the lungs and digestive organs, with certain leukaemias and myelomatosis (see page 148) being important here also. Cancer of the prostate gland is even more strikingly connected with the age of a man, but some other tumours, like sarcoma and even cancer of the cervix of the womb are more usually found in rather younger people.

There are some hereditary factors involved, and some cancers are caused by harmful agents like tobacco and industrial chemicals, most of which take a long time to produce their effects. It follows that older people will have had more time for this to have happened. Taken all in all, an ageing population (see Chapter 1) will have more cancer than a youthful one. In some very old patients cancers move forward less fast, and some – a very few – seem to diminish in size. These facts all need to be considered when one is planning what to do for any one sufferer.

This is not the place for a discussion of the characteristics of individual cancers and their management. The care of the terminal illness of such patients will be mentioned again in Chapter 16. Certain special facts about cancer in later life are nevertheless worth mentioning. First, cancer of the breast is common and very often it is missed, though hardly ever so where nurses are having to wash patients regularly. At home many of these cancers go undetected, and one cannot avoid the conclusion that the women know of the lump, more than suspect what it is, but decide to say nothing either because of embarrassment or, more likely, because they are afraid to hear the truth and undergo treatment. Many many tragedies have happened this way, from ignorance or fear. One patient of the author's developed a breast cancer over 20 years previously; it gradually spread and ulcerated the skin, became infected and finally spread to half the entire chest wall. This patient must have known what it might be, but she concealed it all this time. Asked if her husband had noticed nothing she replied, "He never saw it, but he did sometimes complain of the smell." Sadly, it killed her soon afterwards.

Cancer of the lower bowel is also very common, slow to develop, and able to produce unexpected signs; but it is not usually a very invasive kind of tumour and could be treated in the early stages. Many a cancer of the rectum has gone to a stage of inoperability because the patient was too shy to mention rectal symptoms, thought that rectal bleeding was "just the piles", or because no nurse or doctor happened to make a rectal examination for symptoms of "diarrhoea" or constipation.

Cancer of the bones is common, and most cases are secondary to other tumours arising in the breast, the thyroid or the prostate gland. They are often the cause of sudden fractures which happen without much physical damage; they even take place in bed. These are called spontaneous or "pathological" fractures, but they heal, strangely, almost as fast as fractures from direct injuries.

Cancer of the skin is common in old people but slow to develop and not very likely to spread far or fast, save where there are multiple secondary cancers in and under the skin from other growths. Primary skin cancers often occur in the parts of the skin exposed to sunlight, and are especially noticed in old farm workers. There is one special type which is exceedingly common, called a basal cell carcinoma or "rodent ulcer"; it is a small raised area near the eyes, mouth or nose, and often with a small dark scab on it which forms again after bleeding. This skin cancer will respond at once to treatment and heal with scarcely a mark. If however it is not treated it can slowly eat away half the face, with terrible disfigurement. Anyone, therefore, who sees anything suspicious of this type on an old person's face, should point it out and most strongly advise she reports it to her doctor who will refer her for X-ray or radium treatment.

It goes without saying that the earlier a tumour is discovered, the better the chance of treatment. All cancer starts somewhere, probably from a single cell. If we could discover it at that stage it would be treatable and curable. There is still a great deal of fear and reticence about cancer, which prevents its early detection. All people, old or young, should be repeatedly encouraged to report pains, lumps, bleedings, losses of weight, and other such symptoms. Old people often do not like to "trouble" their nurses or doctors with "little things"; possible cancer signs or symptoms are not little things.

The treatment of cancer is first, perhaps, surgical. Surgery may be possible for older patients, and surgical advice should almost always be taken unless it is clear there already is secondary spread of the tumour. Many times, however, it is too late for surgery, or the operation would be too much for the patient to stand, or too mutilating. Yet this should not be assumed just because the victim is of a certain age. If surgery is not possible to cure or to relieve symptoms, deep X-ray or radium therapy (radiotherapy) may be worth a try. Certain cancers, especially those of the skin, and some lymph gland tumours melt away under the influence of X-rays. Some other tumours turn out not to be radio-sensitive, and the patient does not get any benefit.

Another line of treatment is drugs which kill cells or tissues (so-called cytotoxic drugs). They especially attack tumour cells. They are effective for certain cancers, but on many others they have little real action, and only help to put off the evil day for a while. Courses have usually to be long, and the drug may make the patient feel very ill – perhaps even more ill than the disease itself. Many older patients, if quietly asked, would say that such treatments are not worth the upset they cause; besides, the cytotoxic drugs have adverse effects on blood-forming tissues, and may make the patient anaemic. Certain cancerous diseases of the glands may be helped by these drugs. Other notable cancers, i.e. of the prostate and some cancers of the breast, are held in check for many months or years by using hormones like oestrogens, or testosterone, which do not have a serious effect upon the patient's general well-being. In general we might say that for older people "heroic" methods with cancer are not advisable. They and their families are not hoping to grasp at every straw, though young people in similar circumstances probably would be doing so.

Chapter 13

PRACTICAL NURSING OF ELDERLY PEOPLE

This chapter is written with a sense of humility. The author, not being a trained nurse but a doctor, has from time to time been professionally in the hands of nurses himself, for years has been watching them at their work, and has reason to be grateful to them both on his own account and much more on behalf of his patients. Nursing and doctoring are not entirely separate arts, and all doctors can learn from nurses. In geriatrics perhaps more than anywhere else the care of patients is a team responsibility. A doctor who practices this art successfully must have taught himself what his nursing colleagues' problems really are in order to be able to help them. He could never with a clear conscience say, "That is your job; it's no business of mine; I don't understand it anyway". The following pages are, therefore, addressed to those who nurse in old people's wards, as personal observations and suggestions, but no more. No attempt has been made to cover the ground completely, for nurses are taught their skills by their own tutors and their seniors. Where modifications of technique might be necessary because of the nature of the older patients and their diseases, these have been mentioned. The reasons for possible modifications may be found in many places in this book.

Much of what follows relates to the nursing of patients in hospital, but the principles remain the same in home nursing, even though the equipment may not be so satisfactory and sometimes harder to come by. It is possible with persistence and using a little guile to obtain vital gear – even hospital-type beds – for the home nursing of elderly invalids. Nursing of elderly people is a difficult job and nurses must have the right tools for doing it. The author has the impression that reorganization of the Health Service has resulted in an improvement in facilities made available for nursing people at home, and that equipment and transport are easier to come by. There was need of this improvement.

The Approach to Patients
From all that is known about the limitations of older people (see

Chapter 2) it is clear that we must approach them face to face, at the right height, speaking clearly but not necessarily very loudly, looking into their eyes (see Plate 1), and giving them time to consider the answer they wish to give to what has been said. The best position for doing this for most patients who are in bed or in chairs is kneeling on one knee; this position is hard on the stockings and the trousers but by far the best for making real contact with patients. Plain, simple, adult language with a little touch of humour sometimes is the recipe, with a reassuring pressure of one's hand when things are difficult. "Talking down" to elderly people as if they were children is deplorable tying their hair up in "little girl" ribbons is equally unacceptable. Psychologists recognize that some old people, if dealt with in this way and not allowed to do things for themselves, exhibit psychological regression: they come to behave like the children their nurses have turned them into, and even can reach the stage of wetting and soiling their beds. The key to success is to be kind and sympathetic always, but always to allow the patient to do what he is able to do without help, insisting on this if one is certain he can do it. This requires particular self-discipline from nurses, whose whole training urges them to help people. It is also difficult to let a patient take his time if doing the job oneself saves a great deal of one's own time – as it usually does! Any other policy is likely to hinder the patient's recovery and reduce his self respect and independence.

As a geriatric patient it is far safer for one to be up than confined to bed (see Chapter 5). The rule should therefore be: every patient is up unless the doctor prohibits it (in most other wards the patient seems to be in bed until the doctor permits her to get up!) The difference is fundamental. In this type of work doctors know experienced nurses will use their discretion when older patients are not fit to be up on a particular day.

It is important that nurses should introduce themselves by name, and do as much as possible to help elderly people orientate themselves. When people are confused in mind the process of introducing oneself may have to be repeated time and time again till the information "sinks in". Old people do not naturally pick up simple ideas about where they are, when the post goes, who is senior and who is junior, or even which way the lavatory is, as younger patients do. Many of them have never been in hospital before, have never had to have intimate things done for them, and are frankly terrified and often resentful – until they have been "brought out" by kindness and patient explanation. They may accept the things we want to do to them, but they like to be told in advance just as younger, more alert people do.

Approaching the Blind

Blind people in their own homes can often manage to get about and do a good deal, unless their blindness came on late and rather suddenly. In

Hospitals and Homes they are in a strange place, amongst strangers, and may be greatly upset and too alarmed to attempt anything. They may hear very well but cannot at first identify who is coming by footsteps. It is a kindly gesture for everyone, from cleaners and paper boys to nurses and doctors, to identify themselves almost every time they pass near by some such phrase as, "Hallo Mrs Robinson; I'm Nurse Johnson". Blind people also need to have their essential belongings always put into the same identifiable place beside their bed or chair, or they feel out of touch with their world. Teaching blind people to move about again in a ward is difficult, but it is possible to say to the courageous ones, "Straight ahead now; there's nothing in your way for five yards". It is best to offer a blind person one's bent arm to take himself, and lead him gently that way – not pulling him forward or propelling him from behind. If the patient is partially sighted or hemianopic (see page 124), then everything must be done from the better side, and the locker must also be on that side. Approaching hemianopic people from their blind side evokes no response until one appears in front of them, when they may be quite startled.

Approaching the Deaf

The deaf are unfortunate and often arouse exasperation, whereas everyone will sympathize with the blind. These trends ought to be compensated for by able health workers, to redress the balance. Every effort must be made to communicate with the deaf by careful articulation of words, offering the chance of lip reading, writing words down, and making signs. All nurses and doctors ought to learn the simple alphabet of sign language. Hearing aids are vital if the patient has been able to learn to use one, but so often they are hanging loose, or are not switched on, or have flat batteries! Some patients can hear with the stethoscope put into their ears while one speaks into the "bell" of the instrument, and many patients can use a flexible ear trumpet even if they cannot master the electronic type of hearing aid. There should be several trumpets in every geriatric ward. Some patients show a remarkable "selective deafness", and some can lip read very well. It pays to be very careful of one's own quiet, unguarded comments! Various special high-grade amplifiers with a microphone and good headphones have been evolved in recent times. They are excellent for person-to-person contact with many deaf people, when the ordinary hearing-aid is of little use. No geriatric ward or residential home should be without such equipment.

CONTINUITY

One of the greatest problems in geriatric medical work is obtaining continuity of care and the passage of important, detailed information. A great deal of medical, psychiatric and social detail is needed in the early stages of the admission, and when rehabilitation is going on just as much detail is needed about the patient's precise capability or disability. Against this background doctors and senior nursing staff know that many of the nurses in this branch of medicine are married and can only work part-time. Part-time nurses and sisters are the pillars which support many geriatric hospitals, but it may sometimes mean that a ward cannot claim even to have one sister as its regular guiding mind. It is difficult then to be sure that the information regularly gets through, back and forth, and continuity is preserved, especially if the patient can say very little herself. Regular recording methods like the Kardex system are therefore vital in all wards, so that all instructions and all progress can be carefully recorded, and hand-over sessions at the changes over of nursing staff must be on a detailed patient-by-patient basis, preferably combined with an actual visit to each individual's bedside by the two nurses concerned. In these days of formal nursing training this may seem to be a glimpse of the obvious, but nurses' hours are shorter, their holidays are longer, and the problem of passing correct and detailed information to the whole geriatric team remains – a problem. It is also valuable to record, after consultation between therapists, doctors and ward staff, and have these records available for everyone to see the precise capabilities of each patient. If Mrs A. can feed herself, it will set the clock back if Nurse B. hand-feeds her because she is new to the ward and does not know that she can.

Observation and Charting

The medical staff in geriatric departments usually have large numbers of patients. It is not uncommon for a department to be responsible for 400 or 500 beds in several hospitals. The doctors cannot see their patients as often as they would wish, and must rely heavily on the opinions and observations of the nurses, who spend much more time with each individual than they will ever do. Particularly important is the observation of the adverse effects of drugs, and the many little "attacks" to which old people are so liable (see pp. 54–57). Nurses can help greatly by recording in detail what they saw, the temperature, pulse and respiration as well as the blood pressure, so that the facts can be put into the medical records. Charting the temperature continuously in geriatric wards is largely a waste of time and need not be done except in cases of severe illness or hypothermia – when it needs to be done hourly. Pulse and respiratory rate charting are much more valuable as pointers to serious disease, and doctors would expect that all geriatric nurses will quickly develop an instinct about a rise in respiratory rate. This matter is not for basic (and sometimes rather casual?) recording twice a day, but it should be at the back of one's mind every time one looks at an elderly patient for any reason whatever. Quick detection and reporting of a rising respiratory rate, coupled with a jump in the pulse rate, will save lives. Pneumonia in old age can strike like lightning.

Input and output fluid charting is often carefully done. The input should not be difficult, but the output may be totally impossible to record with accuracy. If one knows how much fluid the patient has taken in, then a regular twice-weekly weighing programme will give a clear enough indication of what is taking place, provided everyone is alert (as all should always be) for the over-distended bladder about which the patient has not even complained. Regularly measuring the patient's weight on a pair of sitting-type scales in standard clothing is an essential aid to geriatric care; it is a vital statistic which must be recorded in the medical notes for immediate and remoter follow-up purposes. Recording of bowel actions must be a matter of nurses recording what really did happen; it is not enough to ask the patient what she *thought* happened.

Progressive Patient Care

In one sense any geriatric department which divides its activities into assessment, early treatment, rehabilitation, longer-stay stages, is practising progressive patient care. The patients at one phase require a different kind of, but not necessarily more, or less, care than the others do. Nevertheless the load in any ward is such that it is most efficient for nursing purposes to group together patients who are very ill and at great risk from complications of their disease and their bedfast state, letting others who can partly look after themselves do so, and be closer to the day space and therapy sections. Ideally, of course, the very ill patients should be grouped in single or small wards close to a nurses' station. It is simpler to observe them closely; it is easier for a team to give, say, two-hourly back attention to four patients in adjoining beds than to four people all in different nursing bays. Unfortunately, frequent changes of position in a ward requires much porterage, reorientation for the staff, and a risk of *dis*orientating elderly patients who have just got accustomed to their new surroundings. All the same, it is a wise move always to indicate clearly who are the most "at risk" patients. In some places an estimate of vulnerability or otherwise to pressure sores is given by a code card on the bedhead (see Appendix 3).

NURSING EQUIPMENT

Beds

The beds needed for caring for elderly patients properly should be the best hospital beds available; all too often geriatric departments have received the worst – that is, the discarded equipment of other departments' upgradings. We must recognize that there may not be money enough to supply the best available beds for every elderly hospital patient. At least they should be adjustable in height, for nursing in low beds is impossible for the staff, and trying to get out of beds which are too high is dangerous for patients. Bed heights, like chair heights, are critical for elderly patients learning to be independent. A good back-rest and over-bed chain and handle are needed; so are castors on the beds, and these must be of the locking type.

Safety Sides

In the old days heavy old beds, with high ends and equally high cot sides were the rule for patients who were in any way "difficult to manage". These old monstrosities with their clanking sides and cage-like appearance are quite unnecessary and should be done away with. Any active patient who is determined to get up out of bed will climb over the sides or end, and the danger then is great. Years ago, the author had one patient who climbed on to the end of such a bed at night, dived head first to the floor, and died instantly. Safety sides should be used not to restrain, but to prevent frail or restless old people rolling out of bed. Though sides in position may give a sense of security to the nursing staff, especially at night, the patient is only secure against a rolling-out accident. With a restless patient, determined to climb out, the sense of security is false, and it could be safer to have a very low bed or a mattress on the floor. Modern telescopic temporary safety sides are clamped on to the frame, they are silent in action, safe, and fold down unobtrusively to bed level when not in use, and below mattress level so that it is simple to make the bed. Their vertical spaces are not wide enough for a confused patient to get his head stuck! This type of safety side is acceptable – as no other sort really is. There can be no doubt that "cot sides" give many patients a sense of being imprisoned, besides depriving them of dignity. Senior nursing opinion is hardening against the routine use of sides, even at night, except for the very ill, the unconscious, or the restless, rolling patient. Where adjustable height beds are available (as they should be everywhere) and always at night-time, with the average patient using the lowest position of the bed, but without the sides raised, should be as safe a system as any. This is obviously a matter for discretion.

Bed Cradles

It should be a rule of geriatric nursing practice that bed cradles are used – preferably of the tubular steel, cantilever type (Fig. 11). They should be obligatory for any patient who could possibly get foot drop, and for all stroke cases, or negligence could possibly be claimed. They also help in the prevention of sore heals.

Tables

Tables are best if they are of the cantilever type which can go over a bed or chair, and better still if they will tilt to act as a book rest or writing desk also. Standard bridge-like over bed tables are not very good for older people, except those who might need to lean forward at night because of respiratory distress.

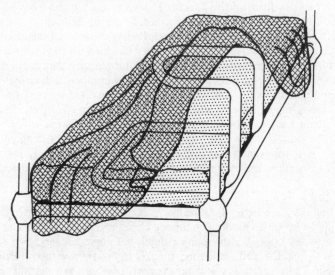

Fig. 11 Use of a cantilever type of tubular steel bed cradle to take the weight of the bedclothes.

Chairs

Chairs for geriatric patients should be of many different types according to the kind of patient and the degree of activity expected. There are too many types to be listed and compared here. Some patients need comfort, maximum support, and to be guarded against falling out. Chairs suitable for this purpose are the high-backed "geriatric chairs", some with footrests and built-in swivelable tables. Other patients need a comfortable, attractive day chair in which they can sit up and take notice, which is easy to get in and out of, and has good, easily grasped arms to grip. The crux of the matter is the height from the floor to the seat, and this must match the leg length of the patient from heel to knee, or be higher still if there is a stiff, straight leg. The minimum height might be 45 cm, the maximum could be as high as 65 cm. The author has for many years had scores of well upholstered, waterproof, simulated-leather dining armchairs made to special order and to varying heights (see Plate 8) and in various bright colours.* There are many other chairs for special

* This is the "Langford" chair of Parker Knoll Limited.

purposes, like tilting chairs, ejection-seat chairs, and large mobile chairs for very heavy, disabled patients. No doubt we shall continue to see many varieties, of varying degrees of usefulness, appearing in the future. There is at present a particular vogue for tilting chairs on castors which have a table in front of the patient. These can be pushed from point to point. An example is the "Buxton" chair, originally devised for the treatment of the common condition of postural hypotension; these chairs are finding a use for the management of very disabled invalids who tend to slide forward out of their chairs. For this latter purpose they are certainly effective, but the price paid is to have a totally immobilized, virtually imprisoned patient. A few ask for their chairs to be tilted because they feel safer; many others bitterly resent being tilted. Tilting effectively destroys any attempt of a patient to move freely and to assist in her own rehabilitation. The practice, regrettably seen in some continuing care wards, of putting most frail old patients into such chairs, tilting them back as a routine, and moving on to the next, simply cannot be defended.

Commodes

Commodes are better than bedpans: almost anything is better than a bedpan. In hospitals modern commode chairs are usually of tubular steel with a barely concealed bedpan or dutch hat container, and two castor wheels to help the staff move them quickly out of sight without having to lift them. The older, heavy wooden-type with wooden arms is still seen in many people's homes; one arm is essential for safety, but it is often best to saw off the other arm which is nearest to the patient's bedside, and then adjust the heights of the commode and the bed so that the patient can slide easily from one to the other.

Sanitary Chairs

A wheeled chair with a lavatory seat in which the frail patient can be taken from her bedside to the lavatory itself is clearly better than anything except an actual journey there which she makes herself, walking. The use of these chairs requires that the doorways and the lavatories themselves should be large enough.

Lavatories

Lavatories can be of the ordinary height, but some should have raised seats for special patients. This can be done with a removable seat-raising device, such as could equally well be used in the patient's own home. It is helpful if the lavatory can be constructed with rails to assist the patient to get up and down, and these rails must be wide enough to allow a sani-chair to go over the w.c. It is most satisfactory, too, if the lavatory itself can be off-centre in the room, so that a nurse can comfortably get round on one side to help with the clothing. (The author's design is shown in

Plate 5.) The number of lavatories is a matter for debate. In the Ipswich Geriatric Department's assessment ward there are eleven lavatories available for fifty ward patients, and two more leading off the dayspace. This, once thought to be lavish, may be considered too few in years to come. Research now suggests that it is necessary to have a lavatory within only a few feet of any bed if incontinence is really to be overcome.

Baths

For practical purposes geriatric patients' baths should be accessible on all sides but with various special aids like the well-known bath seat, bath board, and a hand rail or upright pole. There should be a non-slip mat or special internal, non-slip surface in each bath. Some patients are frightened of lying flat in a long bath and even may think they are going to drown; these may prefer a sitting-type bath which can be "mounted" by a suitable plinth (see Plate 3a). Many other varieties of special baths have been introduced, with varying success, and each has its devotees. The patient can walk into one type (the Medic bath) and sit down, an end plate is lowered, sealed to make it watertight, and the bath quickly filled. In another type, the Ladywell bath, a sitting patient is slid into a long bath on a special sliding seat, the hinged door is closed and sealed. After bathing the patient is slid out again and goes back to the ward still in the sliding device. The most modern tendency, with the coming of the Ambulift (see below), is to use standard long baths, and to raise them an extra two or three feet from the floor, so that nurses can do the job standing at the most convenient working height. The ultimate perhaps is a bath which itself can be raised or lowered, but the cost of these is great.

Showers

A shower bath to most people suggests something under which they stand controlling the tap themselves. Many elderly patients can be *given* a shower, and they enjoy it. They sit in the shower sink on a waterproof stool, holding onto a grab-handle, while a nurse dressed in rubber boots and a waterproof apron (see Plate 3b) holds the rose of a flexible shower pipe in one hand, a sponge in the other and, having carefully adjusted the water temperature by the mixing tap, washes the patient down from neck to foot. There is no climbing or lifting in and out to be done, and no fear of total immersion. The whole process is more hygienic than taking a bath. It seems very likely that many more patients would accept this system if there were more nurses who were convinced of its value – and that will only happen when it comes to be accepted that giving showers to patients is part of the standard training procedure.

Hoists

Devices for lifting patients are used in many wards. In geriatric wards not only are some patients very obese and inert, but may be severely crippled, or in pain, and frightened of being handled. Hoists are of many kinds; the hydraulic hoist on a frame with castors; the wall-mounted hoist; an electric hoist (e.g. the Winchester Hoist) mounted on a gantry, so that an intelligent but very disabled person could take herself unaided from bath to lavatory to wheelchair. Two main sorts of hoists are found to be most practical in geriatric wards. One is the hydraulic hoist where the patient is held in a variety of slings and can be lifted about; the other is the more rigid bath-seat with arms, called the "Ambulift". In the latter the principle is rather like the industrial fork lift; the patient can be placed on the seat while still on her bed, the seat is clipped onto the apparatus which is then pushed down the corridor on its castors in perfect safety (see Plate 4a and 4b), the seat being lowered right into the bath (or onto a mobile frame to turn it into a sanichair), and so the patient goes back to bed without ever having to leave the special seat. This has proved to be an outstanding piece of geriatric nursing equipment, deservedly popular with patients and staff. It has revolutionized bathing techniques for frail or heavy, crippled people who can sit up. It is fast, simple and safe to operate. The apparatus requires enough space round the bath for its spread legs to be guided each side, and the access from wards and corridors must be good.

Hoists can be used by intelligent relatives for nursing very crippled people at home, and the type generally chosen for general adaptability is one of the hydraulic sling-hoist varieties. Smaller, mechanically operated apparatus (e.g. the Medilift) may be better in confined spaces at home. When nurses working in pairs are busy they usually discard hoists as too slow, preferring the direct lift. For patients who are very large indeed, they are nevertheless the only answer.

Clothes and Clothes Lockers

It is not humane to deprive grown men and women of their clothes. Letting them sit in their night attire makes them feel like invalids, and putting on their daytime clothes over nightgear is hardly any better. We should wherever possible let them wear clothes – and their own clothes at that. Dressing may take a long time if one is struggling, but for most patients there is all the time in the world if the room is warm and there is some privacy from curtains. There are many ways of arranging clothes and their fastenings so that disability can be overcome, and there is not space enough here to detail all the possible adaptations. A regular, practical review of clothes suitable for elderly and disabled people needs to be made. The Disabled Living Foundation has made a study of clothing for people with disabilities, much of which would be useful for older patients, disabled or not. When doctors visit elderly people at home and try to examine them, when home nurses try to wash or bath them, they see what extraordinary difficulties are created for patients by totally unsuitable clothing; but these patients seldom like change! There is no reason why the same absurdities should be carried over into the Hospitals and Homes by the authorities, when they are called on to do so by providing patients with thoroughly impracticable attire. The cheapest hospital clothing usually gives the nurses the most trouble in every respect.

The principle should be that the patient ought to be able to get out of her clothes easily, and, perhaps with some help, put them on for herself, and the design and fastenings should help, not hinder.

In some wards it is possible to have a cupboard close at hand and the patient's clothes on hangers ready to be brought to the bedside. To have clothes squashed into old suitcases and stacked away is ludicrous. In some wards large lockers are sometimes provided in which clothes can be hung full-length; but these lockers tend to be bulky and to obscure the nurses' view of the patients. They are probably better kept for long-stay or rehabilitation sections than for assessment wards, where patients may be extremely ill. Ward lockers generally should be interchangeable right-for-left, because the correct placing of the locker for seeing and reaching is vital for any patient who has hemiplegia or hemianopia or if, because of crippling arthritis, she cannot manage with the locker in the place it would normally occupy.

Sanitary Apparatus

Excretory problems are a major preoccupation in all old people's wards. If they cannot use any other methods, then bedpans and urinals have to be used. Such is the pressure of hard work for nurses that their load must not be added to by anything which could be avoided. Disposable systems for bedpans and urinals are essential; their first cost may be high and the running costs are high also, but this sort of expenditure is even more essential and unavoidable in geriatric wards than in others where more patients can attend to themselves.

PRACTICAL METHODS

The Bedclothes

There is no need for special bedclothes for older people, but it should be remembered that they are inactive and often feel the cold. Indeed, ward temperatures need usually to be a little higher (say 21–24°C) for them than for younger people. The objection they often raise to the bedcradles which they must have is that these allow their feet to get cold. The quality of the bed linen must be kind to the patients' elderly and fragile skin. One hospital authority, intent on avoiding any risk of theft, caused its draw sheets to be woven deeply along their entire length with the name of the authority in one inch letters; so this name became printed on the behinds of all their older patients! Draw sheets are not needed for continent patients who spend much of their day out of bed.

Absorbent paper incontinence pads are often used if there is any risk that the patient will be incontinent. If not, then they are pointless. An incontinence pad must be capable of absorbing at least one pint of urine without overflowing, or it will be useless. There has been a vogue for natural sheepskin pads for bedfast patients to lie upon; these are comfortable but expensive and not suitable for those who are incontinent. The synthetic "North" pad is longer lasting, and can be used even with incontinent patients.

Position in Bed

The patient who has to be in bed is really best sitting right up, or lying right down, because the 45° position causes shearing stresses on the buttocks. However, frequent changes of position, using the overbed chain and handle, are best of all. The importance of the bedcradle has been emphasized already. Heel-protecting tubipads and wedgeshaped "Lennard" pads will help to preserve the heels. The latter pads have in fact a double purpose; they can be used with their wedge placed to let the calves slope gently upward and keep the heels free from the bed; they can alternatively be wrapped round an entire limb and strapped in place with the serrated cuts outward, so that a very vulnerable foot is protected in any position whatever (see p. 207).

Lifting

Nurses do not need anyone to remind them of the importance and difficulties of lifting heavy inert old people. The well-known shoulder or Australian lift is ideal, but so often the patient cannot co-operate even with this. The important thing to remember in any lift is that sliding the patient up the bed rather than lifting her clear involves a great risk of tearing her sacral or buttock skin, and a single handed lift is of course a great danger to the nurse's own back than one done with the help of a colleague.

Routines of Turning

An unconscious patient should never be lying on his back; otherwise, for an inert but conscious patient, two hours on one side, two hours on the back, and two hours on the other side is a reasonable routine. So much depends on the vulnerability of the patient to pressure effects (see below, and Chapter 5). Nothing less than two-hourly turning is safe for a very ill patient, and in special circumstances it may be necessary to start one-hourly turning. This is the most basic point in prevention of pressure sores, and all other methods – like ripple mattresses – are subsidiary or bonuses, and not substitutes for this most basic nursing duty. Turning must continue in the night too in any case of doubt. Broken sleep is greatly preferable to a broken back. It is important to see that by means of pillows and positioning of the upper knee in flexion, the patient stays on the side on which she has been placed. There are now many elaborate turning frames, special beds and expensive mechanical contrivances to assist the turning of patients. They are usually found in special units like paraplegia and burns units, but it is unrealistic to suppose that they could be generally supplied to reduce the inevitable necessity of conscientiously turning ill patients in geriatric departments. There is really no substitute for good nurses, in good personal health, using good lifting and turning techniques.

Feeding

Dietary principles in geriatrics are outlined in Chapter 6, but there is a great deal of difference between providing the food and getting it accepted and into the patient's stomach. He has his problems; he may have no teeth; his swallowing may be difficult; he may have a poor appetite and very clear preferences; he may not be able to use his best hand, nor even steady a glass. First, it is vital that the food should be hot from the trolley, in an acceptable form, and in a portion which is not dauntingly large. It must be placed at the right height to be seen, and within reach of the normal active feeding hand, even if this happens to be the non-dominant hand in a stroke case.

Some very desirable foods like oranges cannot be tackled by many old people without help. Some people would like to eat with a knife, spoon and fork as usual, but they may find it impossible: that does not mean everything must then be given to them as a mash to be eaten with a spoon. Some food can be diced into fair sizes for spearing with a fork one-handed. Bearing in mind that many old people literally chew with their gums, it is not hard to see why tough foods end up as "plate-waste".

Cutting off the rind of bacon and the skin of meat and sausages is a labour of love not to be forgotten. A deep plate or a plate bunker will help a one-handed eater, and so will a "Nelson" combined fork and knife. Blind people need deep plates always, for finding food without pushing it over the edge; and it is easy to forget to tell them what is on the plate. All sorts of modifications of standard cutlery are available, and every ward should have a good selection. For self-help drinking through non-spill cups or using a flexible straw may make all the difference. Many patients with swallowing difficulties can be greatly helped by the food being made soft, smooth and liquid. A liquidizer is a vital piece of equipment anywhere where frail or elderly invalids are being nursed.

Many elderly patients have to be fed, but it may be possible to do this for two people at once, sitting between them, and the very act of sitting to feed a patient makes him feel that one has plenty of time, and this is psychologically of great importance. Though "bibs" are, sadly, needed in some cases, they are a comedown for an adult; but even a bib is better during a meal than having a foodstained shirt or frock for the rest of the day. A half-filled cup (filled twice over of course!) is usually better than risking an overfilled one being spilt. There are very few elderly patients who will not benefit from fresh fruit, though it may have to be prepared for them by nurses. A good alternative is a glass of fresh fruit-juice daily.

Fluid Needs

Keeping the fluid intake satisfactory is one of the nurses' greatest problems with all old people. We have all seen the dehydrated old patient with an unused full water jug on her locker top because there are so many other calls on the nurses' time. The need for fluid is not less than 3 pints a day (say 2.5 litres), and with some diseases and especially with fever the need is much greater, particularly if little food is being taken. Yet so many geriatric patients, especially old women, refuse to drink. The problems of dehydration are discussed in Chapter 5. All manner of drinks can be given if the patient is swallowing normally, and "temptation" can be put in his or her way. A promised daily glass of beer or stout will sometimes work wonders. Tap water is of course the standard fluid, but 4.3% dextrose with one-fifth normal saline will cover most needs till the doctors can be consulted whether an intra-gastric drip is needed or not. The ethics of using a naso-gastric tube are discussed on page 257. Some care must be used with salines (and with Bovril, etc.) in the case of patients with heart disease. Most patients – especially the fat ones – are convinced of the "nourishing" properties of glucose-fortified or sweetened fruit drinks. Certainly their fattening value is undisputed; they should always be looked at with suspicion on the lockers of large people, and their relatives should be reasoned with! How often the weight-reducing efforts of the entire geriatric team are frustrated by indulgent or ignorant patients' visitors.

Medicine and Tablets

Most people have become used to the change from the old bottle of "physic" to the modern tablets; but many elderly people have great difficulty in swallowing tablets, and a high proportion of them either forget, or refuse, or hide away their tablets, often because they think they are doing them harm! Worries of this kind need to be talked over. The truth is, either at home or in hospital a great many tablets prescribed for old people are found in the bed or the waste paper basket, or are being quietly hidden away to be put into the lavatory later. Many powerful modern drugs need to be given in accurate dosage, and one duty of nurses is really to see that the drug reaches its destination, or to report the failure of the patient to take the drug. Blank refusal is not uncommon. Naturally, once a drug has been injected, one knows it is in the body, but nobody likes to give injections, especially to old people, if there is any other simpler, safer route. Modern drug formulations have taken into account the difficulties of getting older people to take drugs. So, many are now available in syrup form and it is easier to persuade "difficult" patients to accept these. At home many old people find difficulty in opening drug bottles or reading the labels, and many more are muddled and forgetful. Thus "compliance" in drug-taking at home is often bad, and sometimes it is not much better in hospitals. It seems quite illogical that patients should be handed the correct doses of their drugs and continually supervised by nurses while they are in the wards, but the day they have to return home they may have to manage their drug treatment entirely unaided. Common sense suggests that in the few days before returning home they should be allowed to handle their own drugs and medicines, keep them in their lockers or handbags, and take responsibility for them. One must hope that this will become standard practice in preparing people to go home from geriatric wards, despite the possible objections of pharmacists on safety grounds.

Going to the Lavatory

There is no doubt that the best place for going to the lavatory *is* – the lavatory. This then should be an inviting place, warm enough, with no queue, and with time enough allowed to perform this necessary human function. Patients should have every incentive to go to the lavatory on their own, using sticks or aids and wall bars on passages. The next best thing is the sanichair; the next is the ward commode behind curtains; the worst of all is the bedpan.

Getting out of Bed

Getting out of bed should be encouraged except for frail or very muddled people. Getting out at night without supervision is often risky. The height of the bed is quite vital. Too low a bed is impossible to rise from, and one which is too high means a risk of a fall and a fracture. In particular, older people should go about it by easy stages, sitting with their legs swinging over the side for a start, standing and testing their balance, and then moving away with their stick or aid. These stages are particularly important when postural low blood pressure is suspected (see page 107). These castors on a hospital bed should be locked on at all times unless the bed is just about to be moved.

Getting out of Chairs

Teaching the business of getting out of chairs is a physiotherapy and rehabilitation exercise (see page 110), but it has to be watched and supervised by nurses at all other times. Patients must have chairs with arms for this, and should lean forward first, with feet back, and a thrusting upwards movement used, with both arms and thighs together. Those who are supervising this – nurses, doctors or therapists – can put one precautionary foot in front of a patient's feet and the other behind the leg of the chair, so that it does not slip backwards, until the patient is up and has found her balance. The same process should go on in reverse during sitting down, but so often patients repeatedly forget to reach back for the arms of the chair before they do sit down. The process should not even start till the patient can feel the seat touching the back of her legs.

Walking with Patients

Doctors, nurses, therapists and orderlies all have to walk with patients. A pulling-backwards stance is totally wrong (see Plate 6a): there are two other very satisfactory positions – either behind the patient, walking in step giving her some gentle support under the armpits, or side by side with her using crossed arms like a skating instructor (see Plate 6b), so as to be able to prevent any tendency to backwards falling, which is so often the pattern when older people start walking again after having been in bed.

Nails and Hair

There is no need to emphasize that care with nail cutting and foot hygiene is essential in any old patient, because arterial disease may so easily be present, and so may diabetes. Toenails should be cut square across and well away from the quick. Some very neglected old people have gross, long, hard curved talons (known as "onychogryphosis"), which require the special skill and equipment of a chiropodist.

The hair of many old men, such as it is, is best left to the barber once it has had a wash. By contrast an old woman's hair can still be her crowning glory. Proper hairdressing is a necessary part of therapy and should be one of the services provided by every geriatric hospital. A great deal of positive good and lifting of morale comes from a shampoo and set given by a hairdresser, even at the very end of life, for any woman who has taken care of her appearance. Nevertheless some of this task may still fall to nurses. Nothing is more depressing than to see rows of elderly women with lank, straight hair which they cannot, or will not bother to tidy. Yet nothing achieves more good more quickly in all nursing than a few strokes with a brush or comb, a pin or two, and a word of encouragement like, "How nice you look now!".

Constipation and Faecal Impaction

The causes and problems of constipation have already been discussed in Chapter 5. Nurses have their part in its management, as have all the team, including dietitians. Constipation, and the faecal impaction which often follows, are a serious disturbance to health and can even temporarily upset mental stability. If a restless old person is struggling to get out of bed at night and cannot explain why, the reason may well be a loaded rectum of which he gives no hint. Even diarrhoea is not always what it seems (see page 53) and a full bladder may be resting, distended, on top of a choked rectum. By the time faecal impaction has taken place it is too late for aperients and purgatives: action per rectum is needed. In the general management of habitual constipation, a regular routine of defaecation, plenty of fluids especially at breakfast time, increased physical activity, bulk-producing laxatives, aperients, wetting agents or even gas-producing or lubricating suppositories all have their parts to play. Yet in the end severe constipation often requires repeated enemas, or manual removal may be needed. The crux of the matter is whether nurses are willing to do rectal examinations as often as necessary to be sure what is going on – and that may have to be quite frequently. It should not be too distasteful in these days of plastic disposable polythene gloves. One of the marks of a good geriatric nurse is that she is used to this duty and does not hesitate to perform it.

It is important to remember that not simply one or two enemas are needed in a stubborn case; it may take a whole series of enemas for two or three weeks before the bowel is clear for a fresh start. This exhausts some patients so has to be done with due care. Sometimes a series of suppositories will ultimately produce the desired result. Sometimes, too, an olive oil enema will just soften hard faeces enough for a start to be made. Once the obstruction has been cleared, a regular check has to be kept for recurrences using rectal examination if necessary. The worst cases of faecal impaction have to be relieved by manual removal under anaesthetic.

Contracture Prevention

The worrying thing about contractures of joints is not only that they occur, but that they occur so quickly. A contracture of a knee joint can appear in three days, and take three months to correct. The subject was dealt with on page 46, and the point was made there that prevention of contractures is not just a matter for doctors and physiotherapists. Success depends upon everyone who has any regular contact with patients being prepared to move their limbs through the full range of movement of which they are capable, and to do it often. So, when patients' beds are being made, and when they are being washed, nurses should see to it that their limbs are not being regularly held in one position, and particularly not in distorted positions. Straightening a limb is best done by placing one hand on the joint to act as a pivot and using the other very carefully to straighten out the joint, stretching the shortened muscle groups, but not so forcibly as to cause pain. It is particularly important to do this when there has been a hemiplegia which is moving from a flaccid to a spastic stage. When a contracture begins to develop in an acute phase of arthritis, however, special measures are needed, and it is not wise to move the joints about in any way without advice.

With one exception the risks in moving patients' limbs about are small; if there is any doubt, medical advice can be sought first. The one exception is the shoulder, which could be dislocated by forcible, unskilled movements especially if the arm muscles are paralysed and flaccid. As soon as a contracture seems to be developing the doctors should be told. A contracture, especially if it is severe, may cause extra problems to nurses because of the difficulty of keeping the skin clean and healthy: it is not only the patients who have a great deal to gain from the prevention of contracture formation.

Pressure Sores Prevention

The prevention of pressure sores should be a combined medical and nursing exercise, in which nurses have the greater part to play. The doctor should indicate in which cases the risk is greatest, and do his best to let the patient be as active as possible to reduce the risk, though sometimes she is just too ill for this to be possible. Nutrition, vitamins, blood and iron supplements should occupy his attention too. The causes of sores, the aggravating factors, and the principles of prevention, have all been discussed in Chapter 5. The core of the matter is relief of pressure, and if a patient is very frail indeed, only slight pressure for short periods may be enough to cause a disaster.

Superficial pressure sores, which are rather like abrasions, are usually not serious, but they can be most painful. Deep sores, though not painful as a rule, are dangerous, and the death rate is high when deep, sloughing sores are present – probably because of the combination of a serious illness, which helps to cause the sore, and the sore itself and the fluid and serum loss. It is well known that the majority of deep pressure sores occur in the first one or two weeks of the illness, and this is the time to be specially watchful.

The basis of prevention is relief of pressure – that is, regular turning, which is a pure nursing exercise. Special precautions like bed cradles, tubipad heel protectors and Lennard pads (Fig. 12) have already been mentioned (see page 200). Other aids are supplementary. The best we yet know of are *water beds* (see below, p. 208) and *ripple mattresses*, especially those of the large-celled variety (with cells about 15 cm across), and with a variable pressure range. Two of these can often be connected to one fairly quiet electric motor – which is another good reason for grouping ill patients close together. Ripple mattresses are justified on the beds of all unconscious and post-operative patients or others who are very inert, as well as especially heavy old people, till they begin to move about of their own accord. These mattresses, though they ought to be available, should never lull the nursing team into a sense of false security. There is no certainty in pressure sore prevention except through personal vigilance and hard work. Neither should one forget that pressure sores can occur over any bony prominence whatever, such as the mid-dorsal spine, the scapulae, and the elbows. In very fragile people even the weight of the head on the pillows causes sores to appear on the ears. The main places are of course the sacrum, the greater trochanters and the heels.

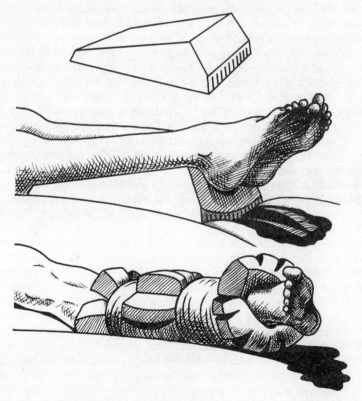

Fig. 12 Use of "Lennard" foam pad (top); to protect both heels (centre); to protect heel and ankle in a restless patient (bottom).

Heel sores are slow to heal, and when they will not heal in a geriatric patient, that patient risks losing a leg.

Regular care of the vulnerable skin is not now so vigorous a procedure as was once considered necessary. A sequence of washing well with a minimum of soap and mildly and generally rubbing the while, followed by drying and powdering, is probably the best. Where the skin might get wet or soiled in incontinence, zinc cream, a waterproof barrier cream, or a silicone spray should help.

Treatment of Pressure Sores

Superficial sores should heal quickly if pressure is relieved at once, and they are kept dry and clean with a dressing. Some nurses like to apply an initial spray of Friar's Balsam (Tinct. Benz. Co.).

To repeat, the treatment of deep sores is first a matter of preventing pressure. If there are sores on two or even three aspects at once (e.g. both trochanters and the sacrum) the problems are immense. Recently there have been developed *water beds*. These have a big, deep plastic envelope, filled with water maintained at body heat by a thermostaticially controlled heater, the whole being contained in a trough on wheels, the size and shape of a conventional bed. The patient simply floats on the surface of the envelope, and his weight is evenly distributed, almost as if he were actually floating in the water. Pressure effects are thus minimised, even over the well-known pressure areas. These beds are a great advance in the treatment of pressure sores, and it follows that they are good for preventing sores in people who are at special risk. They have several disadvantages; (a) they cannot be altered in height; (b) they are cumbersome and very heavy when filled with water – so heavy that they should not be used on upper floors of old buildings without consulting the Works Staff: (c) they are not practical except for patients who are lying down; (d) moving patients "floating" on water beds is difficult for nurses, because there is no firm base for their operations. The earlier models were rather high for nurses below average height, and the edges of the trough were too angular for comfort. It must be remembered that if the water temperature drops, the patient could get into a state of hypothermia. Water beds are normally kept ready connected to the mains supply, even when not immediately in use. Notwithstanding the difficulties of their use, water beds are invaluable. It is not practicable, and it should not be necessary, to have more than a few in a geriatric department.

A much more elaborate bed, the "low air loss" (L.A.L.), bed was evolved for special purposes, and could be of value in the treatment of severe sores. Vertical mattress sections are connected to special air pumps, to feed in warm conditioned air, which slowly escapes upwards. These would seldom be found in geriatric departments, because of their great cost, their maintenance problems, and the special nursing techniques involved. Before the coming of special beds it was sometimes necessary to suspend the whole patient with multiple slings from an overhead frame, or to use sectional "spinal pack" sorbo mattresses, stacked three high and three along, making nine moveable pieces in all, so that the broken skin areas can lie in the gaps.

Deep pressure sores will not respond to any special applications. They ought to granulate from the base if nutrition and asepsis are satisfactory, but they will need packing with gauze if there are any overlapping edges, as so often happens. The black slough can be removed with a scalpel and forceps, a process which is quite painless; alternatively packs of gauze containing a proteolytic enzyme jelly (like Varidase) will help to loosen the adherent sloughs. Some infected sores need paraffin and eusol dressings, and a bacteriological swab may indicate the need for an antibiotic by mouth as well. A recent development in the treating of deep pressure sores, and ulcers generally, has been an absorbent powder made of finely developed plastic grains, sterilised for local application under simple dressings. This substance, "Debrisan", is reported to promote fast healing. It is at the time of writing highly expensive, but the expense of treatment must be measured against the possibility of time saved, and therefore money and resources saved.

Some severe deep sores in a patient with sepsis who is also anaemic will not respond till a blood transfusion is given. There will be much scarring in the healing of deep pressure sores, but this can partly be avoided, and the healing accelerated, by full thickness skin grafting.

It is not necessary to keep a patient with a sore on the back of her heel from walking. Walking short distances on the sole and heel which is covered by a thickly padded dressing may stimulate it to heal, but in bed a Lennard pad will be essential.

Incontinence

A good deal has already been said in Chapter 5 about the basis and causation of incontinence, and the following paragraphs suggest some practical thoughts for the control of this nuisance.

We should never assume incontinence is deliberate unless it is proved to be, and that will be very seldom. Some old people are thought to be just lazy, but considering the discomforts involved in wet beds and clothing, the so-called laziness could very well be a psychological "protect reaction" or else a state of regression (see page 52). Whatever the provocation, it can hardly ever be right to scold an old person for an act of incontinence. Incontinence in unconscious people or severe stroke cases or grossly demented patients is due to a failure of higher cerebral control, as we have seen. Otherwise, it is uncommon for a person who is in full possession of her faculties and alertness to be incontinent unless there is a "local" cause, like a gynaecological disorder, for instance a fistula, or a small "spastic" contracted bladder which is the result of prolonged infection. Nevertheless, some old people are very slow to move, and have urgency of wanting to pass water (precipitancy). It is useless to expect them to be continent if we put them furthest from the lavatory, or if we only have very infrequent "bedpan rounds", or if we fail to answer their calls for toilet attention. It does not take many unanswered calls to make an old person give up hope of getting attention and become indifferent; she may even think incontinence is the accepted standard in that ward! Best of all, of course, she should be encouraged to attend to herself and go out to the lavatory by whatever means she can.

In the control of incontinence the first essential is to discover and record the type of incontinence. Is it stress incontinence? Is it incontinence with overflow? Is it urgency incontinence with a small "irritable" bladder? Does it happen apparently haphazardly and at night, and if so when is the most likely moment? In fact the crucial moment may be the first few minutes after waking in the morning.

Knowing the facts one can institute treatment or a system of "habit-training" – reminding the forgetful to go outside at specified times and not just when the Call of Nature penetrates the mind – which is often too late. Waking old people at night and persuading them to pass urine is a perfectly legitimate exercise to re-establish continence. It is permissible in some cases, but only with medical advice, to restrict fluid completely after 5 p.m.; then the patient is woken last thing at night in order to pass water, and a dry bed may be the reward. With this method it is essential that the patient should have a full quota of fluid during the daytime; otherwise it would be dangerous.

Some drugs like atropine, ephedrine and emepromium bromide (Cetiprin) are supposed to help control incontinent bladders. They may, at the risk of other effects. Some drugs, notably hypnotics, increase the risk of incontinence – and the moral of this does not even have to be stated!

Incontinence aids like absorbent pads or waterproof plastic knickers are not a cure but a help in management. The pants may be a help to people with stress incontinence, or those who want to feel safe when they are out on a trip. If used continuously with people who are totally incontinent they are simply a urinary compress. For men it is easier, for a urine bottle can be left discreetly within reach, provided one is sure the patient can get it into place.

For the regularly and incurably incontinent woman, there are in effect no reliable external appliances, for these devices always leak. Men are more fortunate in that they can have a funnel or pubic pressure urine pouch or disposable condom-type sheath, or a Portex plastic appliance connected to a disposable leg bag or a bedside plastic bag carrier. A few men can manage with a penile clamp, if the springing is just right for their particular needs. All these appliances call for a good deal of co-operation from the patient. None of them are too reliable while the patient is in bed for then gravity cannot operate.

In the most uncontrollable cases the only solution is permanent catheterization for men or women, with a self-retaining indwelling Gibbon or Foley type catheter and closed drainage to a bag. The worry about continuous drainage is always that the bladder, never being allowed to be distended, gradually contracts in size until it would be bound to empty, say, every half-hour in any circumstances. Modern indwelling catheters are not so risky as the older systems were, though the risk of ascending infection is never very far away. Sometimes such patients are prescribed regular urinary antiseptic drugs because of this risk. It may be necessary to start regular bladder washing, and indwelling catheters usually have to be changed every second week.

With a catheter in position it may be possible to re-educate the bladder by clamping off for a specific length of time, then allowing it to drain, then repeating the process (i.e. intermittent drainage). This ensures that the bladder will not have a progressively smaller capacity, as it probably would with continuous drainage. Closed drainage should be the rule anyway – with the catheter connected to a plastic container. It is obvious that a patient is less conspicuous with a plastic leg-bag, worn under trousers or stockings and skirt, than with a plastic bag in a stand on the floor. The latter is perhaps the worst indignity, and if it cannot be avoided, the appliance should surely be hidden discreetly away or at least covered and the tube concealed. A bag on a stand may be necessary for night use, even when a leg-bag is worn by day. Naturally, all patients who have the capability should be expected to empty their own leg-bags, and to transfer the tubing from one container to another if the day and night systems are both necessary.

The answer to incontinence is eternal vigilance, intelligence and ingenuity; above all, making a patient feel a real active human being with proper social obligations to herself and others will greatly reduce the chances of incontinence. Many of the author's ward day-rooms are fully carpeted, and the number of "accidents" is remarkably small.

Colostomy Management

Many older patients have colostomies, some because there was no alternative, and some because (many years ago perhaps) it was considered the only feasible line of treatment, say, for diverticulitis. For a person to have had a colostomy to manage for some time is bad enough, but for an old person suddenly to find herself with such a thing is a severe psychological upset. Many older people whom one might think would learn to manage a colostomy themselves never do so; they think of this as "a nurse's job" and leave the matter there, never being discharged from hospital.

The difficulty is to establish a regular colostomy bowel routine, with one, or at most two, actions a day of the right consistency. It is a question of careful dietary control, with a sufficient use of bulk foods or bulk evacuants, and slowing down of bowel action, if need be, by doses of codeine. A sensible patient knows her limitations exactly; a less sensible one may never get things right.

There are various colostomy dressings, and disposable Chiron bags (and similar devices) with their in-built adhesive patches are ideal. The patient very quickly learns to cut out a hole for the size of the stoma, attach the bag, and close it with its retaining adhesive strip. The difficulty is that aged skin often becomes inflamed with frequent changes of the adhesive ring, and other devices embodying plastic flanges and belts with disposable envelopes to apply are used as alternatives. Some patients just make do with a large sized gauze and wadding dressing under a belt or elastic "Velcro" fastened binder. For a well behaved – once a day – colostomy opening this may suffice, but there is nothing to beat, for convenience, a well fixed "Chiron" plastic bag, except that its disposal is a problem in a private house.

Even self-reliant old people are not very popular in Residential Homes when they have colostomies. There is often an odour which is difficult to get rid of entirely, and there is always the chance of a difficulty arising after, for example, a little excess in the fresh fruit season. However, with a room of her own to retire to and a sympathetic attendant or two, there seems no reason why such a person should not be acceptable in a Home. After all, many manage quite well in their own homes entirely alone.

* * *

At the conclusion of this chapter the author might be allowed perhaps to offer his own opinion that geriatric hospital and home nursing, of all the branches, is *real* nursing. There are interesting technical things to do, but they do not overshadow, as they tend to do in some departments, the real stuff of the job – that of caring for sick people in difficulty and need, according to the very best traditions of the profession, using first and foremost the basic skill and compassion which all people who take up nursing wish to use – because it is in them. Geriatric nursing is hard work; it calls for great patience and optimism; it deals with the whole man or woman and extends out as far as the home. Not all the battles fought turn out to be victories, but by no means all are defeats. Considering we are dealing with people of such an age, we should not be asking for greater success than this. Even in an apparent "defeat" an old person's last hours can be turned into something notable just by the way good nurses shoulder his final burdens for him.

Chapter 14

CARE OF OLD PEOPLE IN THE COMMUNITY

"Home is best". This is not an empty phrase. A great many patients in hospital say it, and mean it with desperate earnestness. It is the phrase hovering on the lips of people when they want to stay at home to be nursed even though they are ill, and most of all when they want to die at home. Home is what most people have worked for, and the place where their roots have gone deep.

In Great Britain the belief is that older people should stay in their own homes for as long as possible. Apart from being what they themselves want, it makes sound economic sense. If it were not for this national policy there would have to be a vast increase in the number of residential homes and hospital wards. Even though the cost of providing help of various kinds for people at home can be high, it is less than the cost of providing other places for them. However if it were not possible to provide enough help; if volunteers ceased to volunteer; if enough paid local helpers could not be recruited, then a fundamental change in national policy would be necessary. In that event old people would have to be herded willy nilly into communal living places or old people's "colonies", to the bitter regret of most of them. It might be administratively a tidy solution, but it is not an acceptable solution.

THE ELDERLY AT HOME

A high proportion of people over 60 are either in their own homes or those of relatives and friends. The figure has been put at about 94%. This may come as a surprise to those who work in hospitals or residential homes, but it is certainly no surprise to people concerned with older people in the community. Since 1948, when Dr. Sheldon of Wolverhampton made perhaps the first serious study of the health and circumstances of older people at home, there have been a large number of surveys. Most surveys by doctors have indicated that though older people felt they were fairly healthy, the doctors considered only one-fifth to one-third were really fit people. Naturally, the older the group, the greater the probabili-

213

ty of unfitness. Indeed – in Chapter 1 there is a telling graph, (Figure 3), which shows how unfitness increases in each succeeding age-group, especially in those decades from 65.

In 1976 Audrey Hunt of the Office of Population Censuses and Surveys carried out a survey on behalf of the Department of Health and Social Security of men and women aged 65 and upwards living in private households in England, to find out how they lived, what they had, and what they wanted most. Interviews were achieved in 1,975 households and involved 2,622 old persons. People in residential homes were not included. At the present time (1979), this is the most up to date study of this vital subject, so it is appropriate to quote from the results, for this helps to put geriatric work generally into a social perspective.

The younger old people aged 65 to 74 and recently retired on the whole had housing and amenities not greatly inferior to younger people, and nine out of ten were able to go out and about without assistance. Thirty per cent of elderly people at home lived alone, and of these the great majority are women (four out of five). The proportion of elderly men who live alone is sixteen per cent as compared with forty per cent of elderly women. The older the group, the more people lived alone.

In 1976 the combined net incomes of nearly half of the married people in the survey was less than £1,500 a year; twenty eight per cent of non-married women and eighty per cent of the non-married men had net incomes of less than £750 a year. This was at a time when the average earnings of adult men working full-time was £3,600 a year. In this survey there was a marked decline in income as age increased. One woman in thirty and one man in twelve had incomes at £2,000 a year or more.

Housing and Amenities

For households where the head was elderly, nearly half owned their own accommodation and nearly one-third rented from a Local Authority – and of the latter, one-third had received rent rebates. As to the date of building of older people's accommodation, one-third was before 1919, one-third between 1919 and 1945, and one-third was more modern. In nine out of ten households there was a separate bathroom. In about one-quarter of the houses older people had to go up or down eleven or more stairs to reach the lavatory from the living-room; twelve per cent had only an outside lavatory. Nearly a third had no heating in the bedroom occupied by old people, and about one-half had no heating in halls or passages and no additional heating in the kitchen. (It was noticeable that the amenities were less satisfactory generally in Greater London, or where there was private renting of accommodation, or where the head of the household was 85 or over). Forty-four per cent of all the households possessed a telephone, but the figure was only thirty-five per cent in households where elderly people were living alone or where the head of the household was 85 or over; and of the latter, only one-quarter had any means of signalling for help. Even then much depended on the vigilance of neighbours. Amongst elderly people living alone, only fifteen per cent possessed a car, but four out of five of all households had gardens, and most of the people were glad to have them.

Employment

One-sixth of the elderly men and one-twentieth of the women were still working, and of these two-thirds were under 70 years old. Nearly half the men would have liked to go on working at the time they were obliged to give up, and most of those still working enjoyed their jobs even though most had had to change to inferior ones when they "retired".

Mobility and Health

Audrey Hunt's survey confirmed a long-held medical opinion that loss of mobility, disabilities and difficulty with looking after themselves rose sharply with increasing age. Five per cent were housebound or bedbound, but at the age of 85 and over that figure was twenty per cent. Of those unfortunate people who were housebound or bed-bound, one-fifth had not been outside their homes for more than three years, and one-quarter were living alone. Special difficulty was found over cutting toenails, bathing, going out of doors alone and using public transport. Between seven and twelve per cent claimed they were not warm enough all the time in bed, or in the living-room, kitchen or out of doors. (The survey was conducted in January and February). Apart from the bed-fast and housebound, seven out of ten of those living alone were able to do all their own shopping, but tasks which were difficult, naturally enough, were those calling for agility and muscular effort.

Visitors

One-quarter of the elderly had received no visits from health or social workers or voluntary organizations for the previous six months. One-third had been visited by a doctor and only one-sixth by a minister of religion. Considering the bedfast and housebound, seven out of ten had been visited by a doctor, one-fifth by a health visitor and thirty-seven per cent by a home nurse. (It seemed likely that vulnerable groups were receiving fewer visits than was desirable).

Social Contacts

Five per cent of all the old people had no surviving close relative except for those, if any, who lived in the same household. Amongst those who were housebound or single the figure was about thirteen per cent. However, forty-two per cent of old people did receive some kind of help from visiting relatives, but five per cent never received any visits from relatives, and twenty-nine per cent received no visits from friends. Many people, especially the bedfast and housebound, would have liked to have had more visits from friends and relatives. Only eighteen per cent went to social centres for the elderly, and the rest often said that poor health prevented them, or that they were poor mixers, or else thought the centres were intended for the lonely or for much older people. The telephone was not much use for social contacts, and amongst those able to use a telephone, there were usually no more than five calls a week. One in seven never received letters from relatives or friends. Ten per cent would not feel able to ask neighbours to help in an emergency, and twenty-five per cent of the bedfast and housebound said the same, yet seventy-two per cent claimed to get on "very well" with their neighbours. Those aged 85 and over and the divorced people were worst off for social contacts.

Transport

Two-thirds had no car in their household, and the ability to use a car fell sharply with age. Two-thirds were aware of special public transport facilities for them in their area, though the nature of these facilities varied widely in different places. For most people the chemist's shop, the pub, the post office and nearest public transport were within ten minutes walk, (one wonders how many country people were included in the survey!). One-half of the elderly people could reach their doctor's surgery within ten minutes, and two-thirds within fifteen minutes.

Interests

Though many had hobbies and interests – no less than younger people – increasing age meant a falling-off in the numbers who kept pets, participated in voluntary organizations, or had individual hobbies. The bedfast and housebound were least able to keep up their accustomed activities and were the least contented, whereas the elderly workers were the most contented.

In general it was ill-health which most people disliked, and loneliness. More wished for volunteers to talk and to be company for them than for any other single form of help. Financial stringency was not often specifically mentioned, but when people were asked for suggestions, financial considerations predominated.

*   *   *

The above is but a brief summary of a survey which went into considerable detail about elderly people and their households. The sample was not perhaps very large, but much trouble was taken to make it as far as possible representative. The conclusions have as much significance for nurses and other health workers as for social workers. They summarise what many working in the community already suspected but could not put into numerical terms. They will give workers in hospitals and homes a greater insight into the likely background of their new arrivals and of those whose return home they are seeking to achieve. The problems of ill-health and loneliness are clearly paramount, and many of these problems might be solved, or prevented even, if everyone was on the alert and if people would just be – more friendly.

SOCIAL NEGLECT VERSUS ILLNESS

There is an idea in the minds of some sociologists that perhaps the problems of old age would all disappear if only people's social conditions were satisfactory. It is tempting to think that most of the diseases of old age could be prevented if pensions were high enough, nutrition was satisfactory, and housing was good. Yet doctors and nurses who spend a large part of their time with old people know that this is just not true – though they wish it were so. In reality the shoe is on the other foot: rather than social breakdown being the cause of the illness, it is much more likely to be the coming of illness which finally causes the breakdown. Many old people live in bad circumstances, neglected and ignored, sometimes in a positively squalid state, but they manage to rub along quite well and cheerfully until an illness strikes them. Then, but only then, the social difficulties make some sort of action urgently necessary.

Most of the illnesses which trouble old people appear without much obvious warning. They are sometimes old maladies breaking out afresh, and many more are due to degenerative processes. Some are the consequence of earlier indiscretions, like a life-time of over-eating. It could be, in years to come, that as a race we learn to eliminate the diseases due to faulty life-styles. The author has written of a certain number of illnesses which he has called "diseases of deprivation". Since deprivations can in theory be made good, so these diseases could be prevented. They include *malnutrition* of all kinds (and even over-nutrition can at times be malnutrition if the obese person has deprived himself of health-protecting in favour of health-ruining food); *deprivation of water* (leading to dehydration); *deprivation of heat* (hypothermia). If one considers the matter carefully, there might also be included here some cases of depression and mental breakdown, (due to *deprivation of affection and incentives*), and a good proportion of *home accidents*. This said, however, there is marked reluctance amongst adults generally to accept health education, and the elderly are not best known for accepting new ideas or liking to be told what is good for them! Here, nevertheless, there could be a most fruitful field for health visitors to work in. The best chance we have for the future is for children in their formative years, at home as well as in school, to be grounded in the rules of healthy living which they might then practise throughout their lives.

The fact remains that however good our social services, however convenient our housing, however high our pensions, these things will not so far prevent artery disease, heart disease, joint degeneration, cancer and a host of other diseases still waiting to be overcome by medical rather than social advances. It is no solution to preventing further breakdowns to start removing everyone at risk to fine new residential homes, for these common diseases will strike there just as anywhere else.

The other side of the coin is, however, that when people are contending with present disabilities or expect future disabilities and increasing frailty as the years pass, satisfactory housing is of paramount importance, and a liberal pension and good local social services will make their lives much easier.

THE ATTITUDES AND RIGHTS OF OLD PEOPLE

Attitudes and outlooks to age and adversity vary greatly. They are part of the man himself, being the results of heredity, upbringing, the buffetings of life, and the presence or absence of plain courage; but sometimes where there used to be great courage it has been sapped by disability, loneliness and neglect. Some people (fortunately for us the minority), are content to take the easiest way, and are quite willing to surrender and go into communal care, which costs them the least personal effort. Many more are ready to carry on at home in spite of the difficulties. The blind are best off in their own houses, knowing the position of every piece of furniture and the number of steps to take for each job to be done. Those who are crippled often find their own ways of overcoming obstacles; often when we take them into hospital we wonder how they possibly managed as they did. Yet when they feel a little better they want to return to their difficult way of living and say so in plain terms. Such courage deserves to be supported, not belittled. We should try to help them get back home, but provide them with more personal help.

Many old people know there will be risks for them at home, and yet still want to take those risks rather than be regimented into a communal way of living. Who are we to say that they may not do this, providing that no one else is being put at risk by it? A difficult set of circumstances might exist where an old person, unsteady on her feet, wishes to return home, but she is known to prefer to use naked lights and there are other people under the same roof.

What person indeed has the right to say that, just because it is not *his* own way, that an elderly client or patient must be prevented from living in rather unclean surroundings, in a general "pickle". All living carries some risks. Even crossing the street is a risk. We cannot guard all people from all risks at all times. If they express different ideas from our own, we shall have done our duty if we have tried to make the risks as slight as possible. We are dealing with adult citizens, not children. On occasions when a mental disorder means the individual is no longer capable of taking personal responsibility, then perhaps other action may be needed. Elderly people have rights, just like the rest of us. They have the right to do as they wish with their lives, to go where they want to (within reason) and to control their own affairs, dispose of their own property (or *not* dispose of it as the case may be), take their own discharge from a hospital if they so desire, and refuse to enter if they do not wish to (but see page 235). It is totally wrong that any old person should be for example taken away to hospital without her consent, or without even having been told about it. Yet this happens from time to time, hospital ward staff are sometimes confronted by a bitter, unco-operative patient who says that the first she has heard of this hospital admission was when an ambulance arrived at her door and the crew said, "You must come with us".

On the other hand, these senior citizens surely have no right to unlimited care from relatives just *because* they are the senior members of the family. They do not have the right to disrupt the entire lives of the younger generation, imposing without mercy on the good nature of their nearest and dearest. Sometimes it happens, indeed, that a submissive younger relative simply has not the strength, knowledge and force of character to control an older relative in the difficult circumstances of an illness.

Again, older people have no right to endless hospital treatment if the need has passed, and no right to occupy a special bed or a special chair in hospital regardless of the needs of other patients.

Besides rights, old people also have certain obligations: they ought for example to behave reasonably to the people who are trying to help them, especially to their nurses. They ought to be considerate towards their fellow patients or residents in homes or hospitals. If they do not behave as they ought, it may occasionally be "sheer devilment", but much more often it is because they are ill, or mentally disturbed, or frightened, or resentful of some imagined neglect or insult. In the well worn phrase, old people ought to try to "grow old gracefully" – but which of us can be sure that we shall have matched up to this requirement when our time comes?

THE ATTITUDES OF RELATIVES AND FRIENDS

There are great numbers of unselfish people who take endless trouble to help and care for their elderly relatives and friends, and they do not always get much thanks for their pains. When illness suddenly comes, the attitudes of these supporters may be crucial. At times the older person's own behaviour and ill-temper makes other people unwilling to help, and no one can blame them for lack of support. It is then that the Hospital or Social Services have to step in.

In other circumstances the younger generation prove to be too sentimental or cautious and do harm that way. Perhaps they put the patient to bed for the sake of "safety", little knowing how hazardous this can be. Or they wait on them hand and foot even when they are still able to do many things for themselves and would be far better if they had to do them. Some old people take advantage of this situation and become more and more demanding, eventually staying in bed continuously as if it were their right. In other words, adopting too helpful an attitude may make a rod for one's own back. The younger generations of families so often say they "have not the heart" to deny an aged mother or father anything. This also is a dangerous attitude. Some make promises they are unable to keep – about looking after their parents "come what may", and then find they cannot. An absolute promise like this is a foolish one ever to make.

Some relatives believe they should never leave an old person alone for a moment, and occasionally a doctor or a Home Nurse issues instructions in those terms, though there is no justification for so definite and so impracticable a suggestion. Other people are frightened of anything going wrong, thinking that they will be blamed by the neighbours, the police, or even the coroner at an inquest. They badly need reassurance that the whole responsibility does *not* rest on them, and they will not be blamed. If they have done their best, more cannot be expected of them

Other relatives take the line that their old people, by virtue of being old, are no longer responsible citizens, so they take all decisions for them and never ask their opinion even about their own affairs. All professional workers should beware of relatives and friends who act like this, for there is a moral responsibility to protect the proper interests of patients and those whose old age and frailty put them at a disadvantage in a battle of wits and words. It is such forceful people who may sell up the home and furniture once the older relative has gone into a hospital, assuming that is the end of the matter, and sometimes without even consulting her!

Sometimes it happens that there is a marked coldness from the younger generation to one of the older, and reluctance to help. There are many possible explanations, but the reason can sometimes be traced to an unhappy childhood in which the parent ignored, dominated or even physically ill-treated the offspring. Apparent neglect or callous indifference by the younger generation could suggest a skeleton in the family cupboard. Expecting affection and help in later life may then be expecting too much altogether! There is a moral here for to-day's parents.

Conflicts
It often happens that what the old person wishes and what the friends

and relatives consider "right" are total opposites, and bring them into conflict. This happens particularly when the question of whether or not the old person should "go away" arises. The elderly person herself may not wish to give up her home, but the family and friends, seeing her deteriorating, say, "Something must be done." Sometimes they do so out of genuine concern, sometimes because they do not wish to be bothered any more, and sometimes they are altogether too cautious. It is a difficult situation, especially if the lives of other people and young children in the household are being upset. Medical opinion and advice is needed, and treatment may help; but all professional workers must be wary of such a situation, and (if anything) err on the side of taking the older, weaker person's part. Sometimes the "Something must be done" is in fact morally the wrong line to follow, and anyway impossible to put into practice legally because one knows the patient or client does not agree. To say as much may not make one particularly popular; but nevertheless it must be said.

THE FAMILY DOCTOR

The General Practitioner carries the immediate responsibility for the medical needs of his patients at home. Because of the fact that there are so many people at home, the family doctor often practises more geriatric medicine than the hospital physician, though he may not call it by that name. He knows that old people make more calls on his time than younger ones, because their problems are so often half social and half medical; they require more consultations per year on average than younger adults. He stands in a special position towards his older patients, because they come of a generation which seldom questioned a doctor's opinion, and will obey it to the letter – though some will not! Even so, the doctor must advise, not dictate. He is often in a difficult position, being the family physician and friend of all the generations of a family, and sees their interests beginning to clash.

Nevertheless the family doctor is in a splendid position to practise prevention of disease if he can find which of his many patients are the most vulnerable. Those who have recently retired, or have been bereaved, or are always lonely, certainly comprise a vulnerable group. Yet so few elderly patients will go to him and report symptoms at a time when they might be cured. There is therefore great scope for Health Visitors working with doctors in a practice or from a Health Centre, as the growing tendency is today, to work out a system of unobtrusive detection of deprivation and illness by a regular, almost "social call' kind of visiting. The social undercurrents of a disease in old people are of the greatest importance and the family doctor sometimes needs prompt help from a Social Worker. Under the recent new organization of social service departments of the major local authorities it should be easier for family doctors to call upon social work support, and there is now, in theory anyway, only one route by which all kinds of official social service help may be obtained. Previously the doctor may have had to telephone separately the home help supervisor, the meals-on-wheels organizer, and others. Similarly, he now has one route to obtain home nursing for his elderly patients as necessary, and the home nursing equipment needed for the job. Both are obtained through the community nursing section of the local Health District of the reorganized National Health Service. In practice the doctor usually forges close but informal links with the social worker in his own locality and with the local home nurse, who in many cases, (especially in country districts), becomes known as the "practice nurse" because of her close professional association with the doctors of that practice. The general practitioner may also need prompt admission to hospital for a patient who cannot be nursed at home; this a good geriatric department should be ready and willing to provide.

COMMUNITY NURSES

It must be apparent to any sensible observer that community nurses (home nurses) have to deal for much of their time with older patients, since most of the latter spend a good deal of their existence at home. The elderly have a high incidence of disease and disability in addition to being often frail and having difficulty with many daily activities which younger people find simple. Many cannot easily get to the doctor's surgery; even less are they able to reach a hospital outpatient department, so it is the home nurse who is the friend and confidante of all her old people, nursing them through their lesser illnesses while trying to ensure these do not become major illnesses through complications. She it may be who supervises the treatment and control of their diabetes, administers their injections, dresses their long-standing ulcers, helps them with their stroke and arthritic disabilities, as well as doing numberless other practical things for them.

A recent analysis of the work of one group of community nurses shows how wide is the range of their duties (see below).

The Pattern of Work of Home Nurses
The Suffolk Area Health Authority has recently sponsored a survey of community nursing which was presented to the Authority by the Area Nursing Officer* in November 1977. The author gratefully acknowledges the Authority's permission to quote from the report items which must be of interest to all nurses, and no less to doctors, social workers and ad-

---

* Miss I. M. Clark, S.R.N., S.C.M., H.V. – Personal Communication

ministrators interested in geriatric work and in the provision of services generally.

This was a survey involving a particular group of community nurses at work in a particular National Health Service area, but the patterns of work revealed should not necessarily be taken as typical of those for all community nurses everywhere. It would be wrong, for example, to use the figures in any way as "norms" for calculating resources or staff needed. These patterns are of interest as they stand, and the age profiles are particularly informative.

Suffolk comprises a large rural community scattered widely around two principal towns about 30 miles apart. The total population at the time of the survey was 489,000, the proportion of retired people being slightly above the national average (17.2 per cent as compared with 16.5 per cent). Naturally most rural health and social workers must expect to travel longer distances to reach their patients or clients than equivalent town and city workers.

Some 180 home nurses in various grades, (S.R.N., S.E.N., students and nursing auxiliaries), participated. After suitable guidance in the method to be used and a brief pilot survey, they themselves recorded on pro formas everything they did professionally in one week in mid-April 1977. The results were then analysed by a computer. The questions under consideration were the number of daily visits, the number of patients seen, their ages, where they were seen, how much time was spent in various activities, (including discussion, liaison and travelling), and what basic nursing and what technical procedures were carried out.

Some results of the survey are as follows:

(a) Over 8,700 patients were seen in the week, with a weekday average of 1,461; about half that number were seen on Saturday, and less than half on Sunday.

(b) Nearly eighty-nine per cent were seen in their own homes, 8.7 per cent in general practitioners' surgeries or health centres, but less than one per cent in old people's homes.

(c) The average time spent with each patient at his home was 21 minutes, with a range of 18–23 minutes.

(d) Amongst the fifteen types of technical procedures recorded, five per cent were post-operative dressings, but thirty-eight per cent were other sorts of dressings. Some fourteen per cent of procedures were insulin injections, and a similar proportion of other sorts of injections. Urine-testing made up ten per cent of the special procedures.

(e) An age profile of patients receiving these technical procedures was made. The present author has calculated the proportion of these procedures used in people aged over 65 as compared with all ages put together. Thus, of technical procedures undertaken, the following proportions were on behalf of older patients:

Post-operative dressings	33%
Other dressings	71%
Insulin injections	86%
Other injections	50%
Urine-testing	77%

(Sum total of all technical procedures on behalf of elderly patients = 66%)

(f) Basic care treatments performed by these home nurses were – assistance with bedpans and commodes, care of the hair, nails and feet, bed-bathing, general care, treatment of pressure areas etc. One would expect that older patients at home would be in particular need of this kind of help, and so it proved. Using once more the dividing line of over 65 years, the proportion of basic care procedures performed for elderly people were:

Assistance with bedpan or commode	89%
Bed-bathing	87%
General care and attention	84%
Treatment of pressure areas	83%
Care of the hair, nails and feet	89%

(Sum of all basic care procedures performed for the elderly = 85%)

(g) Certain extra procedures were called for, and many of these were done on behalf of people over 65, viz.,

Teaching and supervision of patients and relatives	73%
Assessing home conditions and patients' needs	75%

(Sum of all extra procedures performed for the elderly = 59%)

So, it can readily be seen what a great deal of home nurses' time is spent on doing things for older patients, but particularly in basic care – and it is surely natural and commendable that this should be the case. It follows that home nurses have need of, and no doubt quickly acquire, great experience of the needs of the older age-groups, and it must be to their particular advantage to have some kind of special training in geriatric nursing and the physiology, psychology and pathology of ageing.

(h) Some interesting statistics about how time was spent also emerged from the survey. Thus, during the survey week the 180 nurses travelled 27,181 miles on duty, which involved them in 1,643 hours of travelling. This meant about 12 minutes travelling per patient seen, and 3.12 miles travelled per patient seen.

Finally, one can quote from this report the follow observations; those 180 nurses spent 51% of their time with patients, 28% in travelling, and 12% in discussion with other people about patients' problems.

HEALTH VISITORS

Health Visitors have a unique opportunity to be the linch-pin of medico-social services to old people at home. Their training includes a study of the ageing process and of disease in old age, sociology, psychology and case work and this, on top of their nursing training and experience, should fit them as almost no other people are fitted for this special geriatric role. This is not to say that they do not have duties towards mothers and babies, children, young people and deprived families: but in geriatrics there is a practical chance to specialize. Some health visitors are employed by local Health Districts of Area Health Authorities specially to form the link between the hospital and the patient's home, seeing the old person before discharge and doing the vital early follow-up visits without which an immediate relapse might take place, meanwhile asking for the various forms of support she finds still to be necessary, and reporting to the hospital doctors when the patient can come for follow-up out-patient visits. This is a most valuable linking service. More and more health visitors are now being employed by secondment (so-called "attachment") to work with groups of family doctors. Here a most vital function could be to visit the elderly who are vulnerable, taking their names from a practice age-sex register, and in general acting as early detectors of all the insidious diseases which are perhaps starting to appear but which will not be reported by the patient direct. She can keep a skilled eye open, see what food is in evidence, hear what is said and how it is said, feel the patient's pulse, quietly ask about symptoms, and in a hundred other ways watch for the early signs of medical trouble and then arrange for the patient to see the doctor at his surgery, or arrange for him to visit. If there were enough practice-linked health visitors the great problem of undetected illness in old age could at last be solved, and a huge load of misery lifted from elderly shoulders. The other great role of a health visitor in respect of elderly patients is as counsellor and friend as well as health educator, as she is with the other age-groups. There is so much to do in this field that there are many who would like to see the establishment of geriatric health visitors to specialize in this difficult art. For some time to come it seems that there will be too few health visitors in training to make a specialist professional group like this a practical possibility.

SOCIAL WORKERS

It would not be appropriate for a medical author to attempt to show Social Workers the measure of their importance in caring for the elderly at home. Except for the medical and nursing requirements, they are the almost universal providers of all that is missing, and so often badly needed. The purpose of the chapters of this book so far has been to demonstrate in every way possible the effects which illness and disability have upon the domestic circumstances of the elderly, and on those who are devoting themselves to the care of elderly people within their family. If Social Workers were ever to say (and they would not) that sickness and disability is none of their business, then they would be burying their heads in the sand. The present concept is of a Social Worker devoted to the interests of the family as a whole. Not even a geriatric physician would pretend that the older members are the most important units in a family, but neither are they *uni*mportant units. It is easy to find enthusiasms and public support for the care of the young who are afflicted and disabled; it is not so easy to find the same support for the old and disabled. So, particular care is needed to give them a full measure of time and trouble, bearing in mind they gave of *their* best a few years earlier.

A single Social Worker beset on all sides by conflicting pressures may wish he or she had the wisdom of Solomon. He will be able to call upon a large number of facilities. One present difficulty is that these are provided for, but not *equally* provided in all areas. Some Authorities make good provision, and others much less. The solution to the mounting problem of domiciliary care for old people is not so much reorganizing the administration as a simple matter of money – money to provide more services at the right time and place Social Workers (with a great variety of duties).

One can list the services currently open to Local Authorities to provide as follows:

Mental and Blind Welfare Services
Welfare Services for the Deaf and Physically Handicapped
Home Helps (Domestic Help Service)
Nightwatching Service
Special Laundry Facilities
Recuperative Holidays
Chiropody

It should not be too difficult for the social services and health services to work together now for the benefit of patients and clients – since their reorganizations in recent times. There remains a division nevertheless, because the two groups of professionals are responsible to different authorities, and the geographical boundaries of their administrative units are not identical. Except in London there is usually similarity if not total identity between the boundaries of Area Health Authorities and the County Councils. However, the sub-divisions of administration and the boundaries below that level are not the same, and this is certain to cause some difficulties in communication and acceptance of responsibility. Hospital staffs, in particular, drawing patients from a wide area, may find they have to refer their patients' social problems to a variety of different social services officers. There is evidence, from the report of the joint working party of the Department of Health and Social Security and the Personal Social Services Council ("Collaboration in Community Care", published by the Social Services Council, 1978) that much co-operation between senior officers of the social and health services at the administrative and consultative level takes place. Readers of this book will be more concerned to know whether there is (or could be) good co-operation between health and social services at the point where it matters most, i.e. where an individual patient or client is in need. Again, there is evidence that co-operation is generally getting better. Yet doctors, especially family doctors, are independent workers and are quite often dealing with life and death matters. They themselves are accustomed to prescribing treatment immediately and asking for rapid solutions for social crises. Field social workers on the other hand are members of a team organization, which means that they cannot often provide immediate solutions to problems but would have to refer to a more senior social worker at their headquarters. Perhaps doctors and other health workers, thinking that the social problems of their patients are not being dealt with quickly enough, do not always understand the differences between the two organizations. There are also some understandable problems about communicating confidential medical information to non-medical social work staff. On the other side, social service staff may not regard it as necessary to take medical opinion when trying to solve a social problem – or even when arranging admission to a residential home. So, it is obviously necessary that both the social work and the nursing and medical professions should henceforward learn more about each others' outlook and methods of working. In geriatric work their interdependence must surely be specially recognized, not least when arranging for the discharge of frail convalescent patients home after hospital treatment, where the social problems may be truly daunting, and again in the assessing of fitness of former hospital patients to enter residential homes. It is one of the main objectives of this book to draw attention to how diverse and complicated are the physical and mental aspects of older people's cases. Much good might come if medical/nursing and social work staff had some of their early training together, and if part of their instruction came from senior staff from "the other camp".

HOSPITAL SOCIAL WORKERS

Social workers based in hospitals have an honoured place in geriatric work. Hospital doctors dealing with the elderly know that their work would virtually come to a halt if there were not first-class links for the patient with the outside world, and for the geriatric team with the patient's environment. Day by day, hour by hour almost, consultation is needed on hospital premises, even at the bedside, and this must by some means be maintained whatever reorganization might be proposed.

The particular value which hospital social workers have – which may not necessarily be possessed by all social workers – is their understanding of medical and surgical disabilities and the limitations these are likely to impose on people returning home, improved, but not always fully cured. Hospital social workers acquire this special understanding by being involved every day with older people who have several disorders at once, and whose commonest illnesses (like arthritis, heart disease or strokes), are likely to leave persistent problems. They commonly attend and contribute vitally to discussion on hospital ward rounds, or they participate in case conferences after ward rounds, if that method is in use in their particular hospital. They should certainly be present to put their clients' cases in the correct light at any "allocation meetings" were the priorities of admission of hospital patients to residential homes – taken alongside the claims of those waiting in the community – are being considered.

Hospital social workers should have the right of direct access to senior doctors in a geriatric department, because of the vital and sometimes highly confidential nature of the information they have available, which affects patients' prospects of discharge and future happiness at home. They must also be "watch-dogs" over the patients' interests – domestic and sometimes even financial – when they are at a disadvantage by being confined in a hospital ward.

THERAPISTS AT HOME

There are now increasing numbers of occupational therapists and physiotherapists who are employed by local authorities rather than by health authorities. Their function is to treat patients at home for conditions which are not serious enough to require hospital admission. There is bound to be some discussion about whether therapists might not be employed more effectively using hospitals as their bases. Similarly, there is controversy about whether elderly patients with, say, strokes should be admitted to hospital or stay at home (if home conditions are satisfactory). This is no place to examine these complicated arguments. However, therapists employed to work with patients at home play a vital part in advising about adaptations to furniture, fittings etc., to help people face their disabilities. Hospital-based therapists are able to do the same thing for patients whom they have treated in the wards, and they commonly make home visits, taking their patients with them, to this end. Clearly there must be close co-operation between all therapists whoever employs them, about these crucial matters of providing aids and adaptations. It is nonsensical that patients ready to return home should be held up for lack of some simple piece of apparatus or modification to their houses.

VOLUNTARY WORKERS

No one will deny that there is infinite scope for voluntary effort in the care of old people. This goes on day and night when good neighbours help in crises, and in the far more exacting business of helping people over long periods, by doing some of their housework, shopping for them, carrying in meals for those who cannot cook, and generally "keeping an eye on things".

There is also another great body of voluntary help organized through voluntary societies such as, in particular, the local branch of "Age Concern", the British Red Cross Society, the Order of St John and the Women's Royal Voluntary Service, who run the Meals on Wheels service in so many districts with the help of Local Authority funds. In addition these indefatigable organizations arrange the following activities:

Old People's Clubs
Day Centres
Disabled Persons' Clubs
Friendly Visiting Schemes
Holiday Schemes
Boarding out Schemes
Loans of Nursing Equipment, and, temporarily, of Wheelchairs
Chiropody Schemes

On a broader scale, national charities like "Help the Aged" collect large sums of money which are devoted to such schemes as special housing, sheltered housing developments and day care centres. These developments have often demonstrated an unexpected need, and they have resulted in national and local government taking up these ideas more widely themselves. "Help the Aged" has lately become involved in a unique experiment by providing funds to build and equip (at Ipswich in Suffolk) a special rehabilitation centre for older patients within a hospital. Here are, combined, special wards for inpatients and large spaces where inpatients and day patients share the skills of the same therapists and nurses at the same time. The staffing and cost of running this centre is the responsibility of the Suffolk Area Health Authority. So, this is an example on quite a large scale of voluntary initiative and a statutory body within the National Health Service working side by side to fill a particular geriatric need.

Without voluntary effort the burden upon the "official" services would long ago have passed breaking point. There is every indication that more voluntary effort will be needed in every sphere if we are to keep pace with the future trends of old people's needs. Already we see evidence of it in the encouragement of volunteers to help in many Day Centres, Day Hospitals, and also in the physical nursing of older people in geriatric hospital wards themselves. There may be those who can offer a regular hour or two of their time to assist the hospital which has helped them by admitting a sick elderly relative of their own. Such arrangements mean that a good working relationship must be established between the professional nurses and the volunteer helpers. The former ought not to look on the latter as "interfering", but should give them suitable jobs within their capabilities – like feeding helpless patients and helping others to gain mental stimulation – then the ward staff will have more time to use their own special skills.

The one essential thing about voluntary work is that it should be regular. A promise of friendly visiting of a lonely old person means that she will come to rely on the visit as a special event in her day or her week, and her disappointment will be intense if the visitor forgets to come after all. Volunary work in support of a hospital, day centre or club is best arranged on a group basis with an organizer so that any unforeseen circumstance need not leave a task "uncovered".

In the organization of voluntary work, defending the rights and interests of older people and giving them information, there is in most places an active Old People's Welfare Council which does most valuable service, and helps to co-ordinate voluntary activities, while itself being financed by grants and voluntary activities.

SPECIAL PROBLEMS OF HOME CARE

Isolation

Isolation can be experienced in teeming cities and in remote country parishes. It can be isolation by distance, or isolation by temperament and behaviour, when people get cut off from friends by their unwelcoming attitudes or if they have lost old friends and cannot somehow make new ones. About one-fifth of all old people are to some extent isolated; a great many live entirely alone, and the majority of them are widows or spinsters. It would be wrong to assume that they are all deprived or unhappy simply because they are alone; but when illness strikes action is needed. In villages a few tell-tale signs, and the word goes round. In towns the milkman may be the one who first gives the alert. It has happened in cities that isolated people have died and their bodies have not been found for two or three weeks; this does not say much for the community spirit of the local people. It happens sometimes that two old people, man and wife, or sisters perhaps, or two friends, are both frail; each can do something but neither can do everything, and when one falls ill the delicate balance is destroyed and both have to be admitted to a hospital or a Home. A useful description for these pairs of people is to call them "semi-isolates".

Isolation can even happen when a group of old people's bungalows or flats are placed together and no provision is made for any warden or Home Nurse or any younger person to live nearby. Then, though they are all close, no one can help anyone. Planning could hardly be less intelligent than this.

Mobility

Several times in these pages it has been said that mobility is the key to independent living. Immobility results from joint disease, fractures, obesity, heart and lung disease, and from time to time simply because of "bad feet". The latter at least is one factor which we can guard against, with chiropody and timely orthopaedic surgery. One of the worst hindrances to mobility is bad footwear, particularly the use of bedroom slippers at all times of the day. Occasionally people who use them are too lazy to wear anything else, but bedroom slippers more often than not speak of corns or swollen feet and thus indicate the need for specific treatment.

Even so, mobility itself is relative: an old woman can be housebound, yet if all her supplies can be organized, her immobility is not a serious social problem. Living downstairs is the simplest solution to the problem of not being able to climb the stairs; yet how often old people will not accept the logic of this – they are completely set in their ways, they will not compromise, and that is an end of the matter. Old people may be immobile in a ward or in a Welfare Home and yet manage to get about their own homes just by holding onto pieces of furniture placed at the strategic points. Many people with arthritis or following on strokes when asked to walk say, "I cannot; I have been sitting too long". The only answer to this is that they should *never* sit too long! The greater the likelihood of getting "set fast", the more necessary it is that old people should take a turn round the room with the help of whatever walking aid or furniture is at hand.

A great deal can be done to aid mobility and self-help before there is talk of "going into a Home", like putting extra handrails on stairs and in passages, eliminating door sills, fastening grab handles, providing ramps in place of steps, or adapting kitchens. There is no end to the possibilities.

Yet it must be said that some local authorities whose responsibility it is seem unable to take rapid action even when what is needed has been precisely explained.

Feeding

The problems of nutrition in older people have been dealt with in Chapter 6. Nevertheless there are many points to consider on the home front. Meals on Wheels are of the greatest possible assistance to those too old and frail to cater and cook for themselves; but the real need is for a service providing at least one hot meal a day seven days a week. This is not practicable under present arrangements. Many schemes can manage no more than two or three meals a week. Meals on Wheels are run by volunteer staff, but largely financed by Local Authority funds (with a contribution from the patient herself), and the Local Authority usually provides help with equipment and cooking facilities. If daily meals cannot be provided for lack of sufficient volunteers, it is hard to see why the service should not be supplemented by official paid staff.

One of the most sensible functions of a Home Help is that she should so time her visits as to be able to cook a meal for her elderly charge. One great problem for most elderly people living alone is that preparation of a single portion is tedious, yet preparing larger portions and keeping part for another day is risky, particularly when food storage arrangements are primitive – as they so often are. It is sad that the day still seems far away when all elderly people will have refrigerators (and telephones) and will know how to use them. Day clubs and day centres should do much to help old people have one good meal a day, a meal which provides the larger part of the protein and protective foods which they so much need.

Incontinence

Bed-wetting and clothes-wetting are the last straw which so often cause otherwise helpful relatives to ask for a patient's ultimate admission to hospital. Even in hospital this makes a difficult problem to solve, as we have seen. Nevertheless, after a careful diagnosis of the cause has been made – and this is essential – one of the first rules of preventing incontinence at home is to try to keep the patient out of bed, while the next is to provide the wherewithal to be continent. In other words, a commode chair of the right height at the right place – very close to the side of the bed – and of the armchair type but with one arm removed perhaps to make it easier to slide from bed to chair. This at least gives the patient the chance, if she has a mind to be continent. If the incontinence cannot be cured, but the patient wants to go on trying to manage, a great deal can be done with plastic sheeting, with plastic mattress covers and various types of incontinence pants and diapers, and other devices which are mentioned in Chapter 13. Surgical appliances for incontinence in men are fairly practicable with a co-operative patient, but no really reliable appliance for a woman has yet been devised other than catheterization, with all that that implies. Large absorbent paper incontinence pads are a help on beds and chairs, but they must be large enough for their purpose. Disposal of large quantities of wet paper creates difficulties in most small households. Special laundry schemes are of the greatest possible help in the management of incontinence at home, and could be adopted everywhere if local commercial laundries would assist. It is a service which more large-scale hospital laundries might undertake in the future more often than they do now.

Home Accidents to Old People

Accidents at home have already been mentioned in Chapter 5, and we have already seen that the causation of accidents is either the natural process of senescence or of disease, or of the patient's environment. The latter is where prevention has the greatest possibilities. The hazards surrounding some old people in badly maintained houses, with ancient wiring, trailing flexes, old electrical appliances, old oil stoves, lack of fire guards, loose mats, rickety furniture, piles of newspaper and dark stairways with loose stair-rods, old gas geysers in bathrooms – these have to be seen to be believed. It is a useful exercise when visiting an old person's home to make a list of what could be done to improve matters. Any health worker, any doctor or any social worker could do this, and most old people will not object if the subject is broached tactfully. Improvements cost money, but families will often help in practical ways once the hazards have been shown to them. The stairs and the kitchen are the two places where most home accidents occur.

HOUSING PROBLEMS

The effect of bad housing and some of the solutions to the problem of housing of older people have been outlined already in Chapter 3. It has been said, and it will bear repeating, that the proper arrangements for supporting old people hinge very largely on their housing. Accidents can often be prevented if the hazards are all removed. There are many ways to demonstrate this. Wall-mounted fires get rid of trailing flexes, and fixed convector heaters are even safer. Electric power sockets fitted at hip height get rid of the need for the householder to stoop down; double-glazing and roof insulation would greatly reduce the fuel bills as well as the risk of hypothermia; bungalows on all counts are safer than houses with staircases. The list is endless, even when we are considering "normal" housing – apart altogether from the special provision which is possible for the more frail, like warden-serviced housing, with centralized boilers for heating and for hot water.

Most needed of all, and at present apparently often still lacking, is the necessary close co-operation between the local Department of Social Service and the Local Authority's Housing Manager and his staff. Proper housing for the elderly is not a matter to be left to chance and personal whim. It should be a specialist study on its own account.

MENTAL UNRELIABILITY AT HOME

Chapter 11 is devoted to the causes and management of mental problems. A sudden unexpected mental change cries out for investigation and prompt action. Nevertheless, a large number of older people are managed at home with established mental unreliability, and are tolerated by a kindly group of neighbours. If such people are quietly, pleasantly confused there is no difficulty, provided the "supporters" have the right temperament. Even so, some relief by intermittent admission or day hospital care may make an endless-seeming burden much more tolerable. If patients make a nuisance of themselves locally, or are a danger to themselves or are incapable of even avoiding the common hazards of life, then they may be admitted to hospitals – to any suitable hospital, not only to mental hospitals – under the Mental Health Act of 1958.

There has been a recent tendency for authorities and planners generally to suggest that many of these old people who are mentally unreliable need not be in hospitals and homes, and indeed that mental hospitals could be reduced in size. The proposal is that these patients should be cared for "in the community". Much depends on the state of the patient and the amount of home care and help available. With attendance at day hospitals and intermittent hospital admissions, perhaps, and with plenty of supporting services available from Social Services Departments, it is possible that this idea would work. Nevertheless the author, from frequent personal observation of the strain placed on families, single daughters and others by having to care for a restlessly wandering, forgetful and obviously demented old person always at their apron strings, believes that this attempt to put the problem back into the community is unrealistic and often unacceptable, even to sympathetic families. What seems to be needed is many more resources for dealing with this nation-wide problem, and especially, more special homes for the elderly mentally infirm (see also Chapter 15), and more suitable hospitals in the right localities for the elderly severely mentally infirm (known semi-officially as "E.S.M.I." patients), where they can be properly looked after by skilled and sympathetic professional people, helped as far as possible by members of their families working as volunteers.

COMPULSORY ADMISSION TO HOSPITAL

Under the provisions of the Mental Health Act just mentioned, it is possible for a patient who is in need of observation and mental treatment to be admitted, by a proper legal process, even though she will not go voluntarily. Naturally, the voluntary ("informal") type of admission is preferable to all concerned, if the patient can be persuaded. This question is discussed further in Chapter 11.

Certain other people who are *not* mentally ill can be admitted to Hospitals or Homes compulsorily by the use of an Order of a magistrate brought to see the patient by a Community Physician, if the patient is in any danger by neglect or disease, and not receiving from other people the care which is needed. This is a serious step to take, because it deprives the subject of her liberty: it is only used very reluctantly when the situation is desperate. The usual form of order used at the present time remains in force for three weeks and then must be renewed, or the patient must be released. This procedure is provided for under an amendment of Section 47 of the National Assistance Act 1946.

*   *   *

Many mentally abnormal or severely afflicted old people who cannot manage their own affairs, or sell their houses when they want to, or manage their money and generally look after the complexities of business sensibly, have to have their affairs put into the hands of the official Court of Protection. The Court will appoint a "receiver" – often a relative, if any is willing – to act for the patient. In these circumstances a Power of Attorney will not be valid any more, even if it had been granted when the patient was *compos mentis*. The Court of Protection exists particularly to protect the interests of the elderly patient – and some old people most certainly need their financial interests to be safeguarded!

Most often the initiative in applying to the Court of Protection is taken by the patient's solicitor, acting in consultation with the family and the doctor – who provides the necessary medical certificate. However, when the affairs of people in hospitals and homes are obviously not being properly conducted by those at home, and where the patient's or client's interests might be prejudiced, it is the duty of senior people responsible, such as the director of social services or the hospital consultant, to inform the Court of Protection direct and request that it looks into the matter.

DETECTION OF ILLNESS IN THE COMMUNITY

Much thought is being given to the widespread problem of finding out where illness exists, to catch it at the earliest stage so that it can be nipped in the bud or treated without delay. There have been notable experiments like that at Rutherglen near Glasgow and elsewhere, in which people in late middle life and apparently in good health are interviewed and examined, and any likely illness or faulty habit is reported to the patient and his own doctor in time for preventive action to be taken. There have been some less satisfactory schemes in which Local Authorities have set up "old people's clinics" without the guidance of doctors and others who have a special knowledge of senescence and disease in later life. Regular medical examinations at certain ages have also been proposed. There are many problems in such schemes – too complex perhaps to discuss in this small book. The main difficulty is that there would never be enough medical personnel to carry these schemes through on a full scale. The problem of detection will remain, but it can be overcome to some extent by a scheme in which family doctors keep a special watch on those people in their practices who seem most at risk as for example on retirement or after bereavement. The attachment of Health Visitors to practices to help with this vital work has already been advocated as a most hopeful possibility for the future. A good age–sex register in the practice is of the greatest value in this respect.

There are also advocates for "screening" of groups of patients for particular diseases. Screening for diabetes of people has already been tried with success (for example in Bedford), and this might be applied generally, especially to people over the age of fifty. Mass Radiography is a screening technique, but it has largely been abandoned now that tuberculosis is so much less prevalent in the community than it was. Yet tuberculosis is not conquered in old age.

There are many other possibilities for mass screening of older people – for cancer, for anaemia, for heart disease, for urinary infection, and even for foot problems. These would be interesting future developments. Simple screening for foot problems might be the most productive of good health and social competence with the least possible expenditure. Trying to organize such activities at times of economic stress is full of difficulties, but ideas of this kind should perhaps be kept in mind for the future.

Two ethical difficulties also arise in screening: first, what is the risk of making people too conscious of illness so that it becomes a source of worry? Secondly, what does the medical team do, and say, when it detects something which might be abnormal, and yet might not be? Diagnosis, unfortunately, is not yet so exact a science that we can say the only problem with screening programmes is to find money and people to do the work.

Chapter 15

HOSPITALS AND HOMES

In the previous chapter the aim was to concentrate on those activities which, if carried energetically through, would give the best prospect of an elderly patient staying at home where he or she would most like to be, circumstances permitting. Yet, however much we try to keep things as they are, the time has to come in the lives of a number of people when some other arrangement, temporary or more permanent, seems inevitable because of increasing frailty or illness, and sometimes because of loneliness. Nevertheless, only about 5 or 6% of the retired people in Great Britain are in Homes or Hospitals. This is a great tribute to the tenacity of older people themselves in holding on to what they have, to the kindly friends and relatives who help them on a voluntary basis, and to the official staff of Local Authorities and other organizations, whose job it is to give support.

There is in the minds of many old people, and in the minds of many of their younger relatives too, the idea that when "Home" or "Hospital" is proposed, this is a road with no way back. One of the themes of this whole book has been that neither sensescence nor even illness in old age necessarily means irrevocable steps have to be taken about "going away". Yet it is not so very long since this was the normal expectation. Before the Second World War and for some time afterwards, entry to an official "Home" (which in a great many cases was also a Hospital) was expected to be permanent. There was a certain right of entry into these erstwhile Public Assistance Institutions if the medical or social circumstances demanded it, and there was one person, called the "Relieving Officer", a non-medical official, who arranged the details and took the patient along. Some, who were more seriously ill, might first be admitted to the general wards of the local municipal hospital, and transferred later if they did not recover, to the older invalids' wards, invariably known in those days as the "chronic sick" wards. Thereafter there was virtually no prospect of the patient's return, for no one expected to be discharged from these wards, and no active treatment was provided to make it likely. Only death provided the release. Geriatric medicine, as practised now in Great Britain in the National Health Service, has greatly changed the pic-

237

ture. It is our duty, doctors, nurses and social workers alike, to show people that there is nothing inevitable about entering a Home or a Hospital towards the end of one's life, and no absolute permanency about it even if it does happen. It is a humane idea to propose that once a person enters an official Home it is his right to stay there for ever; but circumstances often change, and people's wishes and attitudes change too. Security of tenure is a splendid thing, but absolute security is not a practical possibility. Those who offer it to anybody else may find they have to break their promises. In some countries arrangements exist by which an elderly person expects to move first from independent living to communal living in an official Home, and thence to an Old People's Hospital as further deterioration takes place, after which the final and inevitable end comes a few weeks or months later. It is one way traffic. There is a dreadful inevitability about this system. This is not how we regard the matter now in Great Britain: we cannot always prevent it happening, but at least we can try.

HOMES

PRIVATE HOMES

There are in Great Britain a large number of privately owned homes which go under such varied names as Homes of Rest, Eventide Homes, etc. and which are technically known as "Residential Homes for the Elderly". There are also a number of Nursing Homes. Some are run by voluntary bodies or religious institutions, but the majority are owned by private people, usually with some nursing experience, and fees are charged. In many countries without State organized hospital services these homes provide most of the accommodation available for geriatric patients.

Some of our larger Nursing Homes are like small hospitals and even have operating facilities: they are not likely to accept older patients except for a strictly limited stay. Nursing Homes and Residential Old People's Homes all have to be registered with the Area Health Authority. The standards of staffing and equipment, etc. considered necessary naturally vary as between the two groups, and this is reflected in their scales of fees. But what really constitutes "nursing" for a frail old person is often a matter for discussion. Many straightforward registered homes say clearly that they cannot provide any nursing attention, and may require their residents to find somewhere else in a hurry – as private hotels do – if they happen to fall ill. Most well-run homes can manage to cater for a short illness in one of their residents, but staff are usually short. Staff salaries are the heaviest items in their costs. Some may wonder why it is that the residents prefer this kind of home to one provided by the Authorities. Some old people like to pay their way if they can, and all credit to them. Others like a little more privacy, and like to have more of their own things about them, with less of the communal type of life. Who shall say that they must not, if they are prepared to pay for it?

Some criticism has been levelled from time to time at private homes in recent years. Even though this criticism may sometimes have been justified, we must remember that these homes have for a long time carried part of the weight of care for very frail and friendless old people. If they were not there, the official Homes and Hospitals would be hard pressed to find room for all the applicants. It is not at all uncommon for a trained nurse and her husband to find their vocation running such a small home, and when it is well done this is a valuable service to the community. The fact that these homes seem so often to open and close and change owners shows that it is difficult to make a success of such an undertaking, when so often the crucial factor is the limited amount of money which an elderly pensioner can afford.

LOCAL AUTHORITY RESIDENTIAL HOMES

Part III of the National Assistance Act of 1948 required the then Welfare Departments of the Local Authorities, to provide residential accommodation in Homes for elderly people and any others who have no homes of their own and who require care and attention. At the time of the passing of the Act there were few Housing Associations and no "sheltered housing" schemes (see Chapter 3). The only answer to any old person's failure to survive independently, if she had no private means, was one of these Residential Homes, which are still called "Part III Homes" by many people, after that section of the Act which brought them into being.

The first of these Homes had developed from the old institutions of the Poor Law and the Public Assistance systems. Thirty years ago most of the Homes were no more and no less than parts of the old Institutions. They had been the "House" side, in contradistinction to the Hospital side, but both were run by the same administration and were under the same Matron. When the two parts were separated because of the advent of the National Health Service, local authorities often took over large old private houses and adapted them to have a fairly home-like atmosphere. Now special Residential Homes are built for the purpose, each as a rule catering for 30 to 50 residents. In these new Homes the standard of accommodation, comfort and freedom of action has improved out of all recognition, and the old oppressive ways of the "House" (i.e. the Workhouse) have gone for ever. The natural fear of such places should also have vanished. Even so, the Welfare Homes offer a communal existence of a kind which many mature adult people have never experienced and do not like when they do meet it. Many homes have single bedrooms, but many still have four residents to a bedroom, with standard modern furniture and very little real privacy. For some old people of spirit and an independent turn of mind, this is not at all satisfactory. For others, on the other hand, who are basically people who like to be helped, waited on, and to have a "bit of company" all the time, they are satisfactory. Many of the authorities have managed within the financial restrictions to produce very comfortable, cheerful places with devoted staffs who provide an excellent standard of care and nutrition, and can look after old people even during an illness, provided that it is only a brief one. It is not reasonable or right that they should try to care for an indefinite time for old people who need regular and continuous nursing attention. They are neither equipped nor staffed for this purpose, whereas geriatric hospitals are (or should be). In such circumstances a transfer from Home to Hospital ought to be arranged with the same degree of urgency as would apply if the patient had fallen ill in her own home.

People who are accommodated in Residential Homes are expected to pay for their maintenance according to their means, up to a certain limit: this is the law. There is no legal reason why a very wealthy person should not occupy a place in such a Home if she wished, but the Authorities naturally exercise discretion about priorities for admission, and would feel obliged to give a vacancy to a needy person first. If a resident has no more than her basic pension, she is expected to surrender most of it for her upkeep, but keeps a proportion for her own personal shopping needs. The type of accommodation offered is not affected by whether the resident pays fully or pays no more than part of her State pension.

The better the outside arrangements for helping old people to stay at home, particularly the domestic help and meals services, the less the demand for places in the Homes.

It follows naturally from events that most of the people in Residential Homes are elderly, and some are very elderly indeed. There has in fact been a notable change in the type of residents in the newer Homes even during the 15 to 20 years since they were first opened. They have survived and are now on average a few years older, and are much more frail. This means the Homes need special modifications like handrails on corridors, alterations to baths and lavatories, special types of chairs, and other non-nursing apparatus which geriatric hospitals have themselves developed over 25 years, and about which geriatric physicians would be glad to offer advice from their own experience. Above all, the Homes must now have enough staff of the right kind, together with some people who are willing to be on duty at night, just to keep a watchful eye open and help a frail old person on her trip to the lavatory.

There is no doubt that the problems of managing Residential Homes in the late 1970s are increasing day by day. They are catering for very old people, who have their own ideas and foibles, their strong preferences, their frailty and their undoubted rights – and yet who lack any real objectives or any obligations to care for anyone else, and are kept in remarkably sheltered circumstances. They are certainly a difficult group to care for. Great devotion is shown by the Care Assistants who do this work. Often they are under the possible threat of criticism from relatives which may come from the subconscious feeling that they themselves somehow failed, by having let their relatives "go into a Home". The implications of the changing characteristics of residents in Residential Homes are discussed again at the end of this chapter.

Until quite recently no special training was required or was available for those who have responsibility for running these Homes. Many of the Wardens and Matrons are State Registered Nurses or State Enrolled Nurses, and the increasing frailty and likelihood of illness in their charges makes their nursing training specially valuable. Now there are from time to time comprehensive courses designed for those who are, or who would like to be, in charge of Residential Homes, in which there is guidance on the psychology, the psychiatry, the geriatric problems of old people, and management questions which they might be expected to encounter. Such courses, for example, were started in Ipswich and Portsmouth in 1969.

Fitness for Homes

Deciding whether an old person is fit for a Residential Home is not always easy. It is not helpful to lay down absolute rules, for Homes vary in what they can provide, and their staffs vary in what sorts of people they can manage. Sometimes it depends on what they can tolerate in their residents' behaviour! As a general rule the old person should be able to get about without needing support, though she could have the use of whatever walking aids are necessary; she should be able to wash and dress alone or with a little help and go to the lavatory, and go as far as a dining room to sit up for meals. Many Homes now have lifts, so the capacity to go up stairs is not necessary. Incontinence is naturally not appreciated, but it happens from time to time that Residential Home residents become incontinent, though they can often be coaxed back to continence by habit-training, just as they would be in a geriatric hospital. Patients with catheters and urinal bags or colostomies are often said to be unsuitable – but if they manage their appliances sensibly and hygienically, there ought to be no greater difficulty with them in a Home than there would be in a normal tolerant family. Diabetes, if it were severe or unstable, might be a serious problem for management in a Home, but most elderly diabetics are mild cases and stable, and their diets could be supervised to a sufficient extent in a Home.

Patients who are deaf are not popular, but deafness should not exclude them. Blind patients can often be managed, and some Residential Homes are specifically run for their benefit, though a leaven of sighted people in such a home – people who can help to guide the blind – are a great help to the staff too.

The greatest difficulty is with mentally disturbed residents. A great many are vague, forgetful and a little "odd" in their ways, but not un-manageable if the staff and other residents are good humoured and tolerant. Out-and-out dementia cases, typified by old people interfering with each other and behaving anti-socially should not be in Residential Homes. However the Mental Health Act of 1959 proposed that Local Authorities should provide hostels or homes especially for people who were mentally not fully reliable, but who did not need mental hospital care or regular nursing attention. Such people are semi-officially designated as Elderly Mentally Infirm, ("E.M.I."), patients. There is now a great need for more local authority homes designated, designed and suitably staffed to care for them gently and sympathetically. Those with experience of this problem mostly agree that it is not to the advantage or liking of mentally normal residents to be in regular contact in the same home with mentally disordered residents. There have however been set up some experimental homes on the unitary principle, where a group of people of mixed mental capability live almost like a family, the more able ones caring for the more mentally frail.

A fair test of the suitability of a person for a Residential Home these days is whether she needs regular day by day medical attention or skilled nursing. Community Nurses are able to visit Homes to give patients the same sort of care that they would give them in private houses. As most Residential Homes are in centres of population, this arrangement should solve many of the lesser problems, like doing regular dressings. Further-more, the Home Nurse should welcome this opportunity, because in Homes the conditions of doing her job should be as good as anywhere. Staffs of Homes often take special pride in seeing the residents through their last short illness; but a long-continuing terminal care problem must overtax their resources, and admission to a Geriatric Hospital would be more appropriate.

HOSPITALS FOR THE ELDERLY

Chapter 1 demonstrated what a large number of older people is cared for by all hospital wards and departments except maternity and children's departments. We cannot arrange to exclude all people over a certain age from the general wards of our Hospitals, nor perhaps would this be desirable. The average age of patients in a geriatric department is always high, and may well approach 80–85 years. Various people have suggested that a geriatric department should take *all* medical-type illness over a particular age, such as 75 years, but no patients below that age. In truth, if such age limits were adopted it would make little difference to the kind of patients seen already in any active, sensibly-run geriatric department. Nevertheless, the author prefers not to erect any artificial age barrier, for people should be able to enter a geriatric ward according to their special *need*, and their age is not the most important consideration. Nevertheless, this section is devoted to considering hospitals and wards specially designated for older people, to show what is needed to provide the sort of comfort, care, activity and treatment which the patients' special circumstances demand.

A very brief history of hospitals for the aged in Great Britain will help to explain more recent happenings, and the shortcomings which are still found existing in some places.

In the Middle Ages small local hospitals were maintained by religious foundations and charities, but the Dissolution of the Monasteries in 1536 must have caused many old, ill and needy people to be cast out. Some organization of "outdoor relief" was made as a result of the Poor Law Act in 1601. In 1784 an Act of Parliament proposed that parishes, which were thought to be too small to run efficient institutions independently, should combine into "Unions" to build workhouses. They were not really designed for nursing the sick, but inside them were collected together the old, the poor, frail, ill, even young orphans, all in the same wards – even though it originally had been the idea to separate the ill from the healthy inmates. Early in the reign of Queen Victoria a further Poor Law Amendment Act made it clear that the accommodation provided in these workhouses was to be less lavish than that which the poorest labourer ought to be able to provide for himself and his family outside the place. Anyone can imagine, therefore, how low a standard was provided – because the authorities did not want to encourage people to enter the workhouses and become a charge on the local rates. It was not until 1867 that special arrangements were made to separate those who were ill by putting them into "infirmary blocks", attached to the workhouses. Thus there were to be two parts to most of them; the Infirmary, and the "House" where those who were not ill were to be maintained; the latter had to do the necessary work of the place and other tasks in return for their keep. So, in those harsh days of the 19th century were built many of the buildings which are still the hospitals of the present time. Indeed, some of our geriatric hospitals are now over 200 years old, having been built even before the Act which brought the Unions of parishes into being. Three of these are still in full use – much changed – in East Suffolk!

In many places the geriatric hospital wards are still the old "chronic sick" wards which started as the infirmary blocks of the old institutions, though many had evolved into the old municipal hospitals of the pre-war period.

It was these depressing, ill-equipped and totally inadequate old infirmary wards which were taken over by the National Health Service in 1948. Some were so cramped that no one, not even the nurses, could move freely. Some were large, barn-like places with 50 patients apiece arranged in four rows of beds, with the bedheads of the middle two rows touching. Even after the National Health Service began hospital ward blocks and welfare ("Part III") blocks existed side by side on the same premises just as the "house" and the old infirmary blocks did. But they became the responsibility of different authorities – the Hospital Service and the Welfare Department of the Local Authority respectively.

We can see therefore that the old workhouses were some sort of a starting point for the geriatric hospitals of today, but that is the best that can be said of them. They were bleak, drab, with peeling paint often spread on plain brick walls without plaster, in durable colours of dark brown, dark green or cream, with disgraceful plumbing, high windows, no lifts, no day spaces, no medical apparatus, and the most primitive of nursing equipment. The beds were simple black iron bedsteads just with a wooden chair and perhaps a basket for the patient's clothes, it being exceptional to find even lockers. In those beds lay rows of sad ill old people, almost always in bed, as there was nowhere else for them to be. Most of them were thought to have "chronic" diseases (but seldom was any diagnosis written down). Meaningful medical notes were not usually kept, and treatment consisted of a very few basic drugs. There was no physiotherapy or occupational therapy, and the food was the cheapest obtainable. In every respect the patients were just people waiting for their end. Even so they were devotedly nursed according to the ideas of the day, and this made up partly for the shortcomings of the medical attention. Since no doctors then believed anything medical could usefully be done, no one attempted anything. It was thought to be "just a nursing matter".

With the coming of the National Health Service at last there was a chance to share out the available money for hospitals more fairly. The old "chronic sick" hospitals and wards had started far back in the queue for improvements and equipment, and the nursing staff were very thin on the ground. In some areas, thirty years later, they are still trying to catch up; but in other places great strides forward have been possible, coinciding with the setting up of geriatric departments in charge of specialists, who were able to show what an asset an active policy of diagnosis and treatment could be. These new departments, starting in old premises, demonstrated that they could soon treble or quadruple the number of patients treated without any additional beds, and could continue to do so.

This is the justification for geriatric departments. They recognized a great need, tackled it, and found their system worked.

Needs of Elderly Patients in Hospital

First, the elderly need to feel accepted, welcomed, and where they are by right and not on sufferance. In the old days a family doctor had the greatest difficulty getting an old invalid into a general hospital bed. Because they had degenerative diseases, they were not "interesting cases" and might stay a long while, the big important hospitals did not want to know about them; so the word went round that the hospital had "no empty beds". This feeling of not being wanted even got to the ears of the patient. Now, in good geriatric wards, old people – however old – are accepted whatever their illness, temper, state of continence of cleanliness, or whatever (within reason) their mental state, by people who care about them. It is a profound difference.

An old person needs a place where the speed of activity in the ward more nearly matches his own speed. In the bustle of a very busy "acute" medical or surgical ward he can feel out of place, and is so often put into a corner bed out of the way and kept in bed "for safety's sake". Everything in this book suggests that this is not right. Next, the patient needs to find nurses and doctors who have a special regard for old people, who understand their particular difficulties and will adopt towards them an optimistic and cheerful attitude.

If anyone should need a longer stay in hospital than the average – which is not invariably so with geriatric patients, but there is the possibility – then surely the standard of accommodation should be *better* than that for younger people who will soon be up and away home. Thus, the older patient needs to be able to see out to the world outside, to have a dayroom, to be surrounded by bright, cheerful colours and flowers, to have good furniture of the right height, tables, and perhaps a garden to go into in fine weather. He needs to have the shortest possible distance to get to the lavatory, handrails on corridors, handgrips everywhere possible to hold onto, and plenty of aids and special equipment. He also should dress in his own night things and his own clothes in the day time, and have a place close by for keeping them handy for dressing. Depriving a patient of his own clothes deprives him of part of his own personality. Sending a patient's clothes away when he enters a hospital is a barbarous, senseless practice. We cannot be so mean that we could not provide a suitable place for them to be kept.

A good modern geriatric department will be pleased to show the range of special equipment it has evolved to do its particular job – the special floors, sanitary annexes, furniture, beds, lifting gear, nursing aids and everything else without which everything must be less efficient. Above all, geriatric departments try to create good cheerful, labour-saving conditions of work for their nurses, whom, they recognize very well, have a hard job to do and need great patience. They deserve the best equipment and most cheerful working surroundings it is possible to create.

In cases where old people are not expected to get better and have to remain as in-patients, they still need a kindly atmosphere and every possible aid and a cheerful place where they can live out their remaining lives, and at the very end have a quiet, serene environment so that their passing can be dignified. Why should we accept less than this sort of standard for older people?

The Design and Policies of Geriatric Departments

In Great Britain geriatric departments have evolved in various different ways, according to geography and history, and because of the positions of the hospitals and the capabilities of each. No department has been able to build itself up from nothing in the completely ideal way. Everywhere in geratric circles it is agreed that the first thing to aim at is an accurate diagnosis. Diagnosis in geriatrics means much more than labelling diseases; it means an assessment of the patient's physiological, physical and mental status, his disabilities, and his social background – if that information can be obtained. More will be said about how far it is right to go with diagnosis and treatment in Chapter 16. Accurate diagnosis is impossible without experts, without equipment or without X-ray and laboratory help. Thus, every geriatric department must be centred in a general hospital and have its own wards there. Any department which does not is not a true geriatric department within the modern meaning of that phrase. Next, there is a vital need for treatment, which, besides drugs, means (in particular) rehabilitation in every sense – rehabilitation of body, mind and morale. So, a geriatric department needs ample wards and space for rehabilitation, with access to physiotherapy, occupational therapy, speech therapy and hospital-based Social Workers. Often it is found best to provide therapy in geriatric treatment wards and their day rooms, or in areas very close, so that old patients do not have to be taken long distances to get what they are needing all day long. In many places, especially cities and large towns, the treatment wards are placed alongside the diagnostic and assessment wards. In country districts it is sometimes necessary to have treatment wards in rather more distant and attractive places. Treatment is often a long business. Geriatric departments set no limit to how long treatment goes on if progress is being made. So, if it can be done in hospitals with lawns and gardens and clean fresh air, so much the better. So much depends on where specialist staff is available.

After the treatment stage, however hard we try, there will be a number of patients needing an indefinite stay, because their disabilities are too great to overcome and there is no one at home capable of giving the care required. Care for the dying will be needed too. It is important to be able to sort patients out into groups who suit each other. Patients who are mentally unreliable ideally should not be put with those who are mentally very alert. It is essential to have several wards and day rooms of different kinds and sizes.

Wards and hospitals for long-term care are not to be regarded as inferior hospitals (and their staffs are most certainly not "inferior"). Long-stay hospitals do not need full facilities for diagnosis and treatment, so the cost of running them is naturally less per patient per week than in general hospitals. There is, all the same, a need for geriatric patients at whatever stage to have access to diagnostic departments when changes take place in their condition. This may mean transporting them back to the centre from the outlying longer-stay sections. One of the most important features of the British system is that the team which cared for the geriatric patient at the outset still has responsibility for her at the later stages; then such moves as may be needed in any direction can be dealt with smoothly and efficiently. All the sections of a geriatric department and all its constituent hospitals, even if they are widely scattered, work as a team and must know that they are indispensable to each other. A breakdown or "blockage" anywhere is felt all the way through the organization. This should be hospital teamwork at its very best, linking itself to the larger teamwork of care at home and in, and by, the community.

Day Hospitals

Since 1961 there has been a steady development of day hospitals, slowly at first and now accelerating, so that there must now be well over 200 in Great Britain. From small beginnings and from adaptations of old unwanted wards, these have progressed to being, often, spacious and well designed, comfortable and well equipped and furnished. The atmosphere in these day hospitals is such as to encourage activities, both individually and in groups, and progress towards more and more personal independence, while at the same time ensuring that the medical progress of patients can be observed, nursing procedures carried out, activities of daily living assessed and practised, and physiotherapy given as need be. The idea is simple: patients are brought by car or ambulance, stay all day in a specially built section, having treatment and stimulus. There is physiotherapy and occupational therapy, recreation, any simple nursing attention needed, bathing, a midday meal, encouragement in mental and physical activities, and group therapy, and the patients are sent home again in the late afternoon. Day hospitals need to be hives of activity (see Plate 7), attractive places, with plenty of therapy staff and volunteer workers. They have several purposes combined into one; (a) to provide supervision and observation of frail old patients who do not need to be in-patients continuously; (b) to provide some relief for people at home from continually giving care; (c) to give the patients companionship and the stimulus of activity in a friendly group; (d) to continue treatment begun elsewhere; (e) to prevent unnecessary admissions and re-admissions; (f) to allow earlier discharge from the wards than might otherwise be possible. We can see from this list that geriatric day hospitals are for the treatment and medical and nursing observation of sick people. They must therefore be on hospital premises and the responsibility of the hospital staff to run. Indeed, every self-respecting geriatric hospital should aim to have its day hospital. The bulk of its patients are likely to be those who have recently been in-patients and need further care, but not so much in need of it as to keep them in hospital day and night. Some of the others will be vulnerable people who are kept from being in-patients by the very existence of the day hospital supervision. The purpose of a day hospital is not to be a crèche for old people who are needing supervision or a mid-day meal but no treatment; nor should it be simply a refuge for the lonely, important though such a refuge might be. Day hospitals create certain problems: there are difficulties with transporting older patients, and the radius from which they can come cannot be large; there must be a "flow" of patients, some returning fully to home life in order to make room for new patients. However, there are some who become emotionally dependent on the place and would like to attend indefinitely.

Day Centres are needed as well as Day Hospitals. These Centres should be places to which older people who are not ill or needing regular treatment or nursing attention can come for activity, recreation and companionship. Such an activity should be a voluntary or community undertaking, and ideally day hospitals should be able to pass on to day centres their patients who have recovered sufficiently so that they do not need regular medical and nursing supervision.

Other Activities of Geriatric Hospitals

Geriatric departments like, where they can, to offer a helping hand to other departments whose elderly patients present them with problems. But there can be no question of all the other departments' "unwanted" or "failed treatment" or "social problem" cases being transferred automatically. The geriatric department itself has a very heavy load all the year round and it must be free to select which of the others it can most help. In particular, radiotherapy departments with few beds and very costly cancer-treating apparatus should not be brought to a stop because they cannot arrange for alternative treatment for their frailer old patients. Orthopaedic departments with a heavy load of fractured legs in elderly women may also need special help with rehabilitation or at least a geriatric physician's advice.

Many geriatric departments also care for a large number of patients who might equally well be in mental hospitals because of their demented state. If an elderly "mental" patient is badly disabled as well as being burdened with a physical problem like a stroke, then a geriatric department should be able to care for her. If she is active, interfering, obstructive and able to walk about, then it probably cannot, and should not – a mental hospital would be the proper place, especially since mental hospital nurses have special skills and training.

Some geriatric hospitals also care for so-called "younger chronic sick" or younger severely disabled patients, but this is not a true part of geriatric work. Certainly they must have separate wards, specially built and equipped for their proper nursing and medical care, even if it happens to be the geriatric hospital team which provides this care.

Nearly all geriatric departments try to provide "holiday care" for elderly invalids whose families look after them for the rest of the year but need a real holiday break from the responsibility. This can only be offered, as a rule, between June and October in Great Britain, when the extra pressure of winter illness and its aftermath has been relieved a little. Holiday admissions of this kind are usually booked well in advance and the discharges are also booked. These arrangements must be a matter of mutual trust, and they ought not to be broken unless the patient herself at the crucial moment is too ill to be moved from place to place.

Many patients' relatives and supporters cannot stand the strain of caring week after week for a severely handicapped heavy person. Geriatric hospitals can sometimes arrange to take the patient for a while, sharing the burden. This kind of prearranged re-admission is called the "six-weeks-in-and-six-weeks-out" principle, because these were the times chosen in experimental schemes. Whatever intervals are chosen, the effect in the hospital is to be able to give more help to more people; the patient gets some home and some hospital life, while the devoted family can look forward to its regular rest periods.

Colour in Hospital

The author has experimented for some years in colour schemes in geriatric hospitals aimed at making the wards and corridors exciting and attractive for patients and for their nurses too. In brightly and variously coloured wards somnolent old people will wake up, talk and come to life. In drab places they themselves seem drab and depressed. Schemes with multicoloured doors, each colour indicating a bathroom, ward kitchen or lavatory, help patients to find their way about, and wards with different schemes help them to remember where they are. It is a good policy to lay floors with polyvinyl tiles or bonded sheet in highly coloured striped patterns between the lines of beds and down corridors, to encourage people to walk down them, rather as "zebra" crossings do in the streets.

Such floors are hygienic and last a long time. Bright, bold colours on walls, floors and ceilings cost no more than the dreaded old institutional dark greens and browns, or the pale pastel shades which fade and dirty so easily.

Staffing of Hospitals

Hospitals cannot work efficiently without sufficient staff, and geriatric hospitals are no exception. Yet in days past they achieved near-miracles with so few staff. The geriatric team must consist of doctors, nurses, social workers, therapists of all kinds, dieticians, technical people, and secretarial staff to help with a great load of administrative detail, correspondence and intercommunication work. Voluntary workers have an honoured place too. There is not space here to discuss how many of these groups there should be or how they should work, but the cases of hospital social workers and nurses must be briefly mentioned.

There is no doubt that the work of the whole team would break down if there were no social workers based in the hospitals, fully trained in the medical aspects of old people's problems, and available for very frequent consultations at all levels. Almost all geriatric patients have major social difficulties to face. They have problems of keeping in touch with home and with aged relatives, managing their affairs when they have been snatched away to hospital, and trying to get themselves resettled at home with such help as is available. This is one of the most difficult fields of activity for any social worker, and all the time she must be aware of what state of recovery the patient has reached. This could not be known to a community-based social worker acting at a distance. It must surely be one of the particular functions of hospital-based social workers to keep in touch regularly with the field social worker who has had responsibility for the patient at home – often miles away – and with her family if she has any family. Information should flow in both directions, always with the objective of satisfactorily resettling the patient at home with such support as she needs.

The nursing profession as a whole is perhaps only now coming to realize fully what a very heavy load is borne by nurses in geriatric wards. Many detailed researches have shown that the number of technical nursing procedures is hardly any less in a geriatric assessment ward than it is in an acute medical ward, whereas the amount of basic nursing attention and personal assistance needed with feeding, bathing, dressing and even helping the patients to move about is a great deal more. Only ten to fifteen years ago it was considered that geriatric wards were fortunate if the ratio of patients to nurses was three to one. Current opinions suggest that the need in assessment wards is *greater* than the need in surgical and medical wards, and the ratio should be about 1.1 to 1, whereas in long-stay wards with many very handicapped people at an average of, say, 85 years old, the ratio should certainly not be less than 1.5 to 1. It would be quite irresponsible for the public to criticize the care given to geriatric patients unless it would provide enough equipment and nurses, and the money to pay them, so that work can be done in a humane and dignified manner.

It is encouraging to see how, over the years, the training of nurses has gradually embraced geriatric nursing. At one time student or pupil nurses were often debarred from working in geriatric wards, because of the poor quality of those wards and because the experience to be gained in them (so it was wrongly supposed) was somehow "inferior". Through a stage of optional experience in geriatric nursing, we have come finally to the stage when the subject is a necessary part of the standard curriculum and, further, when special courses in advanced geriatric nursing are being organized by the Joint Board of Clinical Nursing Studies.

THE FUTURE OF RESIDENTIAL HOMES

On page 240 the difficulties of the Residential Homes with their increasing numbers of very old and very frail residents was touched on. It is becoming plain for all to see that there is very little difference between the state of the residents of such a Home and of many of the more active of the longer-stay patients at present in Hospital. The amount of personal attention and nursing-type care they will need is steadily increasing. There are so many very frail and handicapped old people in the community that for an able-bodied "young" person of, say, seventy to find a place in a Home seems hardly fair to the others. If, as the author believes, the present Residential Homes are becoming, and should naturally become, homes for the elderly with handicaps (in practice if not in name), then they should be the responsibility of the Hospital Service authorities. Their staffs would then be able to receive training in all the techniques of skilful handling of disabled old people, and would be interchangeable with hospital staffs, while medical supervision could be the responsibility of local doctors with special links with the geriatric department in the area. Then there would be no disputes as to which department should be responsible for the patients' or residents' care, nor would there be any difficulties about moving from the Homes to Hospitals and back again as the needs of the individual required. The Social Services Department could meanwhile concentrate their efforts on the work which only they *can* do – the providing of domiciliary care needed by the rest of the aged in the community, and the provision of various kinds of sheltered living conditions for those who do not need to enter any institution and might never need to do so if housing was good and domestic help was really well organized.

It has been objected that if the Homes were to become the responsibility of the Health Authority, they might be less home-like and altogether too "clinical". However, good geriatric departments have shown that, especially in their continuing-care sections, they can provide bright, colourful and comfortable places for their patients, with good and practical furniture, carpeted day spaces, and a range of creative and diversional activities for their patients which might be the envy of many existing Homes. They already welcome voluntary activities and Leagues of Friends, and arrange trips out, shopping expeditions and entertainments. They also arrange holiday admissions and intermittent care for some patients – just as Homes do (or should do). The differences between Homes and continuing care hospitals are more apparent than real, and the hospital team knows the advantage of being well accumstomed to the management of great frailty and major disabilities.

The wardens (erstwhile "matrons") of existing Homes are often trained nurses, although this idea is not welcomed by all authorities. It is perhaps significant that family doctors who have patients in Homes seem greatly to appreciate the warden being a nurse. There are numerous incidents and crises, great and small, in Homes full of frail old people, and to have a trained health worker on the staff is a great advantage.

Chapter 16

THE GERIATRIC LIFE: DEATH AND DYING

Health has been described as a state of well-being in which a full life can be enjoyed unhindered by mental or physical disability. If what this definition says is true, then, a physically handicapped person cannot be really healthy however full an intellectual life she may lead, and a physically active but demented person cannot be healthy because she is unable to have a normal intellectual life. So, life for many old people must have lost some of its magic. We know that in nearly every case a young person's life, however ill or handicapped she is, is worth trying to preserve for the sake of what undeveloped potential there is. When we are dealing with old people we are a little less sure of our ground. Of course a great many old lives *are* very well worth preserving, and many elderly people show a truly remarkable capacity to recover from illness. Yet in a good many cases the geriatric physician believes he is witnessing the closing stages of a battle against senescence and disease, even if it is a battle with many skirmishes, after each of which the patient lives again to fight another day. He knows that in the end he will not be able to win. His patient knows this too. Sometimes the old person says, "Let me go; enough is enough". Sometimes he does not say this, but one reads it in his eyes. Working with younger people death, the ultimate reality, can be put out of one's mind for a long time; in geriatrics the thought of death is never very far away.

As has been said earlier, the quality of life is what counts to many people, not life itself. But what *is* quality? For a great thinker to be deprived of his reasoning might be as bad as death; for an outdoor man, a hardworking pensioner, paralysis might be the same. It is important always to use the right standards. We might, if we are busy young people, ask what possible quality life could have cooped up in a Residential Home, or worse still in a ward of a geriatric hospital. Yet some old people, whose ambitions are spent, might find the security of a continuing-care ward, with good food provided, pleasant surroundings, and kindly nurses to attend to their modest wants, a sufficiently acceptable way of spending the last months or years, in spite of disabilities.

The author believes that the older an adult is, the less sophisticated are his real needs. So it could be that a dustman and a duke both aged 100 could have very similar basic needs, the majority of which would be concerned with bodily comforts.

Every person concerned with geriatrics approaches the problems in ways which depend up on his own age, his upbringing, his optimism (or his pessimism), and his compassion for others. It would not be right therefore for the author to state his opinions categorically to nurses and other people, trying to lay down the way they should follow. Nevertheless problems and ethical questions should not be ignored because they are unpleasant to face. This chapter is a personal statement of beliefs, to be accepted or rejected just as the reader wishes. Circumstances alter cases, and all patients are unique. One thing is certain however; there is no room for the confirmed pessimist in geriatrics. Great opportunities do occur for treatment and the lessening of disability; the pessimist will not see or seize them, and that is not fair to the sufferer, especially if she shows the great courage of which so many old people are possessed.

HOW FAR TO GO?

Doctors who work in geriatrics must often say to themselves, "I *think* the diagnosis is such and such: we might prove it by doing so and so; but should we go that far?" Naturally, diagnosis is vital for correct and prompt treatment; so there are many things which could and should be done. The doctor takes a history and examines the patient with care; he should do a rectal examination even in a shy little woman; blood count and blood chemistry, urine examination and simple X-rays, an electrocardiograph – these are all necessary things. Other investigations like an electroencephalogram, a radio-isotope scan of a particular organ, or even a lumbar puncture may be needed and are not as a rule too upsetting. Even a barium meal is very revealing and is acceptable enough to an old person if what is to be done is explained. Yet there are many other investigations which *could* be done, which would normally be done without argument in a younger patient if the case required them, but which for an old patient might be very upsetting and not free from risks. There can be no real justification for elaborate and risky procedures unless they might make a fundamental difference to the kind of treatment used. In geriatrics the quest for scientific truth may have to be abandoned in the interest of being humane. A good example would be the finding of a suspicious shadow in the X-ray of an old man's chest: it looks very like a cancer of the bronchus; a bronchoscopy could prove it, but this is a highly unpleasant undertaking. In such a case, and in an old man, it would probably have been decided already that the whole lung could not be removed even if it was cancerous, and nothing short of removing the whole lung would cure the condition. Therefore this unpleasant bronchoscopy would be unjustifiable; anyway, further simple X-rays would give the truth sooner or later.

The next problem to be faced is how far to go if the treatment is very elaborate and very expensive. One might take the view that life is infinitely precious; but are all lives equally precious? Would one admit an unconscious 98-year-old patient to an Intensive Care Unit? It is exceedingly doubtful if this would be the correct thing to do, and it would not be right if by so doing one were to prevent a young man or woman from benefiting from that special form of care. It is reasonable to say that when drugs and special apparatus are in short supply, the young should have them first. Yet that is not the same as saying that expensive apparatus like cardiac monitors should not be provided to make geriatric management of a case more effective.

Further difficulties may arise if a particular line of drug treatment is unusually expensive. One day something might be discovered which could benefit older patients, but which had to be supplied to large numbers of them for indefinite periods. The question then to be faced would be whether such a line of treatment would be a practical possibility within a National Health Service which does not have unlimited money to spend, and in which certain priorities have to be given.

RESUSCITATION

Resuscitation is a relatively new word in medical practice when it is taken to mean almost bringing the dead back to life, as when the heart has suddenly stopped beating. The question of whether or not emergency resuscitation should be used in the cases of older people is difficult to decide. It would not be acceptable to anyone if we were to make a rule, for example, that no person over the age of 70 should be resuscitated if anything suddenly caused his heart to stop. Choosing any particular age limit would be impossible, and a total denial of our principle that people vary greatly and that actual age is only one consideration. Thus it might be quite possible, and sensible, to restart the heart of an old person by electrical means (the apparatus all being near at hand) if she was already under treatment and close observation for a heart condition, and was otherwise well. The reasons and eventualities would have to be worked out in advance, and everyone would be prepared. On the other hand, sudden "crash call" external cardiac massage might be quite wrong in, say, a patient of 89 in a surgical ward if she was already very disturbed and known to have been mentally abnormal for some time. Besides, the resuscitation of aged people must be very promptly done if it is to succeed fully. There is no gain whatever to the patient if she is left with a paraplegia or total dementia because the emergency resuscitation measures were not applied quickly enough – and this is a very real risk indeed.

Without setting out any instructions, then, or making any age limits, it is a reasonable thing that the staff of any ward with old people in it should occasionally discuss whether or not emergency measures like this should be used for any particular patient. The decision is one which should be taken on an entirely individual basis, and kept private to the people who would be directly concerned.

Quite a number of old people do in fact die suddenly, and for many varied reasons. This does not seem the stark tragedy it would be if it happened in a young mother or the breadwinner of a family. There is a certain rightness about this merciful sort of ending, and the staff of a geriatric ward would seldom feel tempted to take very urgent action. Many of us would wish to die in that fashion: many of us doubtless will.

PNEUMONIA: TO TREAT OR NOT TO TREAT IT?

The last of the problems of "how far to go" is perhaps the most difficult. It concerns whether or not to use a simple treatment if one believes it could bring about a cure, but the patient is already very old or very disabled, mentally or physically. There are many patients who say to the doctor at his first visit in an illness, "I am old, let me go". But that request may come because she feels ill, or has just lost a relative, or has had some other recent tragedy. Yet time is a healer of events, and medicine and nursing are healers of diseases. If that patient felt a little better after treatment and with the passage of time, she could very well change her mind. For this reason, therefore, one could not comply with that first request. This, indeed, is one of the main arguments against euthanasia. Every case is different, and circumstances alter with time too.

In the days before very powerful antibiotic drugs, pneumonia was reckoned to be "the old man's friend". It took him off quite quickly and mercifully. In fact it is the basic cause of death, in the end, of most longer-term invalids. Now, because of these drugs, we can send away the "old man's friend". So, to treat or not to treat is a question which faces a geriatric physician several times a week, especially in the winter months. He can, if his conscience tells him so, *not* give the powerful new antibiotic and let Nature take its course. This is never an easy decision, and it is not right to have any set rules. Very often the doctor will be grateful to discuss with the nurses (who spend much more time with the patient than he does) what sort of a person that patient has seemed to be, and whether she seemed to enjoy her limited life. He may also ask the relatives the same questions, and listen to their opinions in the matter. In the end, though, it is the doctor who must decide. Most doctors do not feel bound to preserve life at all costs. They will not, in the old phrase, "officiously strive" to keep alive, especially if they believe the patient would not be grateful to them for doing so. The quality of the life which the patient might be able to live afterwards is of fundamental importance, and that depends partly on its quality before the crisis arose. In the case of a patient who is new to the geriatric team, so that no one can tell what sort of a life she led, it seems wisest to assume it was a happy useful life, and the logical answer is then to treat the urgent illness without delay.

These are some of the most difficult questions of all to face. The author has several times treated attacks of pneumonia which threatened an old person of 100 during the last five years of her life; she was blind but she was fully alert and enjoyed her life. On the other hand he is faced so often with a much younger patient who is, say, ill, and in pain with arthritis, has a hemiplegia, and has been mentally very disturbed for months. This kind of patient seems to have had no pleasure in anything for a long time. In such a case, therefore, the decision could be quite different.

In the matter of treatment generally we should try to see that the patient at least feels, and is, no worse after we have finished than before we started. Some treatments are probably worse than the illness they are supposed to relieve. Some have very disabling side effects. For example, corticosteroid drugs given over a long period are very distressing to old people and run them into certain dangers. Drugs of the nitrogen mustard type, cytotoxic in action, and prescribed sometimes specifically, but sometimes as a last resort in the treatment of cancer, are so upsetting to frail old people that it is usually kinder not to use them. Anticoagulants and anti-hypertensive drugs are also full of hazards for old people, and this explains why geriatric physicians generally are cautious about starting to use them in any individual case.

TUBE FEEDING

In many geriatric wards one may see patients being fed with nasogastric tubes in position. Nurses are sometimes criticized, but only by non-medical people, who say, "Why do you struggle to keep them alive like this, with tubes?". Some old people are too ill to eat, or are dehydrated and urgently need fluids which they will not swallow. Even worse is the plight of those who have had recent strokes where the swallowing mechanism is faulty; they might choke to death, and many of them are only too keenly aware of this. In such cases therefore the reason for passing the tube in the first place is clear and indisputable. This decision is usually taken by a doctor and a senior nurse in consultation. It may mean that the tube has to be used for many weeks or perhaps indefinitely, and this is a circumstance which has to be reckoned with. Nevertheless failure to use the naso-gastric tube when it is needed could lead to a patient's immediate death, or to pneumonia after aspiration of food. It is unthinkable that any nurse would allow a patient to die in this way if she could prevent it, or let the patient feel in danger of choking, or see a patient die a dreadful death of starvation or thirst when a naso-gastric tube skilfully used would prevent it. These arguments will silence all criticism. In fact, modern tubes can be used continuously for several years and keep a patient reasonably and safely nourished without undue discomfort. "Tubes" look more distressing, perhaps, than they are.

By contrast the misery of a patient who is being fed by a gastrostomy is appalling to see. Many patients have said they would rather die than be kept going in this way, and the operation is performed less and less often now; it could hardly ever be justified in a geriatric patient.

DEATH AND DYING

Doctors, nurses and social workers too who deal mostly with old people are well acquainted with death, yet many may not feel well equipped by their training for dealing with the many problems which arise.

In earlier days, battle, murder and sudden death, not to mention pestilence, brought the possibility of death so much nearer to everyone's consciousness. So it would have been in days when the average expectation of life was only forty-five, as it was only 150 or so years ago. Youth today thinks of death as something too remote – except when encountered suddenly in a car crash – to be considered at all. There even seems to be a general taboo about discussing the subject. Yet the elderly often think of death, since they are so much closer to it. Some of them really *want* to discuss what it means.

In recent years the work of Dr. Cecily Saunders, a trained nurse as well as a doctor, has shed most welcome new light on the subject of managing the dying patient which we should all do well to study.

Geriatric departments ought not to have policies which exclude dying people from admission; to do this would be to deny care to people who might need it most particularly. On the other hand, it is unthinkable that all deaths should automatically take place within hospitals, since the dearest wish of most old people is to die at home with familiar surroundings and faces. Things may change in future years. It could become the natural thing for people to leave this world as they will usually have entered it – through a hospital ward. Certainly the time for this is not yet: hospitals in general and geriatric hospitals in particular could not at present bear the load. The fact is that most deaths still do take place at home, and Home Nurses and doctors devotedly see the matter through with courageous, helpful friends, and give them invaluable comfort and support as they do it. All right-minded geriatric teams with resources enough will arrange high priority admissions for patients who are dying alone or in squalor or in severe pain, or in any other significant distress, and the fact of knowing that they are not able to cure the patient is of no consequence at that stage. There are certain homes where the emotional state of the people round about is quite unsuitable for giving the care needed to a dying person, so she would be best in hospital. A great deal has to be done in the treatment of the symptoms of the dying, as all nurses know. Caring for the dying really well is an art needing great skill and close attention to detail.

In geriatric wards naturally we observe many deathbeds. This does not mean that the wards are depressing places full of dreadful foreboding. The experienced members of their staff come to accept what *has* to be philosophically and are glad to be able to help when, of all the times in anyone's existence, most help is needed. Even in a long-stay ward a familiar face will be sadly missed one day, but the wound heals, memories are mercifully short, the gap is filled, and the limited life of the place seems to go on. Young nurses in geriatric wards have to face these happenings more often, perhaps, than we should like, and they should have our very special consideration and support. Nevertheless, the nursing staff in these wards are not made insensitive and "hard" by a high death rate – which might have a numbing effect on the staff of other wards where deaths are normally much fewer. Where the patient concerned was aged and very handicapped, there is something logical and inevitable in departure, and death is not necessarily the bitter, deeply regretted thing it is in a children's or younger persons' ward.

Death in old age is seldom very dramatic. This is not the same as saying that deaths do not take place suddenly, for often they do – by heart attacks, strokes, or pulmonary embolism perhaps. Quite a large number of people are found peacefully dead in their beds. Some deaths are unexpected; many are half-expected, and many, many more are clearly seen to be coming. The old person gradually begins to fail and sometimes takes many days over the journey, drifting gradually and peacefully into Eternity through a state of coma which is often quite prolonged. Even those who die from strokes or terminal pneumonia are often unconscious for several hours, even though to the untrained eye they may appear to be suffering.

It is one of the most moving and rewarding things for a doctor in geriatric work to watch the skill and compassion of good nurses caring for an elderly person who is slipping away even though in the insensibility of coma.

DISTRESS IN DYING

Though most of the deaths of old people are either sudden or slow and peaceful, about one patient in four or five experiences some pain or distress. The distress happens most often in diseases which cause breathlessness, nausea or vomiting, or difficulty with swallowing. There is not much doubt that the possibility of distress is greater for younger patients, because many of them are deeply worried about domestic matters, such as who will care for their families, and they also become very depressed because they cannot any longer enjoy their lives. Older people have often shed their immediate family responsibilities, their outlook has become naturally more self-centred, and they suffer less from anxiety and depression in a terminal illness. Many of them are mentally very muddled, so that they are not fully aware of what is going on, and this is often a blessing in disguise. Even when they are not confused, older patients seem to possess greater calmness in the face of death. Some, though remarkably few, will say they are frightened by the prospect of dying, but seldom do they show it when the time comes.

However, because some deaths are likely to be painful and distressing, it is our clear duty to watch carefully, and use treatment so that symptoms, particularly pain, are relieved. Surely no one believes now that there is any virtue in a person enduring pain for its own sake? We must be able to reassure patients and their relatives that pain will be relieved; and we certainly have the means to do it.

HOW MUCH TO TELL.

Several helpful pieces of research have suggested that quite a large proportion of patients in their last illnesses suspect that they are dying, or at least know that there is this possibility. The nearer they are to the end, the more they are likely to think so. This is so of dying people in general, though with the elderly there is often confusion and a twilight state, when it would be hard to judge what they are thinking. Geriatric departments often have to help with younger people who have inoperable cancer, so it is important that we should be aware of the general trend.

The next question to face is whether patients wish to know the truth for certain, supposing they suspect it. Do they also wish to discuss it with their doctors or nurses? This is one of the most difficult questions in the practice of medicine. Doctors of the older school used usually to teach that the only thing the patient really wished to hear is something hopeful – whatever he might say about wanting to be told the truth. This is a view which many doctors still conscientiously hold. The worst thing, they would say, is to take away all hope; therefore it may be necessary to tell untruths, or at least to sidetrack the question.

It is quite certainly possible to do a great deal of harm by telling a patient the facts bluntly, at the wrong moment. We are not all strong

enough to bear the truth in this matter. Judging a patient's moral strength
is very difficult, and so is judging the correct moment if he is to be told
the truth. Many patients seem to be totally unaware of the possibility of
dying, and the question of telling them does not even arise. It is as if they
had shut off their powers of deduction. Other people need time to appreciate the possibility of bad news, and this appreciation comes to them
as their lack of progress slowly dawns on them. Very few doctors believe
that it is invariably their duty to tell everyone the stark truth, so that they
can be prepared spiritually and otherwise for what is to come. If they do
believe this is their duty in every case, they perhaps over-estimate their
patients' strength.

Nevertheless if a proportion of people, as we now believe, do suspect
they are dying, it is very likely they will want to talk to someone, and
naturally they would turn to those who are medically ministering to
them. Yet even then they might hold back from asking the vital question,
not wanting to embarrass anyone, because they think that the tradition is
"not to tell". It then becomes a sad little game of bluff.

More and more doctors are now coming to believe that they must
allow dying patients the chance to talk about their fate if they want to; if
asked the direct question in the course of talking, they are prepared to
confirm the patient's belief. Then at least they can learn about the
patient's fears – of pain, of mental breakdown, or whatever these fears
may be – and reassure them of help and a gentle ending amongst understanding people who will be at their side.

With very elderly patients the matter does not arise so very often,
though a few are absolutely certain they are dying, and uncannily can
almost predict it to the day. The best method is to sit with the dying
patient for long enough at a time just talking generally and watching for a
sign that there is a wish to discuss more fundamental things. The author
believes that it really is the doctor in the case who should carry the
responsibility to tell or not to tell; but that is not to say that a nurse
should *never* tell. It could happen, it sometimes does, that it is the nurse
who is asked the dread question, "Nurse, am I dying?" – perhaps quietly,
in the middle of the night, when all problems seem at their worst. Even
so, she need not tell untruths; it would be quite proper for her to say, "I
think that's a question you ought to ask the doctor" – but she must warn
the doctor that the question has been asked. It is always a great help if
doctors and nurses, and even responsible relatives too, can quietly discuss from time to time how much they believe the patient suspects, and
make sure that everyone concerned directly with the case has been told
what is being said to the patient.

The majority of doctors think that it is right to inform a close relative
of the truth whatever they intend to say to the patient. There may be
other relatives to summon, and there will be so many things to decide.

But it is not always the closest relative who should be told first; some are too frail or distressed for the news, and it is best to tell another, stronger person, and let him tell the others in his own good time. We must not forget, either, that telling relatives may put them into a difficult position when they come face to face with the patient himself. Families need all the sympathy, support and help we can possibly give them at this crucial time.

TERMINAL CARE

It can be said that any long-term illness could very well be the patient's last illness, but now we must deal with the closing stages of the battle when the end can be reasonably predicted. The time for active, curative treatment is past, and it would be quite wrong to persuade a patient to enter hospital for final nursing care under the false impression that he was going away to have curative treatment. It might solve the immediate difficulty for the people at home, but this piece of deception leaves the hospital in an impossible position, and the patient, when he discovers, eventually feels grossly cheated and embittered. The phrase "for further observation" is just about allowable as a reason for a move like this. In fact many patients willingly accept hospital care, even though they had hoped to finish their illness at home, because they believe that the hospital doctors and nurses will be able to relieve their pain and suffering more certainly than can be done at home. Many are only too willing to come, at this point; but many more, of course, do not enter hospital even at this stage, and have no need to do so just because the end is near. The moment for admission, if admission is needed, has to be carefully chosen, otherwise the patient might take his own discharge again. A case would not be a terminal case in the hospital's eyes unless nursing care was needed or symptoms were too difficult to control with drugs at home. Sometimes, too, treatment makes the sufferer so much better that he could return home and come into hospital again later. Even if this is not possible the doctor's pronouncement of the word "terminal" does not at all mean that the patient has to stay in bed. Patients should be allowed to do as they please in this matter, and many would like to stay up for much of the time; it all helps morale.

At the terminal stage *the symptoms must be treated* even if curative drugs are not used. Yet many courageous patients will not speak of their symptoms, so it is right to ask tactfully about the likely ones, and report them to the doctors. Drugs must be administered confidently, giving the patient the feeling that his needs are fully understood and that the drug really will be effective. Explanations of why a particular line of treatment, like an aspiration, is used will help a great deal to uphold morale. Sedatives are not needed in every case, though it is important that the patient sleeps soundly, because the night is the time of greatest fear. Alcohol is a valuable drug to use, because it gives most people a sense of well-being. Treating nausea and vomiting is difficult, and chlorpromazine (Largactil) or prochlorperazine (Stemetil) are valuable here.

Perhaps the greatest fear is the fear of pain. This is not the place for a complete description of pain-relieving methods. Much can be done by good nursing, but in the end drugs are needed; then to have the courage to use powerful remedies is the least we can do for the dying person. In terminal illness there is no reason not to use habit-forming drugs. The circumstances are quite different, and no one need be in the least concerned about any habit, or be afraid to increase the size of the dose because of it. In the end very few patients exaggerate their pain; and if they do, does it matter so very much? Just a few nurses instinctively seem to feel that a patient ought not to have painkillers until he is "really in pain". This seems a puritanical viewpoint, and it is surely better by far to give the patient the benefit of any doubt. The modern idea is much more to anticipate pain – to give the pain-killer before the pain is expected to return. It would be a dreadful plight to have to expect agony, or to endure the pain while watching the clock for when the next dose is "due". Therefore regular and sufficient dosage of drugs, precisely prescribed, is what is needed. Nurses' opinions on whether or not a patient is suffering pain are most valuable, but the author believes they should be relieved of the anxiety of deciding when to give the pain-relieving drug. In other words, a doctor should prescribe the exact dose and the exact intervals, varying them as the patient's condition varies, but not prescribing them on a "give as necessary" basis. The only exception would be that if a patient was fast asleep, that dose might be omitted.

Clearly it is best to use mild pain-relieving drugs first, work up to more powerful ones, and ultimately change to opium-type drugs or their modern equivalents, if these are needed. At that stage the dose is the dose required to relieve pain, no matter how large it has to be. Many patients do not like to have their senses dulled. It is our duty to respect the wish to be clear headed for as long as possible. So, it is a mistake to use more drugs than the situation demands; it only makes nursing more difficult and the risks of complications like pressure sores greater. Many patients have the notion that the use of injections means the end is near, and it is kinder to use drugs by mouth for as long as possible; however, vomiting and other problems sometimes require the use of regular injections. The tranquillizing drug chlorpromazine (Largactil) combined with pain-killing drugs makes a very valuable combination, as each seems to help the other. One of the best combinations of all is the "Brompton Cocktail" which utilizes an opium drug with cocaine and alcohol, and this helps many a patient quietly over a difficult stage without causing the depression which opium drugs alone so often bring. If pain is relieved, anxiety usually goes too; and what cannot be entirely relieved with drugs can often be helped by showing kindness and confidence at the patient's bedside, with time for gentle talking, and the ministrations of a priest.

In the end the needs of the dying patient are the needs of all sick creatures – comfort, warmth, cheerful surroundings, companionship, food and drink in a form which is easy to take, help with things when self-help is impossible, relief of distressing symptoms, privacy, and peace. Terminal care calls for imagination, close attention to detail, and resourcefulness. Some relatives of patients have these qualities in good measure; the best nurses have them in abundance, and to watch them at work, easing the path of a dying person, is to see what dedication really means.

APPENDIX 1

Notes:
(1) This list does not set out to be comprehensive; there are many hundreds of drugs, and doctors' tastes in prescribing differ.
(2) Drugs of certain groups are not mentioned, not because they are never used in geriatrics, but because their use calls for special consideration on account of increased risks; e.g. barbiturates, anticoagulant drugs, drugs to reduce blood pressure, corticosteroids, morphine and heroin.
(3) The drugs are grouped according to their actions, but some are used in more than one kind of situation. Full dosage schedules are *not* given, because these depend on the doctor's methods of prescribing for the circumstances. Instead, the common forms in which they are dispensed, or the sizes of tablets are given.
(4) The *official* names are given first, but usually omitting the name of the salt, etc. (e.g. Dihydrocodeine tartrate ("D.F. 118") is listed simply as "Dihydrocodeine"). Commonly used drug firms' names are given afterwards in brackets, but there are sometimes several of these proprietary names for the same drug. Drugs prescribed by their official names are often cheaper.
(5) In general it is best to use drugs by mouth, and though many old people will take tablets, they often find syrups and liquid suspensions easier. In certain circumstances injections are unavoidable, and at least with an injection one can assume the patient has had the whole dose prescribed!
(6) It must be remembered that old people, especially very old and frail people, can react excessively to a dose of a drug which is a standard dose for younger adults.

(1) ALIMENTARY SYSTEM

| Carbenoxolone | ("Biogastrone") | tablets of 50 mg |
| | ("Duogastrone") | capsules of 50 mg |

Cimetidine	("Tagamet")	tablets of 200 mg (or syrup)
Aluminium hydroxide	("Aludrox")	Gel – a liquid. tablets of 750 mg

Laxatives, etc.

Methyl cellulose	("Celevac")	tablets
Standardized Senna	("Senokot")	tablets, granules or syrup
Bisacodyl	("Dulcolax")	tablets of 5 mg (also suppositories)
Danthron, etc.	("Dorbanex")	liquid, 200 mg/5 ml
Dioctyl Sodium sulphosuccinate	("Dioctyl forte")	tablets of 100 mg (or syrup)
Lactulose	("Duphalac")	syrup, 3.35 g/5 ml

Sodium bicarb. and anhydrous sodium acid phosphate	("Beogex")	suppository

For dyspepsia and flatulence

Polymethylsiloxane with aluminium hydroxide	("Asilone")	chewing tablets or suspension

For nausea

Prochlorperazine	("Stemetil")	tablets of 5 mg (also suppositories or injection)
Promethazine	("Avomine")	tablets of 25 mg
Metoclopramide	("Maxolon")	tablets of 10 mg (also syrup or injection)

For diarrhoea

Kaolin mixture B.P.C.		mixture

See also under "infections"

(2) CARDIOVASCULAR SYSTEM

Digoxin	("Lanoxin")	tablets of 0.25 mg
Quinidine		tablets of 200 mg
Propanolol	("Inderal")	tablets od 10 mg or 40 mg
Procainamide	("Pronestyl")	tablets of 250 mg injection 100 mg/ml

Oxprenolol	("Trasicor")	tablets of 20 mg or 40 mg injection, ampoules of 2 mg
Isoprenaline	("Saventrine")	tablets of 30 mg
L-Noradrenaline	("Levophed")	injection, 1 mg/ml, etc.
Metaraminol	("Aramine")	injection, 10 mg/ml
Aminophylline	("Cardophylin")	tablets of 100 mg injection 250 mg in 10 ml suppositories of 360 mg
Diphenoxylate with atropine	("Lomotil")	tablets of 2.5 mg (or liquid)

For angina pectoris

Glyceryl trinitrate		tablets of 0.5 mg
Glyceryl trinitrate (sustained action)	("Sustac")	tablets of 2.6 mg or 6.4 mg
Pentaerythritol tetranitrate	("Mycardol")	tablets of 30 mg
	("Peritrate")	tablets of 10 mg
Oxprenolol	("Trasicor")	see above
Propanolol	("Inderal")	see above

Vasodilators

Thymoxamine	("Opilon")	tablets of 40 mg (also ampoules for injection)
Tolazoline	("Priscol")	tablets of 25 mg
Inositol	("Hexopal")	tablets of 200 mg or 500 mg
Naftidrofuryl	("Praxilene")	capsules of 100 mg (or injection)
Potassium chloride	("Slow K")	tablets of 600 mg

Diuretics

Mersalyl		injections of 2 ml
Chlorothiazide	("Saluric")	tablets of 500 mg
Hydrochlorothiazide	("Hydrosaluric")	tablets of 25 mg or 50 mg
Chlorthalidone	("Hygroton")	tablets of 50 mg or 100 mg
Frusemide	("Lasix")	tablets of 40 mg injections of 20 mg/2 ml
Triamterine	("Dytac")	capsules of 50 mg
Ethacrynic acid	("Edecrin")	tablets of 50 mg
Spironolactone	("Aldactone 'A' ")	tablets of 25 mg
Amiloride, with hydrochlorothiazide	("Moduretic")	tablets of 55 mg

(3) RESPIRATORY SYSTEM

Isoprenaline		tablets of 10 mg (to place under the tongue)
Ephedrine		tablets of 15 mg, 30 mg or 60 mg
Aminophylline	(see under "Cardiovascular System")	
Choline theophyllinate	("Choledyl")	tablets of 100 mg or 200 mg
Beclomethasone	("Becotide")	aerosol, 50 mcg, metered
Salbutamol	("Ventolin")	tablets of 2 or 4 mg (or syrup)
Sodium cromoglycate	("Intal")	inhalation from capsules

See also under "infections"

Note: Old people can seldom master the use of drugs by inhalation or as aerosols, etc. Also, drugs intended to suppress their coughs may be dangerous to them.

(4) NERVOUS SYSTEM

For pain relief

Soluble aspirin	("Solprin", etc.)	tablets of 300 mg
Paracetamol with dextropropoxyphene	("Distalgesic")	tablets
Tab. codeine co.	("Veganin", etc.)	tablets
Dihydrocodeine	("D.F. 118")	tablets of 30 mg
Pentazocine	("Fortral")	tablets of 25 mg injections of 30 mg/ml
Levorphanol	("Dromoran")	tablets of 1.5 mg
Pethidine		tablets of 25 mg

See also drugs for rheumatism, arthritis etc, below

Hypnotics

Chlormethiazole	("Heminevrin")	tablets of 500 mg (also capsules and syrup)
Dichloralphenazone	("Welldorm")	tablets of 650 mg
Glutethimide	("Doriden")	tablets of 250 mg
Nitrazepam	("Mogadon")	tablets of 5 mg
Methyprylone	("Noludar")	tablets of 200 mg or 300 mg

For Parkinsonism

Benzhexol	("Artane")	tablets of 2 mg or 5 mg
Orphenadrine	("Disipal")	tablets of 50 mg
Amantidine	("Symmetrel")	tablets of 100 mg
L-Dopa	("Brocadopa", etc.)	capsules of 250 mg and 500 mg
Levodopa with Carbidopa (10%)	("Sinemet")	tablets "110" or "275"
Bromocriptine	("Parlodal")	tablets of 2.5 mg capsules of 10 mg

Tranquillizers

Chlorpromazine	("Largactil")	tablets of 10 mg, 25 mg, 50 mg or 100 mg also syrup; or injection, 10 mg or 25 mg/ml
Promazine	("Sparine")	tablets of 25 mg, 50 mg or 100 mg (or oral suspension or injections)
Thioridazine	("Melleril")	tablets of 10 mg, 25 mg 50 mg, or 100 mg (also syrup)
Perphenazine	("Fentazin")	tablets of 2 mg, 4 mg or 8 mg
Chlormethiazole	("Heminevrin")	tablets of 500 mg (also capsules, syrup, or injections)
Chlordiazepoxide	("Librium")	tablets of 5 mg, 10 mg or 25 mg (also capsules and injections)
Diazepam	("Valium")	tablets of 2 mg, 5 mg or 10 mg
Haloperidol	("Serenace")	capsules of 0.5 mg tablets, various strengths (also liquid or injection)

Anti-depressive Drugs

Protriptyline	("Concordin")	tablets of 5 mg or 10 mg
Imipramine	("Tofranil")	capsules of 25 mg or 50 mg
Trimipramine	("Surmontil")	tablets of 10 mg or 25 mg
Amitriptyline	("Tryptizol")	tablets of 10 mg, 25 mg or 50 mg

| Phenelzine | ("Nardil") | tablets of 15 mg |
| Tofenacin | ("Elamol") | capsules of 80 mg |

(5) GENITO-URINARY SYSTEM

See also under "infections" (below)
Hormones

Stilboestol B.P.		tablets of 0.1 mg, 0.5 mg, 1 mg, or 5 mg
Ethinyloestradiol B.P.		tablets of 0.01 mg, 0.02 mg or 0.05 mg
Chlorotrianisene	("Tace")	tablets of 24 mg (also capsules)
Testosterone propionate		injections of 25 mg (also implants)
Emepronium	("Ceteprin")	tablets of 50 mg or 100 mg

(6) INFECTIONS

The list of possible drugs is now almost endless
General

Benzylpenicillin	(penicillin G)	injections, e.g. 150 mg/ml
Streptomycin		injections
Benzylpenicillin ⎫ Streptomycin ⎭	("Crystamycin")	vials for ⎰ 500,000 units injection ⎱ 0.5G.
(N.B. Penicillin has several other forms)		
· Tetracycline	("Achromycin")	tablets of 100 mg or 250 mg (also syrup or injection)
Oxytetracycline	("Terramycin")	tablets of 100 mg or 250 mg (also syrup or injection)
Chlortetracycline	("Aureomycin")	capsules of 250 mg (also as syrup)
Chloramphenicol	("Chloromycetin")	capsules of 250 mg (also as suspension or injection)
Ampicillin	("Penbritin")	capsules of 125 mg, 250 mg or 500 mg (also as syrup or injection)

Erythromycin	("Erythrocin")	tablets of 100 mg or 250 mg (also as suspension or injection)
Cloxacillin	("Orbenin")	capsules of 250 mg or 500 mg (also as syrup or injection)
Cephaloridine	("Ceporin")	vials for injection 250 mg, 500 mg or 1G.
Cephalexin	("Ceporex")	tablets or capsules of 250 or 500 mg. (also syrup)
Co-trimoxazole	("Septrin", "Bactrim")	tablets of 480 mg (also suspension)
Doxycycline	("Vibramycin")	capsules of 100 mg (also syrup)
Gentamicin	("Genticin")	injection, 40 mg/ml

Urinary tract infections

Sulphadimidine	("Sulphamezathine")	tablets of 500 mg (also as suspension)
Sulphafurazole	("Gantrisin")	tablets of 500 mg (also as syrup)
Sulphamethizole	("Urolucosil")	tablets of 100 mg (also as suspension)
Nitrofurantoin	("Furadantin")	tablets of 50 mg or 100 mg (also as suspension)
Nalidixic acid	("Negram")	tablets of 500 mg (also as suspension)
Hexamine mandelate	("Mandelamine")	tablets of 500 mg

Bowel infections

Succinylsulphathiazole Neomycin }	("Sulfasuxidine")	tablets of 500 mg
Phthalylsulphathiazole	("Thalazole")	tablets of 500 mg
Succinylsulphathiazole Neomycin }	("Cremomycin")	suspension
Kaolin Streptomycin Sulphaguanidine Kaolin }	("Guanimycin")	suspension

(7) METABOLISM

Anabolic Steroids

Nandrolone	("Deca-Durabolin")	injection of 25 mg/ml or 50 mg/ml
Norethandrolone	("Nilevar")	tablets of 10 mg

Diabetes

Soluble insulin		strength of 20, 40 or 80 units/ml
Protamine zinc insulin		strength of 40 or 80 units/ml
Insulin zinc suspension amorphous	("Semilente")	40 or 80 units/ml
Insulin zinc suspension	("Lente")	40 or 80 units/ml
Tolbutamide	("Rastinon")	tablets of 500 mg
Chlorpropamide	("Diabinese")	tablets of 100 mg or 250 mg
Phenformin	("Dibotin")	tablets of 25 mg or 50 mg
Glymidine	("Gondafon")	tablets of 500 mg
Metformin	("Glucophage")	tablets of 500 mg or 850 mg
Glibenclamide	("Daonil")	tablets of 5 mg

Thyroid diseases

Thyroxine	("Eltroxin")	tablets of 0.05 mg or 0.1 mg
Tri-iodothyronine	("Tertroxin")	tablets of 5, 20 or 25 micrograms
Methylthiouracil		tablets of 50 mg
Carbimazole	("Neo-Mercazole")	tablets of 5 mg

(8) NUTRITION

Calcium Gluconate	("Calcium Sandoz")	tablets equiv. to 1.5G of gluconate . (also as syrup or injection)
Calcium Lactate B.P.		tablets of 300 mg

See also iron compounds (below)

Vitamins

Vitamin A	Halibut-liver Oil Capsules	equivalent to 4000– 5250 units

Vitamin D	Calciferol tablets (strong) B.P.	equivalent to 50,000 units
Vitamin B	Nicotinamide	tablets of 50 mg
	Thiamine	tablets of 3 mg, 10 mg, 25 mg or 50 mg
	Riboflavine	tablets of 10 mg
Vitamin C	Ascorbic Acid	tablets of 50 mg, etc.
Multiple Vitamins – Vitamin Capsules B.P.C.		

(9) BLOOD DISEASES

Ferrous sulphate		tablets of 200 mg
Ferrous gluconate		tablets of 300 mg
Ferrous succinate		tablets of 150 mg
Ferrous fumarate		tablets of 200 mg
Iron dextran	("Imferon")	injection; ampoules of 2 ml or 5 ml
Cyanocobalamin	("Cytamen" etc.)	250 mcg/ml or 1000 mcg/ml
Hydroxocobalamin	("Neo-Cytamen")	250 mcg/ml or 1000 mcg/ml
Folic Acid		tablets of 5 mg

(10) RHEUMATISM, ARTHRITIS AND GOUT

Soluble aspirin		tablets of 300 mg
Phenylbutazone	("Butazolidin")	tablets of 100 mg and 200 mg (also suppositories)
Oxyphenbutazone	("Tanderil")	tablets of 100 mg (also suppositories)
Ibuprofen	("Brufen")	tablets of 200 mg
Indomethacin	("Indocid")	capsules of 25 mg and 50 mg (also suppositories)
Mefenamic acid	("Ponstan")	capsules of 250 mg
Benorylate	("Benoral")	tablets of 750 mg (also suspension)
Colchicine B.P.		tablets of 0.25 mg or 0.5 mg
Probenecid	("Benemid")	tablets of 500 mg
Sulphinpyrazone	("Anturan")	tablets of 100 mg
Ethebenecid	("Urelim")	tablets of 500 mg

(*also corticosteroid drugs in certain circumstances*)

APPENDIX 2

ASSESSING MENTAL STATES

There are many systems of "scoring" patients' mental capabilities. None is entirely satisfactory, and for research purposes and for accurate measurement of improvement or deterioration much more elaborate systems are necessary. However, the following simple system, evolved by Professor H. M. Hodkinson in 1972 ("Age and Ageing" Vol. 1, p. 233), is useful and quite quick to apply. It depends largely on memory.

(N.B. Mental test scoring can only be used with patients who co-operate, who are not dysphasic and who are able to hear the questions.)

1. Age
2. Time (to nearest hour)
3. Address for recall at end of test – this should be repeated by the patient to ensure it has been heard correctly: e.g.: "42 West Street"
4. Year
5. Name of Hospital
6. Recognition of two persons (doctor, nurse)
7. Date of Birth
8. Year of First World War
9. Name of present Monarch
10. Count backwards from 20 to 1

Scores below 7 indicate a significant amount of mental aberration. The maximum score is 10.

APPENDIX 3

PREVENTION FOR PRESSURE SORES

A method of judging, from the patient's condition, how great is his chance of developing a pressure sore unless proper preventative nursing measures are applied.

The work of Prof. A. N. Exton-Smitt and his colleagues (as described in the *British Medical Journal* 1967, Vol. 1, p. 934) shows that it is possible to predict which patients will be most in danger by giving them a "score" related to certain of their abilities, as follows:

A. General Condition		B. Mental State		C. Activity	
Good	Score 0	*Alert*	Score 0	*Ambulant*	Score 0
Fair	Score 1	*Confused*	Score 1	*Walks with help*	Score 1
Poor	Score 2	*Apathetic*	Score 2	*Chairfast*	Score 2
Bad	Score 3	*Stuporose*	Score 3	*In bed all day*	Score 3

D. Mobility in Bed		E. Incontinence	
Full	Score 0	*Continent*	Score 0
Slight limitation	Score 1	*Occasional Incontinence*	Score 1
Very limited	Score 2	*Usually incontinent of urine*	Score 2
Immobile	Score 3	*Doubly incontinent*	Score 3

Interpretation (a) The best score is 0, the worst is 15. The higher the score, the greater the risk of pressure sores.

(b) Experience of the method indicates that *scores of 7 and upwards indicate a severe risk*; preventative measures should be concentrated most on patients with high scores.

(c) Scoring is best done in the first place by a doctor (e.g.

on admission), but it can equally well be done by experienced trained nurses.

(d) Scoring should be repeated at intervals; the score will vary according to progress.

INDEX